T0188656

Chronic Pelvic Pain

Chronic Pelvic Pain

EDITED BY

Paolo Vercellini

Associate Professor of Obstetrics and Gynecology
Istituto "Luigi Mangiagalli"
Fondazione IRCCS Ca' Granda
University of Milan, Italy

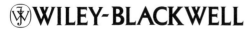

A John Wiley & Sons, Ltd., Publication

This edition first published 2011, © 2011 by Blackwell Publishing Ltd

Blackwell Publishing was acquired by John Wiley & Sons in February 2007. Blackwell's publishing program has been merged with Wiley's global Scientific, Technical and Medical business to form Wiley-Blackwell.

Registered office: John Wiley & Sons, Ltd, The Atrium, Southern Gate, Chichester, West Sussex, PO19 8SQ, UK
Editorial offices: 9600 Garsington Road, Oxford, OX4 2DQ, UK
                       The Atrium, Southern Gate, Chichester, West Sussex, PO19 8SQ, UK
                       111 River Street, Hoboken, NJ 07030-5774, USA

For details of our global editorial offices, for customer services and for information about how to apply for permission to reuse the copyright material in this book please see our website at www.wiley.com/wiley-blackwell The right of the author to be identified as the author of this work has been asserted in accordance with the UK Copyright, Designs and Patents Act 1988.

All rights reserved. No part of this publication may be reproduced, stored in a retrieval system, or transmitted, in any form or by any means, electronic, mechanical, photocopying, recording or otherwise, except as permitted by the UK Copyright, Designs and Patents Act 1988, without the prior permission of the publisher.

Designations used by companies to distinguish their products are often claimed as trademarks. All brand names and product names used in this book are trade names, service marks, trademarks or registered trademarks of their respective owners. The publisher is not associated with any product or vendor mentioned in this book. This publication is designed to provide accurate and authoritative information in regard to the subject matter covered. It is sold on the understanding that the publisher is not engaged in rendering professional services. If professional advice or other expert assistance is required, the services of a competent professional should be sought.

The contents of this work are intended to further general scientific research, understanding, and discussion only and are not intended and should not be relied upon as recommending or promoting a specific method, diagnosis, or treatment by physicians for any particular patient. The publisher and the author make no representations or warranties with respect to the accuracy or completeness of the contents of this work and specifically disclaim all warranties, including without limitation any implied warranties of fitness for a particular purpose. In view of ongoing research, equipment modifications, changes in governmental regulations, and the constant flow of information relating to the use of medicines, equipment, and devices, the reader is urged to review and evaluate the information provided in the package insert or instructions for each medicine, equipment, or device for, among other things, any changes in the instructions or indication of usage and for added warnings and precautions. Readers should consult with a specialist where appropriate. The fact that an organization or Website is referred to in this work as a citation and/or a potential source of further information does not mean that the author or the publisher endorses the information the organization or Website may provide or recommendations it may make. Further, readers should be aware that Internet Websites listed in this work may have changed or disappeared between when this work was written and when it is read. No warranty may be created or extended by any promotional statements for this work. Neither the publisher nor the author shall be liable for any damages arising herefrom.

Library of Congress Cataloging-in-Publication Data

Chronic pelvic pain / edited by Paolo Vercellini.
    p. ; cm. – (Gynecology in practice)
  Includes bibliographical references and index.
  ISBN 978-1-4443-3066-3 (pbk. : alk. paper)
  1. Pelvic pain.   2. Generative organs, Female–Diseases. I. Vercellini, Paolo. II. Series: Gynecology in practice.
[DNLM: 1. Pelvic Pain. 2. Chronic Disease. WP 155]
RG483.P44C46 2011
618.1–dc22
                          2010036365

A catalogue record for this book is available from the British Library.

This book is published in the following electronic formats: ePDF 9781444391831; Wiley Online Library 9781444391855; ePub 9781444391848

Set in 8.75/11.75 by Toppan Best-set Premedia Limited
Printed and bound in Malaysia by Vivar Printing Sdn Bhd

01   2011

Contents

Series Foreword

In recent decades, massive advances in medical science and technology have caused an explosion of information available to the practitioner. In the modern information age, it is not unusual for physicians to have a computer in their offices with the capability of accessing medical databases and literature searches. On the other hand, however, there is always a need for concise, readable, and highly practicable written resources. The purpose of this series is to fulfill this need in the field of gynecology.

The *Gynecology in Practice* series aims to present practical clinical guidance on effective patient care for the busy gynecologist. The goal of each volume is to provide an evidence-based approach for specific gynecologic problems. "Evidence at a glance" features in the text provide summaries of key trials or landmark papers that guide practice, and a selected bibliography at the end of each chapter provides a springboard for deeper reading. Even with a practical approach, it is important to review the crucial basic science necessary for effective diagnosis and management. This is reinforced by "Science revisited" boxes that remind readers of crucial anatomic, physiologic or pharmacologic principles for practice.

Each volume is edited by outstanding international experts who have brought together truly gifted clinicians to address many relevant clinical questions in their chapters. The first volume in the series is the volume on *Chronic Pelvic Pain*, one of the most challenging problems in gynecology. Following volumes cover the subjects of *Disorders of Menstruation*, *Infertility*, *Contraception*, *Sexually Transmitted Diseases*, *Menopause*, *Urinary Incontinence*, *Endoscopic Surgeries*, and *Fibroids*, to name a few. I would like to express my gratitude to all the editors and authors, who, despite their other responsibilities, have contributed their time, effort, and expertise to this series.

Finally, I greatly appreciate the support of the staff at Wiley-Blackwell for their outstanding editorial competence. My special thanks go to Martin Sugden, PhD; without his vision and perseverance, this series would not have come to life. My sincere hope is that this novel and exciting series will serve women and their physicians well, and will be part of the diagnostic and therapeutic armamentarium of practicing gynecologists.

Aydin Arici, MD
Professor
Department of Obstetrics, Gynecology, and
Reproductive Sciences
Yale University School of Medicine
New Haven, USA

Preface

Chronic pelvic pain (CPP) is a common gynecologic problem that may negatively affect health-related quality of life. Prevalence figures for CPP in the general female population vary greatly according to several variables, including definition, country, and socioeconomic status. Overall, CPP has an estimated prevalence of 38 per 1,000 in women aged 15–73 years, a rate higher than that of migraine (21 per 1,000) and comparable to that of asthma (37 per 1,000) and chronic back pain (41 per 1,000). CPP is the single most common indication for referrals to gynecology clinics, accounting for 20% of all appointments in secondary care, and constitutes the indication for 12% of all hysterectomies and over 40% of gynecologic diagnostic laparoscopies. In a Gallup poll of 5,325 US women, 16% reported CPP, 11% limited their home activity, 12% limited their sexual activity, 16% took medications, and 4% missed at least 1 day of work per month.

An estimated $274 million is spent annually on the management of this condition in the UK National Health System, and $881 million a year on its outpatient management in the United States. Direct and indirect costs may total over $2 billion per year. CPP may cause prolonged suffering and disability, with consequent loss of employment, family conflicts, repetitive unsuccessful treatments, and serial ineffective surgical procedures.

In women, several causes of CPP are recognized, although in a not negligible proportion of patients, a definite diagnosis cannot be made. Different neurophysiologic mechanisms are involved in the pathophysiology of CPP. Pain may be classified as nociceptive or non-nociceptive. In the former, the symptom originates from stimulation of a pain-sensitive structure, whereas in latter, pain is considered neuropathic or psychogenic. The patient's history is crucial and is generally of the utmost importance for a correct diagnosis, being sometimes more indicative of the condition than several diagnostic investigations. The main contributing factors in women with CPP can still be identified by history and physical examination in most cases.

Many disorders of the reproductive tract, urologic organs, and gastrointestinal, musculoskeletal, and psychoneurologic systems may be associated with CPP. Indeed, CPP is a symptom and not a disease, and rarely reflects a single pathologic process. When multiple factors are present, treatment of only some of them will lead to incomplete relief and frustration for both patient and clinician. Therapy for CPP, different from that of acute pain, generally requires acceptance of the concept of managing rather than curing the symptoms. Gaining women's trust and developing a strong patient–physician relationship is of the utmost importance in determining the long-term outcome of care and may reveal itself to be no less important than drugs or surgery.

Given this background, we deemed it of interest to review, with the collaboration of authoritative experts in the field, the pathophysiology and etiology of CPP, as well as the various proposed therapies targeted at both general pain relief and the treatment of specific disorders associated with CPP. Our aim is to define a rational approach to the differential diagnosis and long-term management of this distressing condition. Specific clinical situations, such as CPP in the adolescent woman, dyspareunia, and CPP without obvious pathology, have been included, as has an evaluation of the effects of complementary treatments and definitive surgery.

I warmly thank the colleagues that have dedicated their precious time in order to offer readers a concentrate of their vast knowledge, and trust that this book will provide a practical guide to effective patient care for gynecologists, limiting the number of undue procedures that women undergo and avoiding prolonged suffering. Finally, I wish to express my gratitude to the Editor, who, since the the very beginning, has stimulated, supported, and coordinated this initiative with uncommon devotion and efficiency.

Paolo Vercellini
June 2010

Contributors

A. Arici, MD, Professor, Division of Reproductive Endocrinology and Infertility, Department of Obstetrics, Gynecology and Reproductive Sciences, Yale University School of Medicine, New Haven, Connecticut, USA

David Ashley Hill, MD, Associate Director, Department of Obstetrics and Gynecology, Florida Hospital Graduate Medical Education, Florida Hospital, Orlando, Florida, USA

Stefano Bianchi, MD, Professor and Head of Department of Obstetrics and Gynecology, Fondazione IRCCS Ca Granda Ospedale Maggiore Policlinico, University of Milan, Italy

Yitzchak M. Binik, PhD, Professor, Department of Psychology, McGill University; Director, Sex and Couple Therapy Service, McGill University Health Center, Montreal, Quebec, Canada

Ying Cheong, MD, MRCOG Senior Lecturer in Obstetrics and Gynaecology and Subspecialist in Reproductive Medicine/Surgery, University of Southampton, Southampton, UK

J. Quentin Clemens, MD, FACS MSCI, Associate Professor of Urology; Director, Division of Neurourology and Pelvic Reconstructive Surgery, University of Michigan, Ann Arbor, Michigan, USA

Liza Marie Colimon, MD, Fellow, Division of Advanced Gynecology and Minimally Invasive Surgery, Department of Obstetrics and Gynecology, Florida Hospital Graduate Medical Education, Florida Hospital, Orlando, Florida, USA

Michael P. Diamond, MD, Associate Chair and Kamran S. Moghissi Professor of Obstetrics and Gynecology; Director, Division of Reproductive Endocrinology and Infertility; Assistant Dean for Clinical and Translational Research, Wayne State University School of Medicine, Detroit, Michigan, USA

Tommaso Falcone, MD, Professor and Chairman, Department of Obstetrics and Gynecology, Cleveland Clinic, Cleveland, Ohio, USA

Cindy Farquhar, MD, Postgraduate Professor of Obstetrics and Gynaecology, Department of Obstetrics and Gynaecology, University of Auckland, Auckland, New Zealand

Luigi Fedele, MD, Professor and Head of Department of Obstetrics, Gynecology and Neonatology, Fondazione IRCCS Ca Granda Ospedale Maggiore Policlinico, University of Milan, Italy

Colleen Fitzgerald, MD, Rehabilitation Institute of Chicago and Feinberg School of Medicine at Northwestern University, Chicago, Illinois, USA

Giada Frontino, MD, Assistant, Department of Obstetrics, Gynecology and Neonatology, Fondazione IRCCS Ca Granda Ospedale Maggiore Policlinico, University of Milan, Italy

Alessandra Graziottin, MD, Director, Center of Gynecology and Medical Sexology, H. San Raffaele Resnati, Milan, Italy; Consultant Professor, University of Florence, Italy; President, Alessandra Graziottin Foundation, Milan, Italy

Jennifer Gunter, MD, FRCS(C), FACOG, DABPM, Director, Pelvic Pain, Kaiser San Francisco, San Francisco, California, USA

Fred Howard, MS, MD, Professor and Associate Chair in Obstetrics and Gynecology, University of Rochester School of Medicine and Dentistry, Rochester, New York, USA

John Jarrell, MSc, MD, FRCSC, Professor, Department of Obstetrics and Gynecology, University of Calgary, Calgary, Alberta, Canada

Jennifer L. Kulp, MD, Instructor, Department of Obstetrics, Gynecology and Reproductive Sciences, Division of Reproductive Endocrinology and Infertility, Yale University School of Medicine, New Haven, Connecticut, USA

Georgine Lamvu, MD, MPH, Medical Director of Gynecology; Director of the Fellowship in Advanced Gynecology and Minimally Invasive Surgery, Department of Obstetrics and Gynecology, Florida Hospital Graduate Medical Education, Orlando, Florida, USA

Marta Meana, PhD, Professor, Department of Psychology, University of Nevada, Las Vegas, Nevada, USA

David L. Olive, MD, Medical Director, Wisconsin Fertility Institute, Middleton, Wisconsin, USA

Nicole Paterson, BSc, MSc, MD, Department of Obstetrics and Gynecology, University of Calgary, Calgary, Alberta, Canada

Kristen Pozolo, BS, Clinical Research Coordinator, Northshore University HealthSystem, Evanston, Illinois, USA

Elizabeth E. Puscheck, MD, Professor of Obstetrics and Gynecology, Wayne State University School of Medicine/Detroit Medical Center, Detroit, Michigan, USA

Andrea J. Rapkin, MD, Professor, Department of Obstetrics and Gynecology, David Geffen School of Medicine at UCLA, Los Angeles, California, USA

Brett A.H. Schultz, DO, MBA, Fellow, Minimally Invasive Gynecologic Surgery, Department of Obstetrics and Gynecology, St Elizabeth Medical Center, Utica, New York, USA

Sangeeta Senapati, MD, MS, Clinical Assistant Professor of Obstetrics and Gynecology, Pritzker School of Medicine, University of Chicago, Chicago, Illinois; Northshore University HealthSystem, Evanston, Illinois, USA

Manvinder Singh, MD, Associate Professor, Department of Obstetrics and Gynecology, Wayne State University School of Medicine/ Detroit Medical Center, Detroit, Michigan, USA

Tevy Tith, MD, Resident, Department of Obstetrics and Gynecology, David Geffen School of Medicine at UCLA, Los Angeles, California, USA

Frank Tu, MD, MPH, Clinical Assistant Professor of Obstetrics and Gynecology, Pritzker School of Medicine, University of Chicago, Chicago, Illinois; Northshore University HealthSystem, Evanston, Illinois, USA

Aarti Umranikar, MRCOG, MFFP, Specialist Registrar in Obstetrics and Gynaecology, Southampton University Hospitals NHS Trust, Southampton, UK

Daniela Wittmann, LMSW, CST, Clinical Social Worker and Sexual Health Coordinator, Department of Urology, University of Michigan Medical Center, Ann Arbor, Michigan, USA

Neurobiology of Chronic Pelvic Pain

Jennifer Gunter

Kaiser San Francisco Medical Center, San Francisco, California, USA

Introduction

The International Association for the Study of Pain defines pain as an unpleasant sensory and emotional experience associated with actual or potential tissue damage, or described in terms of that damage. Chronic pelvic pain is defined as pain in the pelvis present for at least 2 weeks out of every month for at least 6 months.

Chronic pain is much more than noxious nociception; it is a complex condition with sensory, adaptive, and affective components. While acute pain has biologic utility, chronic pain does not appear to confer any evolutionary advantage.

Many of the complexities of chronic pelvic pain are born from the complex neuroanatomy of the pelvis and corresponding responses of both the peripheral and central nervous systems; therefore a thorough understanding of the neurobiology is essential.

> ### ☆ TIPS & TRICKS
>
> All structures in the pelvis should be considered as potential pain generators. In addition to the uterus and adnexa, it is also important to consider the bladder, the bowel, muscles of the pelvic floor, the skin, and both the peripheral and central nervous systems as potential pain generators. When evaluating a patient with chronic pelvic pain, make a list of all the potential pain generators in the painful area and consider the possible contribution of each one. Remember that, for many patients

with chronic pelvic pain, there may be more than one pain generator in addition to changes in the central nervous system that enhance pain (central sensitization).

Nociception and pain

The nociceptors of somatic structures (e.g. muscle, skin, and bone) are undifferentiated nerve endings of myelinated A-delta and unmyelinated C fibers.

Mechanical, chemical, or thermal stimulation results in an influx of sodium across the sodium/ potassium ion channels resulting in depolarization, which converts the noxious stimulus into an electrical impulse. The wave of depolarization is transmitted along the afferent sensory neuron, where it triggers the release of excitatory neurotransmitters at the synapse with second-order neurons in laminae I–V of the dorsal horn of the spinal cord. Some afferent nerves travel up or down for several segments in the spinal cord before making contact with second-order neurons, while others synapse at their level of entry.

The muscles of the pelvic floor and the skin of the vulva are innervated by spinal segments L4–S4, although the mons and labia also receive sensory innervation from L1 and L2 via the ilioinguinal and genitofemoral nerves.

Nociceptive input from the uterus and bladder is transmitted via the sympathetic nervous system. The sympathetic afferents also transmit some sensory input from the vagina, pelvic

Chronic Pelvic Pain, First Edition. Edited by Paolo Vercellini.
© 2011 Blackwell Publishing Ltd. Published 2011 by Blackwell Publishing Ltd.

muscles, and skin. Sympathetic sensory axons are either thinly myelinated A-delta or unmyelinated C fibers. The pelvic viscera contain three categories of nociceptors: stimulus specific, intensity responsive, and silent. Visceral nociceptors are unresponsive to stimuli such as cutting and crushing but very responsive to distension, traction, ischemia, and inflammation. The viscera have fewer afferent neurons compared with somatic structures.

Afferent neurons from the pelvic viscera converge with sympathetic afferents from the enteric nervous system forming a series of retroperitoneal plexuses that pass through the sympathetic chain without synapsing. These afferents enter the dorsal roots at T1–L2. Like the somatic sensory afferents, the cell bodies of the visceral afferents are located in the dorsal root ganglia. These sympathetic afferents synapse with second-order neurons, primarily in laminae I, V, and X, on both sides of the spinal cord. Parasympathetic primary afferents travel from the enteric nervous system to the central nervous system (CNS) via the vagus nerve.

Somatic and sympathetic afferents both synapse on the second-order neurons of the spinothalamic tract. There are three types of spinothalamic tract neuron in the dorsal horn: low-threshold mechanoreceptors, high-threshold nociceptors, and wide dynamic range neurons (WDRs).

WDR neurons are found in laminae I, II, V, and VI of the dorsal horn. They are multireceptive, gathering somatic input from A-delta and C fibers, with some input from A-beta fibers (touch), as well as input from visceral afferents. This convergence of both somatic and visceral afferents on the same second-order neurons results in a loss of visceral specificity, contributing to the vague and poorly localized qualities of visceral pain. Convergence is also responsible for the phenomenon of referred pain.

The second-order neurons receiving afferent input cross over to the contralateral side of the spinal cord and ascend to the brain as part of the spinothalamic, spinoreticular, and spinomesencephalic tracts. When depolarization in these ascending tracts reaches the thalamus, excitatory neurotransmitters are released that trigger depolarization of third-order neurons. These neurons are the final step in relaying nociceptive input to the somatosensory cortex, where nociception is translated into pain. As each somatic afferent has cortical representation, somatic pain is well localized; however, there is no direct visceral representation in the somatosensory cortex.

SCIENCE REVISITED

Visceral pain is typically poorly localized because viscera have no direct projections to the cerebral cortex. Well localized pain is more likely to be somatic or neuropathic in origin.

Once pain is perceived by the brain, descending pathways are activated at many levels including the cortex, thalamus, periaqueductal gray matter, nucleus raphe magnus, and locus coeruleus–subcoeruleus complex. Inhibitory pathways descend in the dorsal column and stimulate inhibitory neurons in the dorsal horn, which synapse on both the primary sensory afferents the second-order dorsal horn neurons. These descending pathways release endogenous opioids, which have an antinociceptive effect, as well as inhibitory neurotransmitters such as gamma-aminobutyric acid (GABA).

Mechanisms of chronic pelvic pain

The nervous system responds dynamically to pain—this is an integral part of the pain response system. When peripheral nociceptors receive a noxious stimulus of sufficient intensity, the subsequent depolarization displaces magnesium from its binding site on the N-methyl-D-aspartate (NMDA) receptors. The open NMDA receptors are now free to bind the neurotransmitter glutamate, which increases the excitability of second-order neurons. The clinical effect is that, after an initial noxious stimulus, less input is required to trigger second-order neurons. This phenomenon is termed wind-up and is a normal response with a biologic purpose: creating hypersensitivity after injury increases the likelihood that the area will be protected from reinjury.

It is this ability of the nervous system to adapt in response to nociceptive input that is the

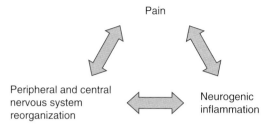

Figure 1.1 Cycle of chronic pain.

foundation for the mechanisms of chronic pain. Maladaptive responses and reorganization in both the peripheral and the CNS increase both somatosensory burden and nociceptive excitability, resulting in a self-sustaining cycle of pain and neurogenic inflammation (Figure 1.1).

Peripheral sensitization

Peripheral sensitization is a heightened response of primary afferent nerves to nociceptive input. It plays a prominent role in the genesis and maintenance of many pelvic pain syndromes. Peripheral nociceptors may become sensitized by inflammatory neurotransmitters such as calcitonin gene-related peptide (CGRP), substance P, histamine, prostaglandins, and bradykinin. Local inflammatory changes may also activate silent nociceptor, upregulate of sodium channels, as well as trigger other genomic changes resulting in ectopic activity at the nociceptors or cell body. Endometriosis and interstitial cystitis, two conditions associated with chronic pelvic pain, have pronounced local inflammatory changes possibility facilitating peripheral sensitization. Nociceptor sensitization has been described in women with vulvodynia.

Abnormal or excessive sprouting of peripheral nerve terminals at the site of injury or disease can also increase sensitivity to excitatory neurotransmitters, resulting in depolarization at a lower threshold or even spontaneous firing of nociceptors.

Changes in the peripheral nerves can also occur proximally at the site of synapse in the dorsal horn with second-order neurons. After peripheral nerve injury, there is greater loss of smaller C fibers than larger diameter A-beta fibers, so surviving A-beta fibers sprout new branches, making connections to second-order neurons vacated by the lost C fibers in the substantia gelatinosa (lamina II). As a result, A-beta fibers may take on a primary nociceptive role. For many patients, this is an important contributor to allodynia, the perception of light touch as pain.

Sympathetically maintained pain

Sympathetically maintained visceral pain is an important component of chronic pelvic pain for many patients. Like their somatic counterparts, sympathetic nociceptors may become unregulated and sensitized by injury or ongoing neurogenic inflammation, lowering the threshold for response to sympathetic stimuli such as stretching and distension. Another important mechanism of sympathetically mediated pain is activation of silent nociceptors. This phenomenon has been described in chronic bladder pain.

Abnormal sprouting is also a mechanism of sympathetically mediated pain. This may occur in neuromas at the site of injury and also in the dorsal root ganglia, where the somatic and sympathetic afferents run in close proximity. Abnormal sympathetic sprouting is reported in endometriosis implants.

Estrogen may affect vulnerability to sympathetically mediated pain. Estrogen alters micturition thresholds in rats, and in humans the menstrual cycle influences bladder pain and urgency. In animal studies, the proliferation of sympathetic neurons in the lower reproductive tract is affected by estrogen, with a significant decrease noted in ovariectomized rats.

Central sensitization

Central sensitization refers to the changes in the CNS that facilitate, enhance, or distort pain. It is largely mediated by WDR neurons.

WDR neurons are found in lamina V. They receive input from four types of presynaptic afferents: C, A-delta, A-beta, and sympathetic. They are particularly sensitive to changes in stimulus intensity and do not normally respond to non-noxious or subthreshold stimuli. Under abnormal conditions, the WDR neurons begin to respond inappropriately to low-threshold A-beta input and may even begin to discharge spontaneously. They can also develop abnormal synapses, sprouting into other areas of the dorsal horn in response to injury and neuroinflammatory changes. Other central changes that contribute to central sensitization are recruitment of previously silent synapses in the dorsal horn and activation of glia.

Neuroinflammatory transmitters, such as CGRP, tachykinins, and glutamate, mediate changes in the dorsal horn that lead to central sensitization. Activation of NMDA receptors by glutamate, also plays a major role in the excitability of WDR neurons. Input from inhibitory interneurons (largely mediated by GABA and glycine) is also decreased, further enhancing WDR output.

Some nociceptive inputs are more likely to lead to central changes. Muscle pain is a more potent inducer of the intraspinal changes of central sensitization compared to skin. This is an important consideration as high-tone somatic dysfunction of the pelvic floor, localized myalgias, and fibromyalgia are common among patients with chronic pelvic pain. Visceral pain is also a highly effective mechanism for inducing central sensitization, producing more dorsal horn excitability when compared to cutaneous tissues.

Neuroinflammation in the spinal cord, which facilitates central sensitization, is also a key mechanism behind the multiorgan system involvement of chronic pelvic pain. Close neural connections in the sacral spinal cord are essential for the complex coordinated visceral functions of the pelvis. However, these intimate connections also allow neuroinflammation to spread from involved to uninvolved neurons via the dorsal horn. Once the end terminal of the previously uninvolved afferent is stimulated in the dorsal horn, the excitatory neurotransmitter substance P travels in a retrograde fashion down C and A-delta fibers, leading to increased expression of sodium channels and sensitization distally at the terminal nociceptors. This phenomenon is seen in animal models: rats with surgically induced endometriosis demonstrate a reduced bladder capacity, vaginal hyperalgesia, and increased visceral pain compared to animals who were subject to a sham procedure.

These central connections do more than allow pain to spread from organ system to organ system; they also allow the spread of pathology. In the murine model, an attenuated Bartha strain of pseudorabies virus (PRV) can be used to initiate a neuroinflammatory response in the spinal cord, leading not only to bladder pain, but also to inflammatory bladder pathology. As PRV is incapable of antidromic spread down either sensory or motor neurons, this effect is not mediated directly by the PRV itself but rather indirectly via neuroinflammation that spreads between shared spinal segments. This centrally-induced peripheral neurogenic inflammation is then translated into mast cell activation in the lamina propria of the bladder, resulting in local cystitis. If a hypogastric neurectomy is performed, the effect on the bladder is prevented.

Therefore, both pain and pathology can be triggered solely by central neurogenic inflammation, explaining the presence of not only of chronic pain, but also end-organ disease in multiple somatic and visceral structures.

Loss of inhibitory control

The affective processing of pain is mediated by neurotransmitters and involves input from the periaqueductal grey, amygdala, anterior cingulate cortex, and anterior insula. Both descending spinally projecting neurons and inhibitory interneurons inhibit neurotransmitter release from primary afferents, modulating nociceptive input. Important neurotransmitters in descending modulation include mu-opioids, GABA, neurokinin 1, and norepinephrine.

Altered activity of the descending pathways has an important role in the maintenance of chronic pain states and can be a mechanism by which changes in mood, anxiety, and depression influence common pain via shared neurotransmitters.

Other systemic factors

Systemic immune activation

Abnormal activation of the systemic immune system may have a role in the pathogenesis of some pelvic pain syndromes. Concomitant inflammatory and autoimmune conditions are significantly more common with interstitial cystitis. Patients with interstitial cystitis are 100 times more likely to have inflammatory bowel disease (Crohn's disease or ulcerative colitis) and 30 times more likely to have systemic lupus erythematosus than the general population.

Sjögren syndrome, present in 0.6% of the population, has a prevalence of up to 28% among patients with interstitial cystitis, and the incidence of other rheumatologic disorders, such as rheumatoid arthritis and fibromyalgia, is also significantly higher. Women with endometriosis have a higher incidence of atopy, allergies, and asthma. It is conceivable that widespread inflammation from a rheumatologic or other source may trigger the neurogenic inflammation of chronic pain. Alternatively, there may be a common genetic component.

✋ CAUTION

For women, cyclic pain does not necessarily imply endometriosis. Cyclic pain is a common phenonomenon as estrogen and progesterone have a complex relationship with pain. The best example is menstrual migraines, which are clearly not an endometriosis-related phenomenon. Exacerbations of bladder and muscle pain with the menstrual cycle are common.

Depression

Depression, anxiety, and catastrophizing all have a role in the neurobiology of chronic pain. Chronic pain can lead to mood disorders but the reverse is also true, that negative mood and emotion can exacerbate pain. Patients with depression are three times more likely to develop chronic pain, and patients with chronic pain have a higher incidence of major depression and generalized anxiety disorder.

Depression lowers both somatic and visceral pain thresholds, possibly via changes in neurotransmitters such as norepinephrine, serotonin, and substance P or by activation of the hypothalamic–adrenal–pituitary access. Depression and hostility are also known to have an effect on circulating levels of inflammatory markers, and markers of chronic inflammation, such as interkeukin-6, are elevated after an immune challenge. These changes may facilitating end-organ inflammation in conditions, as well as stimulate or enhance both peripheral and central neurogenic inflammation.

Selected bibliography

Berkley KJ, Hubscher CH, Wall PD. Neuronal responses to stimulation of the cervix, uterus, colon, and skin in the rat spinal cord. J Neurophysiol 1993;69:545–56.

Chen H, Lamer TJ, Rho R et al. Contemporary management of neuropathic pain for the primary care physician. Mayo Clin Proc 2004; 79:1533–45.

Fields HL, Basbaum AI, Heinricher MM. Central nervous mechanisms of pain modulation. In: McMahon S, Koltzenburg M, eds. Wall and Melzack's textbook of pain, 5th ed. St. Louis: Elsevier; 2005. pp. 125–42.

Giamberardino MA, Berkleyt, KJ, Affaiti G et al. Influence of endometriosis on pain behaviors and muscle hyperalgesia. Pain 1995;61: 459–69.

Gunter J. Neurobiology of chronic pelvic pain. In: Potts J, ed. Genitourinary pain and inflammation. Totowa, NJ: Humana Press; 2008. pp. 3–17.

Moshiree B, Zhou Q, Price DD, Verne GN. Central sensitization in visceral pain disorders. Gut 2006;55:905–8.

Powell-Boone T, Ness TJ, Cannon R, Lloyd LK, Weigent DA, Fillingim RB. Menstrual cycle affects bladder pain sensation in subjects with interstitial cystitis. J Urol 2005;174: 1832–6.

Roberts M. Clinical neuroanatomy of the abdomen and pelvis: implications for surgical treatment of prolapse. Clin Obstet Gynecol 2005;48:627–38.

Robinson DR, Gebhart GF. Inside information – the unique features of visceral sensation. Mol Interv 2008;8:242–53.

Salter MW. Cellular neuroplasticity mechanisms mediating pain persistence. J Orofasc Pain 2004;18:318–24.

Siddall PJ, Cousins MJ, Neurobiology of pain. Int Anesthesiol Clin 1997;35:1–26.

Sinaii N, Cleary SD, Ballweg ML, Nierman LK, Stratton P. High rates of autoimmune and endocrine disorders, fibromyalgia, chronic fatigue syndrome, and atopic diseases among women with endometriosis. Hum Reprod 2002;17:2715–24.

Wesselman U. Neurogenic inflammation and chronic pelvic pain. World J Urol 2001;19: 180–5.

Wiech K, Tracey I. The influence of negative emotions on pain: behavioral effects and neural mechanisms Neuroimage 2009;47:987–94.

Winnard KP, Bmitrieva N, Berkley KJ. Cross-organ interactions between reproductive, gastrointestinal, and urinary tracts: modulation by estrous stage and involvement of the hypogastric nerve. Am J Physiol Regul Integr Comp Physiol 2006;291:R1592–601.

The Differential Diagnosis of Chronic Pelvic Pain

Fred M. Howard

University of Rochester of Rochester School of Medicine and Dentistry, Rochester, New York, USA

Introduction

Chronic pelvic pain (CPP) is a common condition in women. Its prevalence in the general population may be as high as 15%. In about 4% of women, CPP is of sufficient severity that it causes them to seek medical care. CPP has a prevalence that is comparable to the prevalence of migraine, asthma, and low back pain in women. It is the fourth most common benign disorder evaluated in gynecologic practices. In spite of being a common condition, the evaluation of CPP remains a complex and perplexing diagnostic problem.

> ### ⬡ SCIENCE REVISITED
>
> The following are important definitions:
> - *Pain*: an unpleasant sensory and emotional experience associated with actual or potential tissue damage or described in terms of such damage.
> - *Chronic pelvic pain*: noncyclic pain of 6 or more months' duration that localizes to the anatomic pelvis, anterior abdominal wall at or below the umbilicus, lumbosacral back, or buttocks and is of sufficient severity to cause functional disability or lead to medical care.

At least one of the difficulties in the diagnostic evaluation of CPP is the common assumption that it is a symptom of a single disease or disorder. Although this is sometimes true, in many cases CPP (like other chronic pain disorders) is due to inflammatory or neuropathic changes of the central and/or peripheral nervous system. This may be at least one reason that so many patients with CPP have more than one pain-related diagnosis. In such cases, it is clinically more productive to view CPP as a diagnosis, not a symptom, and to view other pain-related diagnoses as pain generators.

> ### ★ TIPS AND TRICKS
>
> General guidelines for the evaluation of chronic pelvic pain:
> 1. Take a thorough history.
> 2. Perform a pain-directed physical examination—a "pain-mapping" examination (Tables 2.1–2.4).
> 3. Laboratory and imaging studies should be obtained specifically to confirm or refute those pain-related diagnoses derived from the history and physical examination.
> 4. Laparoscopy has a limited role as a diagnostic modality.
> 5. Those diagnoses with level A evidence of association with chronic pelvic pain should always be considered first.

Women suffering from CPP are a heterogeneous group, and the possible pain-related diagnoses are numerous and varied (Table 2.5). There is a

Chronic Pelvic Pain, First Edition. Edited by Paolo Vercellini.
© 2011 Blackwell Publishing Ltd. Published 2011 by Blackwell Publishing Ltd.

Table 2.1 Components of the standing physical examination of the woman with chronic pelvic pain and general problems or diagnoses that may be suggested based on these components of the examination

Standing examination	Possible problems diagnosed
Gait	Short leg syndrome Herniated disc General musculoskeletal problems
Posture with and without forward bending	Typical pelvic pain posture Scoliosis One-leg standing
Standing on one leg with and without hip flexion	Laxity of the pubic symphysis Laxity of the pelvic girdle Weakness of the hip and pelvis
Iliac crest symmetry	Short leg syndrome One-leg standing
Groin evaluation with and without Valsalva maneuver	Inguinal hernia Femoral hernia
(Incisional evaluation with and without Valsalva maneuver)	Incisional hernia
Pubic symphysis evaluation, including trigger points	Peripartum pelvic pain syndrome Trigger points Osteitis pubis Osteomyelitis pubis
Hip and sacroiliac evaluation, including trigger points	Arthritis of hip Trigger points
Buttocks (gluteus and piriformis) evaluation, including trigger points	Piriformis syndrome Pelvic floor pain syndrome Gluteal trigger points
(Fibromyalgia tender point evaluation)	Fibromyalgia
(Pelvic floor relaxation evaluation)	Enterocele Rectocele Cystocele Uterine descent

Table 2.2 Components of the sitting physical examination of the woman with chronic pelvic pain and general problems or diagnoses that may be suggested based on these components of the examination

Sitting examination	Possible problems diagnosed
Posture	Levator ani spasm Pelvic floor pain syndrome
Palpation of the upper and lower back	Trigger points Myalgia Arthritis
Palpation of the sacrum	Trigger points Sacroiliitis
Palpation of the gluteal and piriformis muscles	Trigger points Myalgia
Palpation of the posterior superior iliac crests	Peripartum pelvic pain syndrome
Basic sensory testing to sharpness, dullness, and light touch	Herniated disc
Muscle strength testing and deep tendons	Herniated disc

Table 2.3 Components of the supine physical examination of the woman with chronic pelvic pain and general problems or diagnoses that may be suggested based on these components of the examination

Supine examination	Possible problems diagnosed
Posture for lordosis or pelvic tilt	Lordosis Pelvic tilt Abdominal weakness Stiffness of the lumbar spine
Active leg flexion, knee to chest	Low back dysfunction Low back pain Abdominal muscle weakness Deconditioning
Obturator and psoas sign testing	Shortening, dysfunction, or spasm of the obturator or iliopsoas muscles or fascia
Head raise and leg raise	Herniated disc Abdominal muscle weakness Deconditioning
Light abdominal palpation	Referred visceral pain Nerve entrapment Neuropathy
Gentle pinching	Referred visceral pain Nerve entrapment Neuropathy
Head maneuver	Referred visceral pain Nerve entrapment Neuropathy
Dermographism evaluation	Referred visceral pain Nerve entrapment Neuropathy
Single digit palpation	Trigger points Myofascial pain Hernias Nerve entrapments
Abdominal wall tenderness test	Abdominal wall pain Visceral pain
Groin and abdominal evaluation with and without Valsalva maneuver	Inguinal hernia Spigelian hernia Epigastric hernia Diastasis recti
(Incisional evaluation with and without Valsalva maneuver)	Incisional hernia
Pubic symphysis evaluation	Trigger points Osteitis pubis Osteomyelitis pubis
Traditional abdominal examination for distension, masses, ascites, bowel sounds, shifting dullness, vascular bruits, deep tenderness, guarding, or rigidity	Acute disease

Table 2.4 Components of the lithotomy physical examination of the woman with chronic pelvic pain and general problems or diagnoses that may be suggested based on these components of the examination

Lithotomy examination	Possible problems diagnosed
Visual inspection of the external genitalia	Inflammatory and infectious diseases Vulvar abscess Trauma Fistula Ulcerative disease Pigmented lesions (neoplasias) Condylomas Atrophic changes Fissure
Basic sensory testing to sharpness, dullness, and light touch	Nerve entrapment Neuropathy Spinal cord lesion
Cotton-tipped swab evaluation of the vestibule	Vulvar vestibulitis
Single-digit palpation of the vulva and pubic arch	Trigger points
(Colposcopic evaluation of the vulva and vestibule)	Neoplasia
Sims retractor or single-blade speculum examination of the vagina and pelvic muscles	Enterocele Cystocele Rectocele Uterine descensus
Cotton-tipped swab evaluation of the cervical os, paracervical, and cervical tissues	Trigger points
(Cotton-tipped swab evaluation of the vaginal cuff)	Trigger points Neuroma
Single-digit pelvic examination of the introitus	Vulvar vestibulitis Vaginismus Trigger points
Single-digit pelvic examination of levator ani	Pelvic floor pain syndrome Trigger points
Single-digit pelvic examination of coccygeus	Pelvic floor pain syndrome Trigger points
Single-digit pelvic examination of piriformis with and without abduction	Piriformis syndrome
Single-digit pelvic examination of anterior vaginal urethral and trigonal evaluation	Chronic urethral syndrome Urethritis Cystitis Interstitial cystitis Trigonitis Urethral diverticulum Vaginal wall cyst
Single-digit pelvic examination of the cervix, paracervical areas, and vaginal fornices	Trigger points Endometriosis Cervicitis Repeated cervical trauma Pelvic infection Pelvic infection Ureteral pain

Table 2.4 (*Continued*)

Lithotomy examination	Possible problems diagnosed
Single-digit pelvic examination of the uterus	Adenomyosis Pelvic congestion syndrome Pelvic infection Premenstrual syndrome Adhesions
Single-digit pelvic examination of the coccyx	Coccydynia
Single-digit pelvic examination of adnexa	Pelvic congestion syndrome Endometriosis
Bimanual pelvic examination	See text
Rectovaginal examination	See text

Table 2.5 Diagnoses that may be pain generators or etiologies of chronic pelvic pain in women by level of the evidence

Gynecologic

Level A
- Endometriosis
- Gynecologic malignancies
- Ovarian retention syndrome
- Ovarian remnant syndrome
- Pelvic congestion syndrome
- Pelvic inflammatory disease
- Tuberculous salpingitis

Level B
- Adhesions
- Benign cystic mesothelioma
- Fallopian tube prolapse after hysterectomy
- Leiomyomas
- Postoperative peritoneal cysts

Level C
- Adenomyosis
- Atypical dysmenorrhea
- Adnexal cysts
- Cervical stenosis
- Chronic ectopic pregnancy
- Chronic endometritis
- Endometrial or cervical polyps
- Endosalpingiosis
- Intrauterine contraceptive device
- Ovulatory pain
- Residual accessory ovary
- Spilled retained gallstones
- Symptomatic pelvic relaxation

Urologic

Level A
- Bladder neoplasm
- Interstitial cystitis/painful bladder syndrome
- Radiation cystitis

Level B
- Detrusor dyssynergia
- Urethral diverticulum
- Urethral syndrome

Level C
- Chronic urinary tract infection
- Recurrent, acute cystitis
- Recurrent, acute urethritis
- Stone/urolithiasis

Gastrointestinal

Level A
- Carcinoma of the colon
- Constipation
- Inflammatory bowel disease
- Irritable bowel syndrome

Level B
- Celiac disease
- Diverticular disease

Level C
- Chronic intermittent bowel obstruction
- Colitis

(*Continued*)

Table 2.5 (*Continued*)

Musculoskeletal	Others
Level A	**Level A**
• Abdominal wall myofascial pain (trigger points)	• Abdominal cutaneous nerve entrapment in a surgical scar
• Chronic coccygeal or back pain	• Somatization disorder
• Faulty or poor posture	• Prior pelvic surgery
• Fibromyalgia	**Level B**
• Neuralgia of the iliohypogastric, ilioinguinal, pudendal, or genitofemoral nerves	• Porphyria
• Pelvic floor tension myalgia	• Shingles
• Peripartum pelvic pain syndrome	• Sleep disturbances
Level B	**Level C**
• Herniated nucleus pulposus	• Abdominal epilepsy
• Low back pain	• Abdominal migraine
• Neoplasia of spinal cord or sacral nerve	• Bipolar disorders
• Piriformis syndrome	• Familial Mediterranean fever
• Rectus abdominis pain	
Level C	
• Compression of lumbar vertebrae	
• Degenerative joint disease	
• Hernias: ventral, inguinal, femoral, spigelian	
• Muscular strains and sprains	
• Spondylosis	

Level A: good and consistent scientific evidence of a causal relationship to chronic pelvic pain.
Level B: limited or inconsistent scientific evidence of a causal relationship to chronic pelvic pain.
Level C: causal relationship to chronic pelvic pain based on expert opinions.

tendency for patients and clinicians to assume that most women with CPP have a gynecologic etiology for their pain. There are data suggesting, however, that this is not the case, and that gastroenterologic and urologic disorders may be more common than gynecologic disorders. Also, most clinicians look for one diagnosis to account for CPP, but, as noted above, many women with CPP have more than one pain-related diagnosis. For example, data from a primary care database showed that, of patients with a diagnosis, 54% had more than one diagnosis. In our center, a tertiary referral practice specializing in CPP, 72% of patients have more than one diagnosis. Studies of patients with endometriosis suggest that up to 65% may also have interstitial cystitis/painful bladder syndrome (IC/PBS).

Reproductive system diagnoses

The number of reproductive tract diagnoses that approach level A evidence of association with CPP is relatively small (Table 2.5). Endometriosis is by far the most common of these diagnoses (Chapter 4). CPP subsequent to pelvic inflammatory disease (PID) is also common—published data suggest that one third of women develop CPP after PID—but it is usually diagnosed as severe adhesive disease at the time of evaluation for CPP (see Chapters 5 and 7). Ovarian retention syndrome, ovarian remnant syndrome, and pelvic congestion syndrome are less commonly diagnosed, and their classification as having level A evidence is somewhat controversial. Tuberculous salpingitis is rare in developed countries but still must be considered in the differential diagnosis. CPP as a manifestation of gynecologic malignancies is a late manifestation and will not be covered in this discussion.

As previously stated, it is most appropriate to evaluate patients for these seven diagnoses with higher levels of evidence to support an association with CPP before considering the diagnoses with lower levels of evidence (Table 2.5).

Endometriosis

Definition

The presence of tissue with the histologic appearance of endometrial glands and stroma located outside the uterine endothelium or myometrium (see also Chapter 4 for more on this condition).

History

Endometriosis is a disease of women of reproductive age; most women with endometriosis-associated pain are 20–45 years of age at the time of diagnosis. However, it has been reported in girls as young as 10 years and may be a more common cause of pain in teenagers than is generally recognized. It may also occur in postmenopausal women, particularly if they are on estrogen replacement. About 70% of women with endometriosis and CPP are nulligravid.

Most often, patients with endometriosis-associated pelvic pain initially have pain at the time of menses, followed by the development of premenstrual and midcycle ovulatory pain. This history precedes the presence of CPP in at least 90% of women with endometriosis-associated pelvic pain. Dyspareunia is present in 40–50% of women with endometriosis-associated pain. Intestinal involvement occurs in about 10–20% of women and may cause tenesmus, dyschezia, constipation, diarrhea, low back pain, and, rarely, hematochezia or symptoms of bowel obstruction. Urinary tract involvement occurs in 10–20% of women with endometriosis and often causes no bladder symptoms, although frequency, pressure, dysuria, or hematuria occasionally are present.

Abnormal uterine bleeding, particularly intermenstrual bleeding, may occur in women with endometriosis.

Physical examination

Some women have persistent areas of tenderness in the pelvis consistent with sites of endometriosis, but in many women with endometriosis-associated pelvic pain, the physical examination is completely normal. In some, there is tenderness only during menses. For this reason, it is sometimes helpful to do the examination during the first day or two of menstrual flow in women with suspected endometriosis.

Some specific findings that suggest endometriosis are: a fixed retroverted uterus with posterior tenderness; tender nodularity of the uterosacral ligaments and cul-de-sac; narrowing of the posterior vaginal fornix; asymmetrically enlarged, tender ovaries that are fixed to the broad ligaments or pelvic side walls; and lateral cervical deviation.

Diagnostic studies

At the present time, an accurate diagnosis of endometriosis can only be made by histologic confirmation. This is usually accomplished through biopsies at the time of diagnostic laparoscopy. Many gynecologic surgeons believe it appropriate to exclude or diagnose endometriosis solely on the basis of visual findings. However, recent studies have clearly shown that endometriosis presents with a variety of appearances, which may make laparoscopic visual diagnosis inaccurate in many cases.

A preoperative ultrasound seems prudent before a laparoscopic evaluation for CPP, specifically to evaluate for possible endometriomas and colorectal or bladder involvement. About 15–20% of women with endometriosis have endometriomas, generally ranging in size from 2 to 8 cm, so they are not always palpable on examination. However, it is important to recognize that only 60% of chocolate cysts are endometriomas.

In patients in whom intestinal endometriosis is suspected, endoscopic evaluation of the intestinal tract is usually normal, as most patients have involvement of the serosa or muscularis and not the mucosa. Imaging studies are more useful in identifying colonic involvement preoperatively. The choice of ultrasound, computed tomography (CT) scans, or magnetic resonance imaging (MRI) scans appears to somewhat depend on the expertise of the radiologist and gynecologist with each modality.

In patients with suspected urinary tract involvement, cystoscopy and intravenous pyelography or CT of the kidney, ureters, and bladder may be indicated. MRI and ultrasound imaging may also be useful.

Ovarian retention syndrome

Definition

The presence of persistent pelvic pain or dyspareunia attributed to one or both ovaries that were deliberately conserved at the time of hysterectomy (also called residual ovary syndrome).

History

Often there is a history of pelvic surgery prior to hysterectomy in patients with ovarian retention syndrome. The time of onset of symptoms and presentation following hysterectomy is quite varied, ranging from less than 6 months to greater than 20 years. Patients also often have a history of pelvic pain prior to their hysterectomy. If the prehysterectomy pain was due to another pain-associated disorder, such as pelvic congestion, pelvic adhesions, or endometriosis, persistent or recurrent pain due to that diagnosis must be considered. Another possible explanation for persistent pain after hysterectomy may be the pre-existence of inflammatory or neuropathic pain. A history of unilateral versus bilateral ovarian preservation at hysterectomy does not seem to influence the subsequent development of ovarian retention syndrome.

The intensity of pain may vary in a cyclic pattern in some patients, but this is not a consistent finding. Pain is usually unilateral in patients with one retained ovary, and may be unilateral or bilateral in patients with both ovaries. The pain can also radiate to the lower back and down into the legs. Deep dyspareunia occurs in at least one fifth of patients with ovarian retention syndrome. It is usually not a solitary complaint, but when it is the only symptom, pain with intercourse usually is located directly at the site of the retained ovary.

Physical examination

The abdominal examination usually is normal, although there may be tenderness to deep palpation in the lower abdomen. Pelvic examination reveals tenderness at the vaginal vault or upon palpation of the ovary. Pelvic examination may also reproduce the pain of dyspareunia at the retained ovary or ovaries.

Diagnostic studies

A diagnostic approach using gonadotropin-releasing hormone (GnRH) agonists has been suggested based on the theory that, since functional ovaries are an integral part of ovarian retention syndrome, suppressing their function should produce an amelioration of symptoms. Published evaluations of this approach are limited but suggest it may be predictive of successful pain relief after oophorectomy.

Laparoscopy may also be used as a diagnostic test and has the advantage of being diagnosti-

cally and therapeutically beneficial. At laparoscopy, the surgeon is able to identify any pathology of the retained ovary. Conscious laparoscopic pain mapping may be useful in cases where the diagnosis is not clear.

Ovarian remnant syndrome

Definition

The presence of pelvic pain with a persistence of ovarian tissue inadvertently not removed at the time of intended extirpation of one or both ovaries, with or without hysterectomy.

History

Ovarian remnant syndrome occurs due to persistence of ovarian fragments unintentionally left in situ during oophorectomy, so by definition there is always a past history of unilateral or bilateral oophorectomy. Most often there is a history of hysterectomy and bilateral salpingo-oophorectomy, but the syndrome may occur in women who have a history of bilateral or unilateral oophorectomy, with or without hysterectomy. A history of prior surgery for treatment of an ovarian remnant should make the physician highly suspicious of recurrent ovarian remnant syndrome.

A patient with ovarian remnant syndrome may present any time from a few months to 5 years or more after her oophorectomy. It is a disorder that occurs in the reproductive years. Patients usually present with chronic abdominopelvic pain. Most often pain occurs in the lower abdomen and pelvis and is ipsilateral to the remnant, although it can be diffuse or variable in its location. Deep dyspareunia is sometimes also present. Patients may complain of flank pain in the rare cases that have ureteral obstruction due to the remnant. Since most of the patients have undergone multiple surgeries, including a hysterectomy and bilateral salpingo-oophorectomy, the possibility of a gynecologic cause is usually not recognized, and they often suffer for years before their diagnoses are made.

The absence of hot flashes in a woman with a history of bilateral oophorectomy who is not using hormonal replacement therapy is an important signal to investigate carefully for ovarian remnant syndrome. However, more than 70% of women with ovarian remnant syndrome do not have hot flashes in spite of not receiving hormonal replacement therapy. In a patient who has undergone bilateral oophorectomy without hysterectomy, cyclic vaginal bleeding in the absence of hormonal replacement therapy is suggestive of endogenous ovarian estrogen production by an ovarian remnant.

Physical examination

Tenderness to deep palpation may be present and is usually on the same side as the remnant. Ovarian remnants are usually too small to be palpated abdominally. At pelvic examination, inspection of the external genitalia and vagina usually reveals signs of estrogen effect, with normal-sized labia and moist, well-cornified vaginal mucosa. Pelvic palpation may reveal tenderness in one or both fornices. Bimanual pelvic examination may reveal a palpable mass, although its absence does not preclude the diagnosis. If a mass is palpable, it is usually tender and small (less than 5 cm) and located on the pelvic side wall or at the lateral vaginal apex.

Diagnostic studies

A follicle-stimulating hormone (FSH) level less than 40 mIU/mL and an estradiol level greater than 30 pg/mL in a patient who has not had hormonal replacement therapy for at least 2–3 weeks are diagnostic in most cases. However, premenopausal levels of FSH and estradiol are present in only 50% of women with an ovarian remnant, so postmenopausal levels cannot be used to exclude the diagnosis.

When ovarian remnant syndrome is suspected and FSH and estradiol levels are postmenopausal, the GnRH agonist stimulation test is useful. GnRH agonists initially stimulate gonadotropin production and therefore ovarian estrogen production. This observation is used in the GnRH agonist stimulation test, in which a baseline level of estradiol is measured and a GnRH agonist (e.g., depot leuprolide, 3.75 mg intramuscularly once, or leuprolide 1 mg a day for 3 days subcutaneously) is administered, followed by a repeat measurement of estradiol four 4–7 days later. If hormonally responsive ovarian tissue is present, a significant rise in estradiol occurs. This test will not be reliable if exogenous hormones are being taken.

Imaging studies are important both diagnostically and preoperatively. Vaginal ultrasound shows a pelvic mass in more than 50% of cases. The diagnostic accuracy of ultrasound may be improved by pretreatment with clomiphene citrate. A 5–10 day course of clomiphene citrate, 100 mg daily, appears to stimulate follicular formation in up to 90% of cases, and this may permit easier sonographic visualization. Not all ovarian remnants have functional follicles, so this technique is not always helpful.

CT scanning, particularly with intravenous contrast to evaluate the urinary tract, can be extremely useful. If there is ureteral dilatation, hydronephrosis, or ureteral deviation, it is likely the ovarian remnant will be directly over the ureter.

In some cases, the diagnosis of ovarian remnant can only be made at the time of surgery, and even then it can be difficult. Laparoscopy is an inconsistent diagnostic tool as dense adhesions frequently hide the ovarian remnant. If diagnostic laparoscopy is used in the evaluation of a patient with a suspected ovarian remnant, the surgeon must be prepared to perform extensive and potentially complicated adhesiolysis. The most common locations are along the pelvic side wall and the vaginal cuff. In both of these locations, the remnant is likely to be on the ureter (Figure 2.1) On the left pelvic side wall, ovarian remnants are often covered by an adherent rectosigmoid

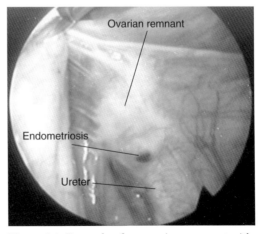

Figure 2.1 Example of an ovarian remnant with endometriosis located over the ureter.

colon. Further complicating the operative diagnosis is the fact that ovarian remnants may be bilateral and there may be multiple remnants unilaterally.

Pelvic congestion syndrome

Definition

A syndrome characterized by pelvic pain, pelvic varicosities, and pelvic venous congestion with delayed emptying of the pelvic veins.

History

Pelvic congestion syndrome remains a controversial disorder. Substantial research suggests that when the diagnosis is accurately confirmed by the triad of pelvic pain, pelvic varicosities, and pelvic venous congestion with delayed emptying of the pelvic veins, it is a legitimate diagnosis and is responsible for pelvic pain in a substantial number of women. Using this triad of diagnostic criteria, one study found that pelvic congestion syndrome could be a source of pelvic pain in up to 40%, and potentially the only source in 30%, of women with CPP.

Symptoms of pelvic congestion syndrome are usually limited to the reproductive years. Pelvic pain is generally described as dull, aching pain in the pelvic area, similar to the quality of pain described in the legs of people with symptomatic leg varicosities. Pain is exacerbated by physical activity. A typical characteristic of pain of pelvic congestion syndrome is that it varies in its location. It is also most severe premenstrually, which has been termed "congestive dysmenorrhea." Occasionally, acute paroxysmal exacerbations of sharp pain may occur, at times severe enough to result in emergent evaluation, and may lead to mistaken diagnoses such as acute appendicitis or PID.

Deep dyspareunia is another consistent symptom of pelvic congestion syndrome, occurring in 70–80% of patients. Postcoital pelvic aching, lasting in some cases up to 24 hours, also is typical of pelvic congestion syndrome and occurs in about 65% of cases.

Physical examination

Abdominal palpation reveals tenderness at the ovarian point in about 75% of women with pelvic congestion syndrome. The ovarian point lies at

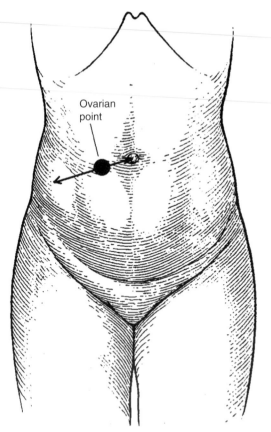

Figure 2.2 The ovarian point; tenderness at this location is commonly found in women with pelvic congestion syndrome.

the junction of the upper and middle thirds of a line drawn from the anterior superior iliac spine to the umbilicus (Figure 2.2). On inspection of the external genitalia, superficial vulvar and paravulvar varices may be observed but are not consistently present. Palpation of the cervix frequently elicits pain and tenderness on movement. The uterosacral ligaments and the parametrium are often also tender to palpation. Uterine and adnexal tenderness to palpation is characteristic of pelvic congestion syndrome.

Diagnostic studies

Pelvic venography is the current "gold standard" diagnostic test for pelvic congestion syndrome. Although invasive, it provides a detailed picture of the pelvic venous anatomy, accurate measurements of venous diameters, assessment of venous dysfunction and delayed emptying, and grading of the degree of venous plexuses. A variety of techniques has been used, but the most common techniques are selective retrograde ovarian venography and transuterine venography.

Transuterine venography is the method best validated for accurate diagnosis. Water-soluble contrast medium is introduced into the uterine venous system via injection into the myometrium of the uterine fundus. This is facilitated by using a special single-lumen needle and metal sheath (a reusable system is available from Rocket Needle, Rocket Co., London, United Kingdom; a disposable system is available from Cook Women's Health, Bloomington, Indiana, United States).

The needle is passed through the cervix via a special concentric sheath that covers all but the final 0.5 cm tip of the needle. With the patient on her back and ideally in a slight reverse Trendelen-burg position, 20–30 mL of the contrast medium is injected. The first image is taken immediately at the end of injection, followed by a second image 20 seconds later, a third image at 40 seconds, and a fourth image at 60 seconds (Figure 2.3). The procedure is painful and may require heavy sedation and/or general or local anesthesia to perform. Beard and colleagues have described a venogram scoring system based on the maximum diameter of the ovarian veins, time of disappearance of contrast, and degree of congestion of the ovarian plexus (Table 2.6). Using a score of 5 or more as diagnostic of pelvic congestion syndrome, a sensitivity of 91% and a specificity of 89% was report. The specificity of transuterine venography has been substantiated by Soysal et al.

Selective ovarian venography can either be performed via a jugular venous approach or via the more commonly used transfemoral approach

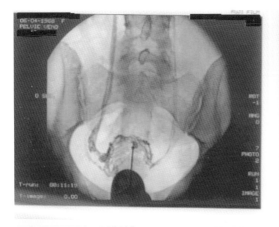
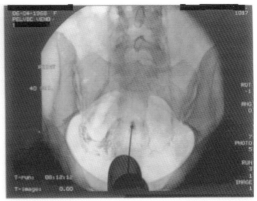
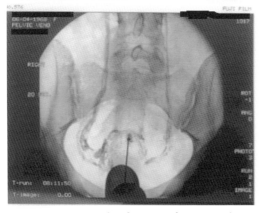
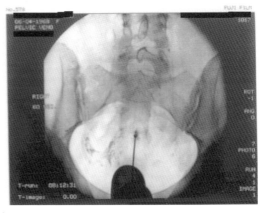

Figure 2.3 Example of a normal transuterine pelvic venogram.

Table 2.6 Scoring system for assessing transuterine pelvic venography

	Score		
	1	2	3
Maximal diameter of ovarian veins (mm)	1–4	5–8	>8
Time to disappearance of contrast medium after end of injection (seconds)	0	20	40
Ovarian plexus congestion	Normal	Moderate	Extensive

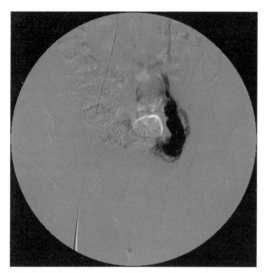

Figure 2.4 Example of left ovarian varicosities as demonstrated by retrograde ovarian venography.

(Figure 2.4). The technique is performed under local anesthesia, often with sedation. Special Teflon catheters are passed under fluoroscopic guidance into the ovarian veins, and nonionic, water-soluble contrast medium is injected. The diagnostic criteria recommended are a maximal ovarian vein diameter of 10 mm or more, congestion of the ovarian venous plexus, filling of veins across the midline, or filling of vulvar and thigh varicosities. These criteria are not as well validated or standardized as those for transuterine venography. Other imaging studies such as ultrasound and MRI can demonstrate pelvic varicosities but have not been validated for the diagnosis of pelvic congestion syndrome.

Laparoscopy is one of the most common diagnostic studies performed by gynecologists for pelvic pain, but it is not a reliable way to diagnose pelvic congestion syndrome, even though pelvic varicosities can sometimes be visualized. It is important to realize that neither the identification of varicosities nor negative findings at the time of laparoscopy is sufficient to make a positive or negative conclusion regarding the diagnosis of pelvic congestion syndrome.

Pelvic inflammatory disease

Definition

An acute infection of the upper reproductive tract, most often used to signify infection of the fallopian tubes (acute salpingitis), but it may be infection of the endometrium (endometritis), ovaries (oophoritis), or peritoneum (peritonitis). CPP is a frequent sequela of PID, occurring in 30% or more of all cases, and has historically been called "chronic PID." This is, however, a misnomer as there is usually no evidence of persistent infection in these cases.

History

The estimated incidence of acute PID is 14 per 100 women, and about 30% of women develop CPP after PID. This makes post-PID CPP a very common occurrence, even though it is not a common diagnosis in most of the published series of CPP. This is probably due to the fact that post-PID CPP does not have any unique characteristics and often there is not a clear history of prior PID. In general, pain is diffuse and not localized. Dyspareunia and dysmenorrhea are frequently components of the pelvic pain symptoms. Sometimes a past history of PID can be elicited, supporting, but not proving, the diagnosis. A history of several episodes of acute PID makes it much more likely to be the source of CPP, as up to two-thirds of women develop CPP after three or more episodes of acute PID. It is important to distinguish recurrent acute PID from CPP as a sequela of PID.

Physical examination

Many times with post-PID-associated CPP, there is both lower abdominal tenderness and uterine and adnexal tenderness. Occasionally a tubo-ovarian complex can be palpated as an adnexal mass. If adhesive disease is severe, the uterus may be fixed in its position, often retroverted, and tender on attempts to move it.

Diagnostic studies

As a sequela of PID, CPP is very highly correlated with fallopian tubal damage and adhesions. Unilateral or bilateral hydrosalpinges may be identified by imaging studies and suggest prior PID as a possible etiology of CPP. Laparoscopy is diagnostically accurate if the pelvic pathology is clearly consistent with previous PID. For example, hydrosalpinges, tubal clubbing, fimbrial occlusion, and perihepatic adhesions are relatively specific to prior PID. Pelvic adhesive disease, however, is not specific to prior PID and may be due to prior surgery, appendicitis, inflammatory bowel disease, or endometriosis.

Genital tuberculosis

Definition

Upper genital tract infection with *Mycoplasma tuberculosis*, especially involving the fallopian tubes and endometrium.

History

Genital tuberculosis usually presents with infertility (45–70% of cases) and amenorrhea or abnormal bleeding (25–45% of cases), but in about 25% of cases pelvic pain is the presenting symptom. Genital tuberculosis is not common in the Western world but has increased with the increase of HIV. A history of exposure to tuberculosis may be obtained, but more often the patient is unaware of her prior exposure. Pulmonary symptoms are usually not present.

Physical examination

Diffuse pelvic tenderness is sometimes present. In some cases, a pelvic mass can be palpated. If adhesive disease is severe, the uterus may be fixed in its position and tender on attempts to move it.

Diagnostic studies

Imaging studies may show evidence of hydrosalpinges. Hysterosalpingography often reveals tubal occlusion and may show uterine synechiae. Laparoscopy reveals granulomatous changes in the pelvic peritoneum and often significant adhesive disease involving the fallopian tubes and ovaries. Chest radiographs are usually normal. Tuberculosis skin testing is usually positive. Specimens obtained by endometrial or laparoscopic biopsy will usually test positive for tuberculosis by polymerase chain reaction or culture for acid-fast bacilli.

Urinary system diagnoses

Urologic pelvic pain-related diagnoses account for about one third of the diagnoses in women with CPP. The list of diagnoses with level A evidence of association with CPP is short, and IC/PBS is by far the most common of these.

Interstitial cystitis/painful bladder syndrome

Definition

Pelvic pain, pressure, or discomfort related to the bladder, associated with the persistent urge to void or urinary frequency, in the absence of urinary infection or other bladder pathology.

History

"Interstitial cystitis" is the term used historically for this syndrome, but because pain or discomfort is the essential criterion of the disorder, it has been suggested that "painful bladder syndrome" or "bladder pain syndrome" may be better names. In this chapter, the name "interstitial cystitis/painful bladder syndrome" (IC/PBS) will be used.

Pelvic pain, urinary frequency, urinary urge, and nocturia are the characteristic symptoms of IC/PBS. Symptoms may be episodic and thought to be due to urinary tract infections, especially early in the course of the disease. This may lead to multiple misdiagnoses as urinary tract infections. A history of empiric treatment of recurrent urinary tract infections without documentation of positive cultures is common in women with IC. Symptoms may exacerbate perimenstrually and be attributed to endometriosis. Symptoms may be continuous, with intermittent flares related to diet, intercourse, and menses. Symptoms may be severe and incapacitating, with disabling pain and urinary frequency every 10–30 minutes. Clearly, IC/PBS may present as a wide spectrum of disease severity and symptoms.

Our clinical experience is that women with IC/PBS do not experience urinary urgency and frequency because of the fear or sense of becoming incontinent, as do women with overactive bladder syndrome. Rather, their urgency is related to the feeling of pressure or pain when there is urine in their bladders. This discomfort sometimes, but not always, improves with voiding. Dysuria, or pain during voiding, is not a characteristic symptom.

Dyspareunia is also a common pain symptom with IC. Pain with intercourse appears to occur from both pelvic floor muscle and bladder tenderness, but may additionally occur with entry due to associated localized vulvodynia (vulvar vestibulitis or provoked vestibulodynia).

A voiding diary is often helpful. This may capture important information about the type and volume of fluid intake, as well as voiding patterns. For example, many women with IC severely restrict their fluid intakes to minimize high voiding frequencies. If this information is not obtained, the clinician may incorrectly assume such patients do not have urinary urgency and frequency.

IC should be considered in patients with persistent pelvic pain after hysterectomy. An observational study of 111 patients with CPP that persisted after hysterectomy suggested that 88 (79%) had IC/PBS. Clearly, this study suggests that pelvic pain after a hysterectomy may be due to IC/PBS, but it also suggests that gynecologists should take care to exclude IC/PBS before proceeding to hysterectomy in patients with CPP.

There are several questionnaires available to assist in screening and diagnosis of IC/PBS. The most commonly used are the O'Leary–Sant, Pelvic Pain and Urgency/Frequency Symptom Scale (PUF), and University of Wisconsin Index.

Physical examination

The physical examination in women with IC/PBS can be normal. Some women may have anterior vaginal wall tenderness under the trigone and bladder base and suprapubic pelvic tenderness, probably due to bladder allodynia or hyperalgesia. Many women with IC/PBS may also have significant tenderness of the pelvic floor muscles. Especially during episodes of acute exacerbation of pain, levator ani or piriformis muscle tenderness may be present. At the time of the examination, it is important to try to exclude findings consistent with urethral diverticula, adnexal pathology, endometriosis, and uterine abnormalities.

Diagnostic studies

Urinalysis and urine culture are necessary tests to exclude urinary tract infections or significant hematuria. Urine cytology (or cystoscopy) is recommended if the patient has a history of smoking or has significant hematuria.

Cystoscopy with hydrodistension with general or regional anesthesia has long been considered the "gold standard" diagnostic test for IC/PBS. Identification of a Hunner ulcer is pathognomonic, but this is not a common finding. More often, cystoscopy with hydrodistension shows glomerulations, which are mucosal hemorrhages that have a characteristic appearance upon second filling of the bladder. Recently, the value of cystoscopy has been questioned. At least 10% of patients who clinically have clear evidence of IC/PBS have normal findings at the time of cystoscopic hydrodistension. Another problem is that glomerulations have been observed in asymptomatic control patients after hydrodistension with up to 950 mL water.

The potassium sensitivity or Parson's test (PST) is performed by instilling 40 mL sterile water into the bladder for 5 minutes, followed by instilling 40 mL of a 0.4 molar solution of potassium chloride (40 mEq in 100 mL water) into the bladder for 5 minutes (the water being drained before instilling the potassium chloride solution). A positive test is when the patient has a change of two or more on the pain or urgency scale with the potassium chloride solution versus the water. The PST can flare severe symptoms in patients with IC, so we recommend that all women with a positive test receive a "rescue cocktail" after the potassium chloride solution has been drained. A number of different solutions have been used as rescue treatments. Two of the most common are 20,000 IU heparin mixed with 20 mL 1% lidocaine or a 15 mL mixture of 40,000 IU heparin, 8 mL 2%

lidocaine, and 3 mL 8.4% sodium bicarbonate. The "rescue cocktail" usually reverses the urgency and pain brought on by the potassium chloride.

The PST can also have an educational benefit for the patient. This may especially be the case for patients who have been given different previous diagnoses, such as vulvodynia or endometriosis. If the instillation of the potassium chloride solution reproduces or exacerbates their usual pain, such as introital burning pain (often a site of referred pain with IC/PBS) or pelvic cramping pain (that may have been attributed to endometriosis), this reaction provides reassurance to them that their pain is of bladder origin. If the pain is relieved with the rescue cocktail, the reassurance and insight into the origin of their pain is even greater.

Patients with high pain levels may not be able to discern a change with the intravesical PST or may not be able to tolerate the discomfort caused by the test. The instillation of an anesthetic agent into the bladder has been suggested as a possible diagnostic test in such cases. The "rescue cocktail" described above also provides an opportunity for the patient and clinician to see if the patient's symptoms are abated by this anesthetic challenge.

Researchers have worked tirelessly to find a simple urinary biomarker that would be specific for IC, but none is currently in widespread clinical use.

Finally, it should be stated that IC/PBS can in many patients be diagnosed based on clinical findings without invasive diagnostic testing.

Gastrointestinal system diagnoses

Although gastrointestinal symptoms are very common in women with CPP, the list of diagnoses with level A evidence of possible etiologic association with CPP is quite short. Irritable bowel syndrome (IBS) is by far the most common diagnosis in women with CPP, but chronic constipation is also relatively common. It is important that inflammatory bowel disease and carcinoma be excluded.

Irritable bowel syndrome

Definition

A common functional bowel disorder of uncertain etiology characterized by a chronic, relaps-

ing pattern of abdominopelvic pain associated with bowel function or with constipation and/or diarrhea.

History

IBS is probably the most common diagnosis in women with CPP, with symptoms consistent with the diagnosis in at least 40% of women with CPP. IBS is most commonly defined by the Rome III criteria: recurrent abdominal pain or discomfort at least 3 days per month in the last 3 months, with a symptom onset at least 6 months prior to diagnosis, and associated with two or more of the following: (1) improvement with defecation, (2) onset associated with a change in frequency of stool, or (3) onset associated with a change in form (appearance) of the stool (Table 2.7).

A screening questionnaire may be helpful in identifying patients with IBS (Table 2.8). Pain quality varies among different patients and may be described as cramping, burning, dull, sharp, steady, bloating, or knife-like. Abdominal pain is most often in the left lower quadrant, but may be located in the middle or right lower abdomen as well. Although the location of the pain may vary from person to person, it generally remains fairly consistent over time in a given patient. Eating commonly precipitates pain. Characteristically, the pain of IBS resolves during sleep. Awakening and noting pain is not the same as being awakened by pain, and it is important to try to have the patient make this distinction if possible. IBS symptoms often exacerbate during menses, and this correlation should not be assumed to mean the pain is of gynecologic origin.

Most patients with IBS have abnormal defecation. The defecatory abnormalities generally can be categorized into one of three predominant patterns: constipation predominant (IBS-C), diarrhea predominant (IBS-D), or alternating constipation and diarrhea (IBS-M).

There are symptoms that should serve as "red flags" that organic disease (especially inflammatory bowel disease or carcinoma) is possible and therefore must be excluded (Table 2.9). A history of unexplained weight loss, anorexia, early satiety, narrow pencil-thin stools, anemia, hematochezia, or melena is not consistent with IBS and mandates exclusion of malignancy, serious infection, or inflammatory bowel disease. Persistent

Table 2.7 The Rome III diagnostic criteria for irritable bowel syndrome (IBS)

Recurrent abdominal pain or discomfort* on at least 3 days per month in the last 3 months,** associated with two or more of criteria 1–3 below:
1. Improvement with defecation
2. Onset associated with a change in frequency of stools
3. Onset associated with a change in form (appearance) of stools

Symptoms that support but are not essential to the diagnosis of IBS:
- Abnormal stool frequency
  - Greater than three bowel movements per day
  - Less than three bowel movements per week
- Abnormal stool form
  - Lumpy or hard stool
  - Loose or watery stool
- Abnormal stool passage
  - Straining
  - Urgency
  - Feeling of incomplete bowel movement
- Passage of mucus
- Bloating or feeling of abdominal distension

*Discomfort means an uncomfortable sensation not described as pain by the patient.
**Criteria fulfilled for the last 3 months with a symptom onset at least 6 months prior to diagnosis.

watery diarrhea, diarrheic stool volumes of over 200 mL per day, or bloody diarrhea suggests a serious organic disorder, such as inflammatory bowel disease or bacterial or parasitic infection. Nausea and vomiting also suggest a disorder other than IBS. Constitutional, nongastrointestinal symptoms such as fatigue, myalgias, arthralgias, fevers, chills, and sweats are not usually reported by patients with IBS except in occasional severe cases. Such symptoms may suggest coexisting fibromyalgia, chronic fatigue syndrome, arthritis or hypothyroidism. A family history of inflammatory bowel disease, celiac disease, or gastrointestinal malignancy increases the chance of these diseases in the patient thought to have IBS.

In addition, symptoms of IBS generally start in late adolescence or early adulthood. Onset in later life is less common, and an onset in patients older than 60 years of age should raise the concern of other diseases, such as colon cancer, diverticulitis, and inflammatory bowel disease. Finally, even though the symptoms of IBS are chronic, they tend to be variable in severity. Pain and bowel dysfunction that are of a steadily progressive nature suggest a diagnosis other than IBS. Also, as a chronic disorder, IBS usually has an onset of symptoms that is gradual and vague,

and it is unusual for the patient to be able to relate an exact date of onset of symptoms.

Physical examination

The physical examination in patients with IBS is usually normal. Generally, they do not appear seriously ill. Abdominal inspection may reveal mild to moderate distention. On palpation, tenderness may be elicited. If present, it is most often in the left lower quadrant but may be generalized. Rebound tenderness occasionally may be elicited but is not a common finding and should serve as a "red flag" for a different and organic illness. Signs suggesting an acute abdomen, with generalized tenderness or board-like rigidity, rebound tenderness, tympanitic bowel sounds, and fever are not consistent with IBS and should lead the physician to evaluate expeditiously for a serious intra-abdominal process.

Rectal and pelvic examinations are important to assess for masses or anal disease, such as hemorrhoids or fissures that could explain some of the symptoms. Often, there is rectal tenderness due to heightened tone, rectal spasm, or visceral hypersensitivity. Severe tenderness, a rectal or pelvic mass, or the presence of blood in the rectum demands detailed diagnostic evaluation.

Table 2.8 Screening questionnaire derived from the Rome III irritable bowel syndrome module and criteria

1. In the last 3 months, how often did you have discomfort or pain anywhere in your abdomen?
   0. Never → *Skip remaining questions*
   1. Less than one day a month
   2. One day a month
   3. **Two to three days a month**
   4. **One day a week**
   5. **More than one day a week**
   6. **Every day**
2. For women: Did this discomfort or pain occur only during your menstrual bleeding and not at other times?
   0. **No**
   1. Yes
   2. **Does not apply because I have had the change in life (menopause)**
3. Have you had this discomfort or pain 6 months or longer?
   0. No
   1. **Yes**
4. How often did this discomfort or pain get better after you had a bowel movement?
   0. Never or rarely
   1. **Sometimes**
   2. **Often**
   3. **Most of the time**
   4. **Always**
5. When this discomfort or pain started, did you have more frequent bowel movements?
   0. Never or rarely
   1. **Sometimes**
   2. **Often**
   3. **Most of the time**
   4. **Always**
6. When this discomfort or pain started, did you have less frequent bowel movements?
   0. Never or rarely
   1. **Sometimes**
   2. **Often**
   3. **Most of the time**
   4. **Always**
7. When this discomfort or pain started, were your stools (bowel movements) looser?
   0. Never or rarely
   1. **Sometimes**
   2. **Often**
   3. **Most of the time**
   4. **Always**
8. When this discomfort or pain started, how often did you have harder stools?
   0. Never or rarely
   1. **Sometimes**
   2. **Often**
   3. **Most of the time**
   4. **Always**
9. In the last 3 months, how often did you have hard or lumpy stools?
   0. Never or rarely
   1. **Sometimes**
   2. **Often**
   3. **Most of the time**
   4. **Always**
10. In the last 3 months, how often did you have loose, mushy or watery stools?
   0. Never or rarely
   1. **Sometimes**
   2. **Often**
   3. **Most of the time**
   4. **Always**

Answers in **bold** type are consistent with the diagnosis of irritable bowel syndrome.

The presence of a fistula or significant perianal disease raises the possibility of Crohn's disease.

Diagnostic studies

The diagnosis of IBS should be symptom-based and the evaluation of each patient individualized. IBS should not be a diagnosis of exclusion, and diagnostic testing usually should not be extensive, difficult, or prohibitively expensive. The history and physical examination are the pre-eminent components of the evaluation. Endoscopy, CT scans, and barium enemas should rarely be necessary. In particular, in the younger patients with obvious symptoms of IBS in line with the Rome criteria and with normal examination findings, usually no diagnostic testing is necessary. For all patients, as a general rule, very minimal testing is needed as long as none of the "red flags" previously discussed is discovered during evaluation (Table 2.5) The major goal of

Table 2.9 "Red flag" symptoms and signs that suggest a diagnosis of organic pathology rather than irritable bowel syndrome

Anemia
Narrow, pencil-thin stools
Rectal bleeding or blood in the stool
Unexplained weight loss
Anorexia or early satiety
Abdominal guarding and rebound tenderness
Persistent watery diarrhea
Diarrheic stool volumes >200 mL/day
Bloody diarrhea
Nausea and vomiting
Fever
Nongastrointestinal symptoms
Initial diagnosis at 60 or more years of age

diagnostic testing in patients with IBS is to identify alternative or concurrent disorders.

In most patient with suspected IBS in whom testing is thought to be warranted, it seems cost-effective to start with a complete blood cell count with differential, chemistry profile, erythrocyte sedimentation rate, and stool testing for occult blood.

If diarrhea is the predominant complaint, three stool samples should be sent for fecal leukocytes, and if positive, for routine culture, ova, parasites, and *Clostridium difficile*. Serologic tests for celiac disease—endomysial antibodies and antigliadin antibodies—should also be ordered in patients with persistent diarrhea. Thyroid testing to eliminate a possible diagnosis of hyperthyroidism may be indicated if there are other symptoms or signs suggestive of hyperthyroidism.

If constipation is the predominant complaint, possible hypothyroidism may be evaluated with a thyroid-stimulating hormone level.

Colonoscopy should be performed in patients of 50 years of age or older. In younger patients, colonoscopy is indicated if they have a strong family history of inflammatory bowel disease or colorectal cancer, if they are anemic, or if fecal occult blood testing is positive. Colonoscopy is generally preferable to barium enema imaging.

If the history suggests lactose intolerance, it can be formally tested with a hydrogen breath test. The breath test is much more sensitive than the blood test.

Musculoskeletal system diagnoses

It is common for physicians, especially gynecologists, to think that all CPP is of visceral origin, but this is not the case. Many women with CPP have somatic pain-related disorders (see Table 2.1). Abdominal myofascial pain syndrome with trigger points and pelvic floor tension myalgia are both very common diagnoses in women with CPP. Pain related to coccygodynia is less common but should be considered, especially if there is a history of a difficult vaginal delivery or a fall on the tailbone. Faulty posture with increased lordosis–kyphosis has been observed in many women with CPP and may play an etiologic role. Fibromyalgia presents with total body pain but may also present with CPP as a component of the syndrome. Neuralgias of the iliohypogastric, ilioinguinal, genitofemoral, or pudendal nerves may present as CPP and especially should be considered in patients with prior abdominopelvic surgeries, pelvic trauma, or metabolic disorders associated with peripheral neuropathies.

Abdominal myofascial pain syndrome

Definition

Chronic abdominal pain of a muscle or group of muscles and fascia that is associated with and/or caused by trigger points. Trigger points are localized and sometimes extremely painful spots found in any skeletal muscle of the body.

History

Pain with abdominal myofascial pain syndrome may be constant or intermittent. Pain is usually worsened by activities such as coughing, turning over in bed, or the lifting of heavy weights that increase tension in the affected muscle groups. Generally, there is an absence of associated visceral symptoms, such as nausea, vomiting, diarrhea, or constipation, and of systemic symptoms, such as fever or chills. Some patients with abdominal myofascial pain syndrome will have a past history of abdominal surgery or injury with physical exertion, but often there is nothing elicited to explain the development of the syndrome.

Physical examination

Tenderness is elicited with relatively gentle palpation of the affected muscle, and especially with single-digit palpation of a myofascial trigger point. A trigger point is always tender and may also show a local twitch response when compressed. Exquisite focal tenderness of the trigger point sometimes is identified by the jump sign—a vocalization by and withdrawal of the patient when the trigger point is compressed. Not uncommonly, trigger point palpation triggers pain within the area of pain referral.

The abdominal wall tenderness test (Carnett test) is often useful in the identification of myofascial trigger points. This test is positive, suggesting that the abdominal wall is the source of pain, when tenderness due to palpation is increased by tightening of the abdominal wall muscles. Clinically, this is most easily done by asking the patient to do a partial sit-up (raise her head off the examination table using her abdominal muscles) while the suspected trigger point is palpated with a single finger, and having her note whether this increases the pain of palpation. Some of the other abdominal wall abnormalities that also will give a positive Carnett test include trauma, hernia, and nerve entrapment.

It is important to methodically evaluate the entire abdominal wall for myofascial trigger points in all women with CPP.

Diagnostic studies

No diagnostic studies are needed to make a diagnosis of abdominal myofascial pain syndrome, but confirmation can be obtained by performing diagnostic trigger point injections (see Chapter 11).

Pelvic floor tension myalgia

Definition

Pelvic pain caused by or associated with pain and tenderness of one or more of the muscles of the "pelvic floor"—levator ani, coccygeus, or piriformis—or their associated fascia or insertions.

History

Symptoms are usually vague and poorly localized. Pain may be diffuse within the pelvis or more localized about the rectum or the anterior pelvis. The pain is most often described as aching, throbbing, or heaviness. Low back pain and radiation of pain to the sacrum at the area of insertion of the levator ani is not uncommon (greater than 80% of patients). Radiation to the hip and down the back of the thigh, like sciatica, may also be noted and is particularly characteristic of piriformis spasm. The pain may be quite severe, and 10–15% of patients experience characteristic episodes of acute, sudden, severe pain in the rectal ("proctalgia fugax") or vaginal ("colpalgia fugax"). This is often described as a knife-like pain going up the rectum or vagina.

Characteristically, the pain of pelvic floor tension myalgia is not worsened by bowel movements (less than 33%), and in only a minority is worsened by coitus (less than 15%). However, dyspareunia is a common symptom. Pain is increased by prolonged sitting or standing in one position. Characteristically, pain from the levator ani starts in the afternoon and becomes progressively worse. When the pain flares, it may be constant for days at a time. As previously noted, it sometimes occurs suddenly with a short duration. The pain may mimic that due to diseases of the reproductive organs, with alterations and cyclic variations due to hormonal influences on the muscles, ligaments, and joints of the pelvis.

Physical examination

If pelvic floor tension myalgia is suspected, the initial portion of the pelvic examination should include a gentle, single-finger palpation of the pelvic floor musculature to assess tone, sensation, and tenderness. The most common finding with pelvic floor tension myalgia is tenderness and spasm of one or more of the muscles of the pelvic floor. Digital pressure on the involved muscle characteristically reproduces or intensifies the patient's pain symptoms. It is not unusual for the tenderness to be unilateral.

The levator ani muscles are easily palpated during vaginal or rectal examination. They lie adjacent to the lateral vaginal walls just above the hymenal ring. The medial margins of the muscles are slightly thicker than a standard pencil, running in an anteroposterior direction, and identification may be confirmed by having the patient contract her pelvic muscles. The anus simultaneously elevates when the levators are contracted. Patients with pelvic floor tension myalgia may not be able to voluntarily contract the levator ani muscles because they are already maximally contracted. The bulbocavernous muscles lie distal to the hymenal ring, allowing them to be easily differentiated from the levators.

The piriformis muscles are somewhat more difficult to palpate. Rectal examination may allow an easier evaluation than vaginal examination. With rectal examination, as one starts in the posterior midline and sweeps laterally and anteriorly, the rectal finger first passes over the piriformis and then the coccygeus and the levator ani muscles. The piriformis originates from the anterior surface of the sacrum and passes from the pelvis via the greater sciatic notch, and it may be palpated along this portion of its course. In the lithotomy position, if the patient is asked to abduct the thigh against resistance as the piriformis is palpated, there is exquisite tenderness of the muscle in cases of spasm or tension myalgia involving the piriformis.

In some patients with pelvic floor tension myalgia, there will also be tenderness of the coccyx, lateral sacrum, or sacrococcygeal ligaments. Coccygodynia is suggested if there is reproduction of the patient's pain when the coccyx is digitally manipulated. This finding may be a way to distinguish coccygodynia from pelvic floor tension myalgia.

Diagnostic studies

The diagnosis of pelvic floor tension myalgia is by clinical history and physical findings. No imaging or laboratory evaluations are needed to establish the diagnosis. However, as pelvic floor tension myalgia may not infrequently occur secondary to other pelvic pathology and pain, other evaluations may be needed to rule out diagnoses such as endometriosis or IC. This is especially true if pelvic floor tension myalgia does not respond to appropriate physical therapy and medical treatment. Evaluation for true coccygodynia (usually localized pain and tenderness at the sacrococcygeal joint due to prior trauma), rare genetic syndromes of familial rectal pain, tumors or cysts of the pelvis or cauda equina (Tarlov cysts), in addition to the more common

pelvic disorders, such as endometriosis or IC, is indicated in such cases.

Anorectal manometry evaluations of women with pelvic floor tension myalgia show that anal canal pressures and electromyographic activity are increased. Anorectal manometry has not been shown to be a reliable test for the diagnosis of pelvic floor tension myalgia, or a predictor of response to treatment.

It is important to also remember that other significant musculoskeletal dysfunctions may be associated with pelvic floor tension myalgia. A thorough musculoskeletal evaluation by a physical therapist or physiatrist is useful in patients with pelvic floor tension myalgia.

Summary

The history and physical examination are powerful diagnostic and therapeutic tools, and it would be difficult to overstate their importance in the evaluation of a patient with CPP. Meticulously performed, they often lead to accurate diagnoses that can be confirmed by a minimal use of any requisite laboratory or imaging testing. It is important to recognize that the examination of the patient with CPP needs to be a "pain-mapping" one. The major goal of the examination is to detect, in as much as is possible, the exact anatomic locations of tenderness and correlate these with areas of pain. At each tender or painful area palpated, the patient should be asked whether this pain reproduces the complaint for which she is being evaluated. This requires a systematic and methodical attempt to duplicate the pain by palpation and positioning.

The diversity of potential pain-related diagnoses demands a multidisciplinary approach to the differential diagnosis of CPP. Although the history is directed to the patient's pain, a thorough review of systems, paying particular attention to the gastrointestinal, reproductive, urologic, neurologic, and musculoskeletal systems, is essential; this can be very time-consuming. Obtaining an appropriate history is greatly facilitated by using a comprehensive pain questionnaire (one is available from the International Pelvic Pain Society at http://www.pelvicpain.org). Even though pain questionnaires can be essential in evaluating women with CPP, they must be used to supplement, and not replace, allowing the patient to tell her story. The physician should not rely totally on a pain questionnaire for the patient's history, but personally should go through at least the most critical portions of the history with the patient. Not only does this allow the chance to obtain more detail about the patient's history, but it also allows observation of her emotional reaction to critical aspects of the history and establishes rapport and trust between the patient and physician.

Finally, it is worth pointing out that chronicity is part of the differential diagnosis of CPP. This has important implications for the diagnostic approach. It is unlikely that a patient with a history of years of CPP and multiple prior evaluations and treatments is going to have a single disease that can be diagnosed and treated to achieve a cure. Yet both patients and clinicians often continue to approach the diagnostic evaluation as if a cure must certainly be available and the right diagnosis and treatment have just been previously missed. Although this may be the case, in fact this is extremely rare. More often, CPP must be considered a diagnosis (i.e., a disease, not a symptom)—and obviously a chronic disease. In such cases, just as patients with diabetes mellitus (and their doctors) must learn to manage their disease so they can lead an optimal life, so must many women with CPP. It is crucial that disorders that worsen the patients' pain and quality of life be diagnosed and treated, but this does not usually result in a cure of CPP, and treatment most often must be considered a lifelong process. Although this approach appears pessimistic, in our experience it allows multimodal approaches to diagnosis and care that lead to very fulfilling and satisfying lives for most patients with CPP.

Selected bibliography

Baker PK. Musculoskeletal origins of chronic pelvic pain. Diagnosis and treatment. Obstet Gynecol Clin North Am 1993;20:719–42.

Driscoll A, Teichman JM. How do patients with interstitial cystitis present? J Urol 2001; 166:2118–20.

Giamberardino MA, Vecchiet L. Visceral pain, referred hyperalgesia and outcome: new concepts. Eur J Anaesthesiol Suppl 1995;10:61–6.

Grant SR, Salvati EP, Rubin RJ. Levator syndrome: an analysis of 316 cases. Dis Colon Rectum 1975;18:161–3.

Howard FM, El-Minawi AM, Sanchez RA. Conscious pain mapping by laparoscopy in women with chronic pelvic pain. Obstet Gynecol 2000;96:934–9.

Mens JM, Vleeming A, Stoeckart R, Stam HJ, Snijders CJ. Understanding peripartum pelvic pain. Implications of a patient survey. Spine 1996;21:1363–9; discussion 1369–70.

Ness RB, Soper DE, Holley RL et al. Effectiveness of inpatient and outpatient treatment strategies for women with pelvic inflammatory disease: results from the Pelvic Inflammatory Disease Evaluation and Clinical Health (PEACH) Randomized Trial. Am J Obstet Gynecol 2002;186:929–37.

Parsons CL, Dell J, Stanford EJ, Bullen M, Kahn BS, Willems JJ. The prevalence of interstitial cystitis in gynecologic patients with pelvic pain, as detected by intravesical potassium sensitivity. Am J Obstet Gynecol 2002;187: 1395–400.

Peters AA, van Dorst E, Jellis B, van Zuuren E, Hermans J, Trimbos JB. A randomized clinical trial to compare two different approaches in women with chronic pelvic pain. Obstet Gynecol 1991;77:740–4.

Sinaki M, Merritt JL, Stillwell GK. Tension myalgia of the pelvic floor. Mayo Clin Proc 1977;52: 717–22.

Slocumb JC. Neurological factors in chronic pelvic pain: trigger points and the abdominal pelvic pain syndrome. Am J Obstet Gynecol 1984;149:536–43.

Steege JF. Office assessment of chronic pelvic pain. Clin Obstet Gynecol 1997;40:554–63.

Sutherland AM. Gynaecological tuberculosis: analysis of a personal series of 710 cases. Aust N Z J Obstet Gynaecol 1985;25:203–7.

Thomson H. Abdominal wall tenderness: a useful sign in the acute abdomen. Lancet 1977;2: 1053–5.

Tu FF, As-Sanie S, Steege JF. Prevalence of pelvic musculoskeletal disorders in a female chronic pelvic pain clinic. J Reprod Med 2006;51: 185–9.

Tu FF, Holt J, Gonzales J, Fitzgerald CM. Physical therapy evaluation of patients with chronic pelvic pain: a controlled study. Am J Obstet Gynecol 2008;198:272 e1–7.

Wald A. Anorectal and pelvic pain in women: diagnostic considerations and treatment. J Clin Gastroenterol 2001;33:283–8.

Walter AJ, Hentz JG, Magtibay PM, Cornella JL, Magrina JF. Endometriosis: correlation between histologic and visual findings at laparoscopy. Am J Obstet Gynecol 2001;184:1407–11; discussion 1411–13.

Psychogenic Causes of Chronic Pelvic Pain, And Its Impact on Psychological Status

Alessandra Graziottin

Center of Gynecology and Medical Sexology, H. San Raffaele Resnati, Milan; University of Florence; and Alessandra Graziottin Foundation, Italy

The good physician treats the disease, the great physician treats the patient who has the disease.
(William Osler, 1849–1919)

Introduction

Pain is like a red traffic light calling for immediate attention to our physical and mental health. When chronic, pain shouts that the key causative factor(s) of the pain have remained unaddressed in the shadow of the untold and/or of diagnostic neglect. Overfocusing on the somatic disease(s) causing chronic pelvic pain (CPP) often leads the physician to forget the patient as a human being with a story to tell, the psychological factor(s) causing chronic stress possibly holding the key to the multisystem disruption that has contributed to the onset and/or worsening of the pain.

However, three major problems arise when discussing the pychogenic causes of CPP. First is the concrete risk that the patient's pain is dismissed as "invented," "all in her head," with a substantial neglect of its biological basis because of the still-persisting belief in Cartesian dualism—that body and mind are two separate entities. As a consequence, only a few physicians respect psychogenic factors as solid biologic contributors to pain. Second, if psychogenic factors work on the etiology and perception of pain, they should do it through a biologic pathway. How can we then recognize the key pathophysiologic steps that translate something "psychological" into a biological contributor of pain? Third, how can we diagnose the subset of patients who really have a powerful and prominent psychogenic component to their pain? And once CPP is rooted in the woman's body, how will it impact on her psychosexual status?

The key points of this chapter are therefore:

- an update of the word "psychogenic;"
- a pathophysiologic, multisystemic description of the biological correlates of psychogenic factors in CPP;
- summary of the evidence supporting the role of psychogenic causes in CPP;
- criteria for a differential diagnosis between a prominent "psychogenic" versus somatic etiology for CPP;
- common diagnostic mistakes in the psychogenic domain, with a focus on iatrogenic factors;
- the psychological and sexual consequences of CPP.

What does "psychogenic" really mean?

"Psychogenic," derived from the Greek *psyche* (mind) and "genic" (meaning caused by), indicates something "generated" in the psychological

Chronic Pelvic Pain, First Edition. Edited by Paolo Vercellini.
© 2011 Blackwell Publishing Ltd. Published 2011 by Blackwell Publishing Ltd.

domain. Psychogenic causes can be intrapsychic or context-dependent:

- *Intrapsychic.* This includes mental disorders, such as psychosis, which may alter both the cognitive processes underlying and self-perception of pain; major depression, which "speaks through the body" and is character-ized by a variety of somatic pain-related complaints; and trait anxiety, in which a genetic predisposition to anxiety disorders and an up-regulated amygdala may increase the neurovegetative arousal response to pain and lower the central pain threshold. Personality disorders may also increase vul-nerability to internal or environmental pain signals. All these disorders are "intrapsychic" but nonetheless have a solid neurobiological basis.
- *Context-dependent, psychological/relational.* Environmental psychogenic factors may act through *active physical damage*, such as in physical or sexual abuse, which may immedi-ately trigger a variety of stress- and trauma-induced physical responses, or *deprivation damage*, as in the persistent emotional neglect of institutionalized children, for example, or the children of severely depressed mothers. In both cases, the psychological factors have a biological correlate, characterized by the neuroimmunoendocrine changes typical of chronic stress mediated through the *corticotropin-releasing factor (CRF) signaling pathways*. This induces a persistent increase in glucocorticoids and a reduced activity of the serotoninergic and dopaminergic neurons and pathways, leading to depression, loss of vital energy, and increased inflammatory activity, with increased levels of inflammatory markers.

In general, intrapsychic and context-dependent factors interact and potentiate each other over time if not adequately addressed from a pharmacologic and/or psy-chotherapeutic point of view. This diagnostic omission or neglect may further increase a woman's vulnerability to peripherally gener-ated pain signals and facilitate the progres-sion to CPP.

> ★ TIPS & TRICKS
>
> Although the word "psychogenic" will be used throughout the text and is often used to describe pain, its close reciprocity to neuroimmunoendocrine correlates should not be forgotten.

How do psychogenic causes translate into physical pain?

The key question here concerns how physical and/or sexual abuse can add to or trigger CPP? If abuse activates CPP, there should be a patho-physiologic mechanism underlying the response to the psychogenic causes. To put psychogenic causes into a proper neurobiological, endocrine and immune context, we need to consider the following.

First, we need an *updated pathophysiologic re-reading of how psychogenic factors translate into biological ones*. The obsolete concept of the dualism of body versus mind (which persists in the clinical setting every time physicians say "Your pain is all in your mind") is therefore to be definitely abandoned in favor of an integrated psychoneuroendocrine and immune view. Indeed, there exists a bidirectional network of interactions between the central and the periph-eral nervous systems (including the pain system), the endocrine system, and the immune system. The existence of these pathways allows stressful life experiences to impact on the immune, endo-crine, and nervous systems, with important implications for health. CPP may be the final result of this complex multisystemic disruption induced by any stressor, from the prominently psychogenic to the strictly biological (see the "Science revisited" box).

One powerful elicitor of changes in the auto-nomic, endocrine, and immune systems is the physical and emotional threat typical of sexual abuse. To detail its psychosomatic correlates is beyond the scope of this chapter, but suggestions for further reading are given in the "Selected bib-liography" at the end of this chapter.

The following example gives an insight into the logic behind this line of thinking. When a child or

⚙ SCIENCE REVISITED

Psychogenic predisposing, precipitating, and maintaining causes of chronic pelvic pain (CPP) may increasingly modify the biologic vulnerability to environmental pathogens or to endogenous noxious substances, inclusive of autoimmunity.

Psychogenic causes of CPP	Biological correlates of psychogenic causes	Biological etiology of CPP
Predisposing *Intrapsychic*: depression, anxiety, paranoia, personality disorders *Context-related*: physical or sexual abuse, chronic emotional distress, alcoholism in one parent, marital conflicts, post-traumatic stress disorders, etc.	**Predisposing** Persistent neurovegetative arousal due to the psychogenic chronic stress leading to: *Corticotropin-releasing factor signaling pathways with:* • Chronic increase of glucocorticoids • Amygdala up-regulation and increased anticipatory anxiety • Down-regulation of the dopaminergic, serotoninergic and opiatergic system • Hyperactivation of mast cell and of the pain system, peripheral and central ↓	**Predisposing** Genetic vulnerability to: • Anxiety and depression (inclusive of its somatic correlates) • Up-regulation and degranulation of mast cells • Allergies and autoimmunity
Precipitating Acute emotional trauma, loss, stress, recurrent abuse	**Precipitating** Increased biologic vulnerability to endogenous and environmental pathogens ↓	**Precipitating** Environmental pathogens (viruses, bacteria, fungi, etc.) Intercourse during vestibular inflammation or in a nonaroused state Endogenous damaging factors (endometrial shedding in endometriosis) Autoimmunity
Maintaining Persistence of predisposing and/or precipitating factors Diagnostic omission/neglect Iatrogenic nocebo effect	**Maintaining** Up-regulation of the inflammatory, nervous, and muscular systems, with chronic inflammation, neurogenic pain, muscle inflammation, and chronic sleep disorders ↓	**Maintaining** Periodic endometrial shedding Recurrent intestinal, vaginal, and bladder infections Chronic inflammation Neuropathic pain
	CPP	

a woman is physically or sexually abused, she undergoes a violent acute stress response, with huge neurovegetative physical and emotional arousal. Indeed, any injurious event provokes autonomic, endocrine, and immune processes as well as sensory signaling. This process will be chronically up-regulated if the abuse is repeated over time, and/or if frequent nightmares of the experience trigger at night the very same abrupt neurovegetative arousal, with all its psychological feelings of fear, anguish, horror, pain, helplessness, and despair. A dysfunctional physical and emotional status, similar to that described as post-traumatic stress disorder (PTSD), may result.

In the brain, this persistent neurovegetative arousal, characterized by a chronic increase in the plasma levels of glucocorticoids and inflammatory molecules, will increase the activity of the amygdala, the crossroads of the four basic emotions command system and a key center for memories with high emotional impact. The up-regulated amygdala contributes to maintain the hyperreactivity of the alarm system even to minor stimuli, through an increase in so-called long-term potentiation of neuronal activity. Moreover, in cases of pain or stress of whatever etiology, the amygdala will immediately activate the maximal alert and arousal response. This contributes to:

- an increase in "free-floating anxiety", which will peak in women genetically predisposed to anxiety disorders;
- a reduction in the central threshold of pain perception;
- reactivation of a neurogenically increased production of pain and inflammatory signals (which can be peripherally mediated through the mast cells).

Meanwhile, identification of the CRF signaling pathway contributes to a deeper understanding of stress-related endocrine (activation of the pituitary–adrenal axis), behavioral (anxiety/depression, altered feeding), autonomic (activation of the sympathetic nervous system), and immune responses present in all the situations where a psychogenic factor induces chronic stress. Furthermore, the chronic increase in glucocorticoids may have specific down-regulating effects on the dopaminergic neurons that mediate the seeking–appetitive–lust system. This will translate into a loss of vital energy, asthenia, fatigue, loss of sexual desire, and, typically, the "anhedonia"—loss of the ability to perceive pleasure and joy in whatever activity—that is complained of by patients with CPP, more so in

the subset of those who have been subjected to previous physical or sexual abuse. In parallel, the down-regulation of the serotoninergic system will contribute to depression, which will further increase the perception of pain signals and the reduction in the central pain threshold.

In the periphery, the neurogenic stress-induced up-regulation of mast cells will increase the vulnerability of different mucosae (intestinal, vaginal, bladder) to the aggression of a variety germs, typical of the so-called "irritable bowel syndrome", or to local noxious substances, such as is seen with endometrial shedding in endometriosis. This vulnerability requires the permitting presence of mast cells as key mediators of the stress response, transforming an environmental stressor into biologic damage, as has been well proven in the mast cell knockout mice. This also contributes to the re-reading of pain under a unifying hypothesis, the so-called "law of pain," suggesting that un up-regulated inflammatory status, involving the inflammatory cells and/or inflammatory molecules such as interleukins and tumor necrosis factor, is the common denominator of acute and chronic pain, independent of its being nociceptive or neuropathic, central or peripheral.

Second, we should also not forget that there needs to be a temporal reading of psychogenic factors as predisposing, precipitating, and maintaining contributors to pain. Compared to a "psychogenic or medical" approach, the "psychogenic and biogenic" approach is more coherent with the real narrative experience in CPP and the biology of pain.

Psychogenic causes of chronic pelvic pain

A huge volume of literature suggests that psychogenic factors are specifically relevant in the clinical history of women with CPP. Table 3.1 summarizes Latthé's (2006) review on controlled trials to provide readers with an overview of the sense of power of such events. For example, anxiety and depression may contribute to and/or increase the perception of pain with an odds ratio (OR), respectively, of 2.28 and 2.69. Paranoia, i.e., the psychotic disruption of cognitive functions and self-perceptions, may predispose to CPP

Table 3.1 Meta-analysis of risk factors associated with noncyclic chronic pelvic pain, focusing on studies of abuse/psychological factors

Factor	No of trials	No of women Cases	No of women Controls	(Cases: Controls)	SMD (99% CI)	OR (99% CI)
Abuse/psychological factors						
Childhood physical abuse***	5	309	960		0.43 (0.24 to 0.62)	2.18 (1.55 to 3.06)
Childhood sexual abuse***	10	592	1472		0.23 (0.08 to 0.37)	1.51 (1.16 to 1.97)
Adult/lifetime physical abuse	5	157	363		−0.05 (−0.43 to 0.33)	0.91 (0.46 to 1.81)
Adult/lifetime sexual abuse***	11	664	966		0.69 (0.51 to 0.87)	3.49 (2.52 to 4.83)
Psychological abuse	1	36	43		0.50 (−0.34 to 1.33)	2.47 (0.54 to 11.24)
Any abuse	6	176	641		0.49 (0.21 to 0.77)	2.45 (1.47 to 4.06)
Disturbed puberty/painful early memories	4	223	71		0.73 (0.31 to 1.16)	3.77 (1.74 to 8.17)
Unsatisfactory relation with mother/spouse	3	135	44		0.77 (0.26 to 1.27)	4.01 (1.60 to 10.06)
Alcoholism in one parent	1	106	36		0.55 (−0.13 to 1.22)	2.69 (0.79 to 9.19)
Divorce in one parent	1	106	36		0.72 (0.11 to 1.33)	3.68 (1.23 to 11.08)
Death in one parent	1	106	36		0.39 (−0.49 to 1.28)	2.02 (0.40 to 10.13)
Disturbed pregnancy	1	32	25		0.95 (0.18 to 1.72)	5.58 (1.39 to 22.39)
Anxiety***	5	178	241		0.45 (0.19 to 0.72)	2.28 (1.41 to 3.70)
Depression**	8	410	376		0.55 (0.34 to 0.76)	2.69 (1.86 to 3.88)
Extroversion	1	35	9		−0.15 (−1.11 to 0.81)	0.76 (0.13 to 4.36)
Hysteria***	2	182	76		0.87 (0.51 to 1.23)	4.83 (2.50 to 9.33)
Neuroticism	1	35	9		0.77 (−0.20 to 1.73)	4.01 (0.70 to 22.99)
Paranoia	1	37	23		1.45 (0.77 to 2.13)	13.89 (4.02 to 48.02)
Borderline syndrome	1	106	36		0.61 (−0.11 to 1.33)	3.02 (0.82 to 11.08)
Current phobias	1	25	30		0.74 (−0.21 to 1.70)	3.86 (0.69 to 21.71)
Post-traumatic stress disorder	1	25	10		0.94 (−0.37 to 2.25)	5.47 (0.51 to 58.84)
Psychosomatic symptoms***	8	303	250		1.15 (0.90 to 1.39)	8.01 (5.16 to 12.44)

OR 0.1 1.0 10.0

SMD −1.0 0.0 1.0

Negative association   *Positive association*

All multiple studies are heterogeneous; ***$P<0.001$; **$P<0.01$. CI, confidence interval; OR, odds ratio; SMD, standardized mean difference. Reproduced from Latthé et al., 2006, with permission.

with an OR 13.89. Similarly, PTSD may increase vulnerability to CPP with an OR 5.47. Finally, eight controlled trials indicate that psychosomatic disruption may predispose to CPP with an OR of 8.01.

Moreover, childhood physical abuse will predispose to CPP with an OR of 2.18. Ten studies suggest that childhood sexual abuse will increase the vulnerability to CPP, with an OR of 1. 51, while 11 trials suggest that adult/life sexual abuse seems to have a stronger predisposing effect, with an OR of 3.49. Interestingly, disturbed puberty or painful early memories further increase the vulnerability to CPP, with an OR of 3.77. An unsatisfactory relation with a spouse may also be consistent with a stressing experience, predisposing to CPP with an OR of 4.01. Environmental psychological/relational factors such as alcoholism in one parent may further contribute, with an OR of 2.69, while divorce in one parent may have an even stronger impact, with an OR of 3.68. *Potential psychogenic factors*

> ★ TIPS & TRICKS
>
> The physician should clarify that the attention to the psychogenic component is meant to recognize potential psychological contributors maintaining or worsening the woman's pain, but that all the physical/somatic factors will *in parallel* be thoroughly and rigorously investigated—and that the physician believes in and cares about the truth of the woman's pain.

> ✋ CAUTION
>
> The word "psychogenic" does not mean that pain is "invented" or "all in the woman's head." Instead, it means that intrapsychic and/or context-dependent psychological-relational factors may: (1) increase the production of pain signals through the chronic stress they cause; (2) increase the vulnerability to pain signals produced in the pelvis through a reduction of both the gate control of painful stimuli at the posterior

horn of the medulla and the central threshold of pain, as well as a chronic increase in glucocorticoids; (3) lead to increased anxiety and depression that may further contribute to increasing pain perception and the vulnerability to pain syndromes, as well as reducing dopaminergic and opiatergic pathways, thus dampening vital energy, sexual desire, and the possibility to enjoy pleasure ("anhedonia").

---

should therefore be investigated in every patient, in a respectful and tactful approach.

Criteria for the diagnosis of psychogenic pain

Key characteristics of psychogenic pain are summarized in Table 3.2. The differences between "prominent" psychogenic and somatic pain have been polarized to ease the reading of the key differences. In real life, however, there is a continuous interaction between the two, and only a very minor subset of patients with CPP have prominent "psychogenic" pain. The vast majority have solid etiologies and frequent comorbidities, often misdiagnosed, neglected, and overlooked for years. The psychological component may have grown as a result of the anguish, the sense of despair, the reactive depression, and the worsening of the clinical picture itself, with more widespread and less differentiated pain. Understanding the psychogenic component, when present, in terms of its various degrees and impacts, is nevertheless essential to address the many contributors of pain in a comprehensive way. In this sense, in the pain clinic's multidisciplinary team, the psychologist/psychotherapist is very important in providing the patient with the right and the setting to give words to her pain, while also feeling well looked after—and therefore reassured that she is being rigorously evaluated—from a strictly medical point of view.

To help in understanding the potential psychogenic components of pain, key questions have been summarized in Table 3.3. The goal is to appreciate *whether the pain is disruptive in an otherwise "functioning" life*, or whether it is the

Table 3.2 Key differences between somatic and psychogenic pain

Somatic pain	Psychogenic pain
The patient describes a more localized pain	The description of the pain site is more elusive
Uses sensory words to qualify his or her pain	The wording to describe the pain is highly emotional
Accurately describes periodic and selective changes in his or her pain	Cannot identify any pattern of pain changes (e.g., circadian, menstrual, premenstrual, ovulatory)
Can identify factors (such as posture, movements, or even foods) that can increase or reduce the pain	Stress is the most cited factor in worsening the pain
Does not report major interpersonal difficulties	Usually reports interpersonal difficulties
Treats pain more as a symptom than as a disease per se	Clinical history indicates other psychosomatic diseases
Repeated consultations are mainly motivated by a feeling of medical inaccuracy in addressing physical symptoms	Has a long history of doctor-shopping, with many examinations, motivated by the need for a second/third/fourth opinion

Modified from Mombelli, 2003.

Table 3.3 Key questions to be asked when considering a psychogenic component of pain

1. How is the patient's life? Is it generally "working" or not?
2. Does the patient suffer from insomnia? What is the general quality of sleep?
3. Is there any stressful event—such as physical or sexual abuse, or emotional neglect—in the patient's life that could have a temporal or symbolic link with the onset or worsening of the pain?
4. How is the general quality of the woman's adaptive coping?
5. What is the patient's opinion about her pain?
6. Do the timing or the characteristics of the pain show any link with other problems (e.g., professional, family-related) in the patient's life?
7. Does the pain carry any real or symbolic advantage?

Modified from Mombelli, 2003.

tip of the iceberg of a variably dysfunctional life. In the latter situation, the psychogenic pain can serve different conscious, or more often, *unconscious*, purposes, such as selected attention, secondary gains, the use of dynamics of power or guilt or avoidance, or just calling for help for previous abuses the patient never found the courage, the words, or the adequate supportive listening to disclose.

The apparently neutral question about the *quality of sleep* is richly informative per se. As a general rule, nociceptive pain gets worse at night, whereas pure neuropathic or psychogenic pain is usually silent during sleep. However, patients with a psychogenic component to their pain, specifically if it is associated to PTSD, report a poor quality of sleep, referred as light and disturbed, with frequent awakening, early waking, a lack of restorative capacity, and a morning sense of being "more tired than the evening before." All these changes are usually related to the hyperarousal typical, for example, of previous abuse and/or PTSD. The key point is that the disruption of sleep pattern is a major biologic stress, which further contributes to the sense of physical and mental exhaustion on top of the parallel increase in inflammatory indexes. Moreover, the recurrence of nightmares, even with a confused content, should alert to the concrete risks for previous physical and/or sexual abuse, with a parallel recurrent hyperactivity of the adrenergic/alertness system that may concur to amplify any signal of pain.

When asking about *stressful events*, it is key to understand whether there is any temporal and/or symbolic link with the onset/site of pain.

Quality of coping is another sensitive area. Patients with a significant psychogenic component to their pain tend to have poor adaptive coping. The way they cope with life difficulties is inadequate; they may feel overwhelmed by even minor events. Catastrophizing coping is the most dangerous in terms of resolution of pain. Even in front of a self-reported pain diary indicating a clear improvement in pain, when asked "How do feel now?," this patient will answer: "Awful, as usual." "But your diary clearly indicates a definite improvement. …" "Yes, but if I get worse again …?" This type of answer may suggest that the woman's life has been increasingly structured around different negative painful experiences, that she is not confident about the resolution of her problem, or that "losing" her pain might cause the loss of secondary advantages or gains.

In this perspective, the patient's opinion about her pain, the presence of guilty feelings, for example for a previous voluntary abortion in a religious patient, the timing or the characteristics of pain, and their potential link with other problems (e.g., professional, family-related) should be gently considered. Finally, the possibility that pain may carry any real or symbolic advantage, for example within the family (to attract the attention of otherwise overbusy parents or partner) or at work, should be evaluated in a psychodynamic evaluation and psychotherapeutic intervention, sometimes extended to the partner, or to parents in case of adolescents. The goal would be to obtain the same attention, or develop healthier family dynamics, with a less self-destructive and painful unconscious strategies.

Common mistakes

Diagnostic neglect

The vast majority of physicians do not routinely ask about previous harassment or abuse, because of fear of posing too intimate a question and feeling not sufficiently trained to work on it, or to avoid the risk for opening a time-consuming Pandora's box of sorrow, tears, and regrets. Only a minority (3% in a Canadian survey on gynecologists and family physicians) ask about previous violence or abuse. the key point here is that *it is difficult to provide an effective intervention if there is no mention of the problem!*

Diagnostic overfocus

When sexual abuse is revealed, many physicians and psychologists alike tend to read everything as a consequence of it, with the risk of missing significant correlated and/or independent comorbidities. The correct thinking should be "and … and" not "or … or." Both the so-called psychogenic domain and the physical one should be explored in a balanced, respectful, informative way.

Inability to read the common neurobiological pathway that blends abuse and CPP

This refers to the complex emotions—fear, terror, anxiety, anguish, physical and emotional pain, panic, depression, loneliness, despair—that are triggered in both physical and sexual abuse *and* in CPP. Specifically, both involve, directly and indirectly, the area of the body with the *highest emotional impact* (the sexual and reproductive, setting aside the sphincter control and continence-related issues), and both have a high symbolic meaning. The human being is a symbolic animal and the reading of life condensed through symbols goes beyond the limits of education, culture or race and becomes universal.

Failure to acknowledge four iatrogenic abuses, inclusive of nocebo effect

First of these is *denial of the biological truth of pain*. Every time a physician states that a woman's "pain is all in her head," he or she abuses the patient's trust, causing further negative emotional states, such as anxiety, depression, sense of unworthiness, loneliness, and despair. The physician can also trigger (further) domestic violence, physical, emotional, and/or sexual, when the family and/or partner is told that the woman is "inventing" her pain. Many partners are frankly furious at the idea of having to keep on traveling and spending money on "doctor-shopping" and not having sex when CPP causes/includes dyspareunia, while it is claimed that the woman is suffering "nothing" and is just pretending she has pain: "If the doctor said that, you must stop complaining once and for all. Shut up! I'm fed up with your pain!"

Next is the *nocebo effect* ("I will damage"). Physicians are all too familiar with the placebo effect, while only a few are aware of the powerful nocebo effect, which includes of their verbal and nonverbal language. Every time we deny the truth of pain, or we state that the situation is more serious than it really is, every time we communicate a negative diagnosis without stressing the space of hope that should be maintained for every patients, particularly in the CPP domain, the nocebo effect is there, whereby the expectation of a negative outcome may lead to the worsening of a symptom. Increasing evidence suggests that the nocebo effect is as neurobiologically based as the placebo one. Specifically, when words (or behaviors) are painful, there is an increase in anticipatory anxiety and a reduction in the serotoninergic, dopaminergic, and opiatergic pathways, opposite to what has been documented when a placebo effect is in play. Recent experimental evidence indicates that negative verbal suggestions induce anticipatory anxiety about the impending pain increase, and this verbally induced anxiety triggers the activation of cholecystokinin, which in turn facilitates pain transmission. Cholecystokinin antagonists have been found to block this anxiety-induced hyperalgesia ("nocebo hyperalgesia"), thus opening up the possibility of new therapeutic strategies whenever pain has an important anxiety component .The practical recommendation here is to be aware of the powerful emotional (and biologic) effect of our wording and to communicate *carefully* and *tactfully*, balancing the description of the severity of the case against the much-needed attention to all that will be done to improve the condition and reduce the pain.

The third iatrogenic abuse is *physical abuse*: 5.8% of my patients with lifelong dyspareunia and vulvar vestibulitis (unpublished data) reported as unique traumatic and abusive experiences in their life the invasive diagnostic or therapeutic maneuvers in the genital area performed, during childhood or early adolescence, by physicians or nurses without care or appropriate analgesia. Examinations such as urethral swabbing, cystoscopy, vaginal swabbing, vaginal examination, sutures of genital minor traumas after injuries received while playing, and manual separation of labial conglutination in cases of lichen sclerosus are recalled as traumatizing, violent, and fear-triggering, increasing the anticipatory anxiety when a "white coat" is approaching the patient's body. Again, a powerful, long-lasting, neurobiologically based nocebo effect is in play.

Finally, there is sexual abuse, when the physician breaks the boundaries of the appropriate doctor–patient relationship, with negative consequences appearing months or even years after the abuse.

Lack of awareness of the first psychological intervention

The first psychological intervention, with a powerful placebo/reassuring effect, that every physician should use in his or her practice, covers the following:

- empathic, respectful listening to the personal history, inclusive of past negative experiences;
- explaining to the woman—and the partner, when present—that her pain is *real*, is not in her head, has a name (the diagnosis), has a number of causes, both psychological and physical, that will be addressed in a balanced way, has a time to improve (the prognosis), and will involve a multidisciplinary approach to accelerate the improvement;
- establishing a good, trusting doctor–patient relationships, which is critically important when CPP is in: "I felt I had finally found the doctor who could take care of me and my problem. For the first time, *I felt I was believed*, and my anxiety melted away." This is an example of a doctor–patient relationship in which the physician becomes the first drug, with a powerful placebo effect, again neurobiologically based, as increasing evidence suggests.

Psychological and sexual consequences of CPP

The psychological and sexual consequences of CPP are modulated by a number of variables, including the duration of pain and the moment the diagnosis of CPP is made during the course of its natural history, its etiology, its severity, the types of comorbidity, the patient's mental state before the CPP developed, and, last but not least, the quality of affective and emotional bonding in the couple/family and the quality of medical support.

Anxiety, depression, loss of vital energy, fatigue, distress, and sleep disorders may increase over time with increasing severity and worsening of the pain. Specifically depressing factors are the feelings that pain is not being considered "rigorously," that its main etiology has been missed, and that physicians are trivializing is as "psychogenic."

Sexuality is among the most neglected areas for patients with CPP. Indeed , the majority of patients with CPP complain of a dysfunctional sexuality:

- loss of sexual desire and poor mental arousal, which may be caused by the comorbidity with depression, or by the negative feedback from the genitals leading to poor genital arousal and complaints of vaginal dryness and/or introital or deep dyspareunia;
- poor genital arousal, with vaginal dryness secondary to spontaneous or iatrogenic (treatment-related) hypoestrogenic states;
- dyspareunia, depending on a number of factors:
  - genital pain, which is the strongest reflex inhibitor of genital arousal and vaginal lubrication. This facilitates microabrasions of the introital mucosa, contributing to vulvar vestibulitis, with hyperactive mast cell, proliferation of pain fibers, and lifelong or acquired hyperactivity of the levator ani;
  - pelvic pain, more often associated with: deep endometriosis, when located within the uterosacral ligament or in the posterior fornix/posterior vaginal wall, or with adenomyosis; pelvic inflammatory disease; irritable bowel syndrome; and interstitial cystitis.

- orgasmic difficulties, specifically during intercourse, when low desire, vaginal dryness, and/or dyspareunia are comorbid with CPP.

In the multidisciplinary approach, the psychosexual consequences of CPP should be carefully evaluated, and an appropriate treatment plan should be proposed and discussed with the woman and, when available, her partner.

Conclusions

Psychogenic factors can be powerful contributors to CPP as predisposing, precipitating, or maintaining factors of chronic stress. One of the currently most credited pathophysiologic readings is that involving CRF signaling pathways. Acknowledging the presence and relative weight of psychogenic factors should increase physicians' diagnostic skills and empower them with the attitude to cure the *woman* with CPP rather than just the disease or its somatic correlates. A multidisciplinary approach, with psychotherapeutic/pharmacologic support (anxiolytics, antidepressants), when indicated, parallel to medical treatment, will enhance the possibility of reducing the emotionally driven stress. Giving words to the emotional side of pain is key in a caring and curing perspective.

Finally, psychosexual consequences should be evaluated and treated accordingly from the medical and/or psychodynamic point of view with a tailored approach. Overall, the caring physician should no longer say "The pain is all in your head" but "*Your psychological suffering (and previous abuses) speaks through your body*. This is why we should give words to your emotional pain, using a psychological approach (when indicated) while curing all the physical causes of your CPP. I want you to feel better, to get better. To reduce your pain in all its components is my priority and our goal."

Selected bibliography

Benedetti F, Lanotte M, Lopiano L, Colloca L. When words are painful: unraveling the mechanisms of the nocebo effect. Neuroscience 2007;147:260–71.

Chapman CR, Tuckett RP, Woo Song C et al. Pain and stress in a systems perspective: reciprocal neural, endocrine and immune interactions. J Pain 2008;9:122–45.

Field BJ, Swarm RA. Chronic pain—advances in psychotherapy. Evidence based practice. Cambridge, MA: Hogrefe & Huber; 2008.

Graziottin A. Iatrogenic and post-traumatic female sexual disorders. In: Porst H, Buvat J, ed. International Society of Sexual Medicine Standard Committee Book. Standard practice in sexual medicine. Oxford: Blackwell; 2006. pp. 351–61. Available from: http://www.alessandragraziottin.it

Graziottin A. Sexual pain disorders: dyspareunia and vaginismus. In: Porst H, Buvat J, ed. International Society of Sexual Medicine Standard Committee Book. Standard practice in sexual medicine. Oxford: Blackwell; 2006. pp. 342–50. Available from: http://www.alessandragraziottin.it

Graziottin A. Mast cells and their role in sexual pain disorders. In: Goldstein A, Pukall C, Goldstein I, ed. Female sexual pain disorders: evaluation and management. New York: Blackwells; 2009. pp. 176–9.

Kemeny ME. Psychobiological responses to social threat: evolution of a psychological model in psychoneuroimmunology. Brain Behav Immun 2009;23:1–9.

Latthé P, Mignini L, Gray R, Hills R, Khan K. Factors predisposing women to chronic pelvic pain: a systematic review. BMJ 2006;332: 749–55.

Mc Donald JS. Pelvic and abdominal pain. In: Ashburn MA, Rice LJ, ed. The management of pain. New York: Churchill Livingstone; 1998. pp. 383–400.

Mombelli F. Dolore psicogeno [Psychogenic pain). In: Panerai AE, Tiengo MA, ed. Le basi farmacologiche della terapia del dolore [Basic pharmacology of the therapy of pain]. Milano: Edi-Ermes; 2003. pp. 527–36.

Omoigui S. The biochemical origin of pain—proposing a new law of pain: the origin of all pain is inflammation and the inflammatory response. Part 1 of 3: A unifying law of pain. Med Hypotheses 2007;69:70–82.

Panksepp J. Affective neuroscience: the foundation of human and animal emotions. New York: Oxford University Press; 1998.

Scott DJ, Stohler CS, Egnatuk CM, Wang H, Koeppe RA, Zubieta JK. Placebo and nocebo effects are defined by opposite opioid and dopaminergic responses. Arch Gen Psychiatry 2008;65: 220–31.

Solms M, Turnbull O. The brain and the inner world. London: Karnac; 2002.

Taché Y, Brunnhuber S. From Hans Selye's discovery of biological stress to the identification of corticotropin-releasing factor signaling pathways: implication in stress-related functional bowel diseases. Review. Ann N Y Acad Sci 2008;1148:29–41.

Endometriosis: Pathogenesis and Management of Pain

Jennifer L. Kulp and A. Arici

Yale University School of Medicine, New Haven, Connecticut, USA

Introduction

Endometriosis is defined as endometrial glands and stroma that are located outside the uterine cavity. It is a common disease that affects 7–10% of reproductive-aged women, and in women who have chronic pelvic pain, endometriosis may be present in 77–87%. Many theories exist regarding the pathogenesis of endometriosis, and it is likely that the etiology of endometriosis is multifactorial. In this chapter, we will discuss the current understanding of the pathogenesis of endometriosis and how this corresponds to patient symptomatology. We will also review current therapies used in the treatment of the condition.

Pathogenesis

Traditional theories of the etiology of endometriosis include retrograde menstruation and celomic metaplasia. Celomic metaplasia may result in endometriosis when undifferentiated cells in the peritoneal cavity differentiate into endometrial cells. During menstruation, shed endometrium may travel out of the fallopian tubes and implant on the pelvic peritoneum and organs. Women with müllerian anomalies that result in menstrual outflow obstruction are more likely to have endometriosis than those who do not have any obstruction. This observation supports the theory of retrograde menstruation resulting in endometriosis. However, some degree of retrograde menstruation may occur in

the majority of reproductive-aged women, yet all do not have endometriosis.

In addition to retrograde menstruation, women with endometriosis may also have altered immunity that allows ectopic endometrium to implant and proliferate. Women with endometriosis have higher rates of hypothyroidism, fibromyalgia, asthma, allergies, and autoimmune diseases when compared to other women in the United States. This lends support to the theory that women with endometriosis may have a dysfunctional immune response. A well-functioning immune system should be able to recognize and destroy misplaced or ectopic endometrial cells. However, this does not occur in women with endometriosis and may be due to defects in humoral and cell-mediated immunity.

Defective cellular immunity is a result of functional deficiencies in T and B lymphocytes. Furthermore, natural killer cells appear to have decreased cytotoxic activity in women with endometriosis. The peritoneal fluid in endometriosis patients contains greater concentrations of activated macrophages, which produce increased amounts of growth factors and cytokines. These factors stimulate the adhesion of endometrial cells to the peritoneum, as well as their proliferation in the peritoneal cavity. The cytokines may also encourage angiogenesis. Ultimately, the immune dysregulation results in decreased surveillance, recognition, and destruction of ectopic endometrial cells and may result

Chronic Pelvic Pain, First Edition. Edited by Paolo Vercellini.

© 2011 Blackwell Publishing Ltd. Published 2011 by Blackwell Publishing Ltd.

in an inflammatory environment that promotes the proliferation of endometriosis.

This impaired immunity, combined with increased inflammation, may also be linked to other defects in the endometriosis implants. These implants produce high levels of estrogen and prostaglandin. Increased prostaglandin synthesis, predominately of prostaglandin E2 and prostaglandin F2α by endometriosis implants likely contributes to pain symptoms both directly and via effects on uterine contractility. Prostaglandins also increase aromatase activity, leading to greater estrogen production by the endometrial implants. High estrogen leads to the survival and proliferation of the endometriosis implants.

The action of progesterone also differs in ectopic compared to eutopic endometrium. Progesterone has an antiestrogenic effect on the endometrium, in part by promoting the conversion of estradiol to estrone, which is a weaker estrogen. Endometrial implants do produce progesterone, but they have lower levels of progesterone receptors than eutopic endometrium, leading to a resistance to the action of progesterone. The resistance to progesterone action results in higher amounts of the more potent estrogen estradiol, and further stimulation of the endometriosis implants.

Some women with endometriosis may have a genetic predisposition to the disease. There is 6.9% recurrence risk for all first-degree relatives of women with endometriosis. Patients with endometriosis who have an affected first-degree relative are more likely to have severe endometriosis than those without one. This genetic component of endometriosis may be due to inheritable allelic differences in drug-metabolizing enzymes that have a role in the development of endometriosis, or be due to polymorphisms in the genes encoding the estrogen receptor and/or CYP17. Women with a genetic predisposition may be more likely to have peritoneal invasion of endometriosis implants after retrograde menstruation occurs. Genetic alterations within the endometriosis implants may allow the lesions to act like malignant cells. Changes in oncogenic pathways may occur, such as inactivation of tumor suppressor genes, which allows for proliferation of the endometriosis implants.

Stem cells may also play a role in the pathogenesis of endometriosis. It is known that nonuterine stem cells can contribute to the regeneration of endometrial tissue. Evidence from animal studies suggests that endometriosis implants may be populated by bone marrow-derived stem cells. Furthermore, the stem cell theory could explain endometriosis found at distant sites such as the lung or nose. The etiology of endometriosis is likely multifactorial. Retrograde menstruation may lead to the initial establishment of peritoneal endometriosis implants, while a dysfunctional immune response and genetic alterations may prevent destruction of the ectopic tissue. Stem cells may allow for progression of the endometriosis lesions once they are established.

> ### ⚘ SCIENCE REVISITED
>
> The pathogenesis of endometriosis is multifactorial, and inflammation is likely to play a role. When the peritoneal fluid of women with endometriosis was examined, researchers found that it contained elevated amounts of macrophages and their secreted products, such as growth factors, cytokines, and angiogenic factors. These greater amounts of macrophages and their secreted factors may lead to the stimulation, implantation, and proliferation of endometrial cells in endometriosis lesions. Also, reproductive organs are surrounded by sterile low-grade inflammation in the peritoneal fluid, and this may lead to scarring, adhesion formation, and anatomic distortion of the reproductive tract.

Symptoms

Patients with endometriosis have a varied clinical presentation. Some women are asymptomatic, whereas others present with generalized pelvic pain or cyclic pain that may be brought on or worsened by their menstrual flow or intercourse. In addition, women with endometriosis may describe pain with urination or bowel movements. Many women with endometriosis suffer from infertility. However, these types of symptom are not specific to women with endometriosis. Although pelvic pain, dysmenorrhea, and menorrhagia are frequently seen in women with endometriosis, these symptoms are also seen in women without the disease. Furthermore, other etiologies of pelvic pain, such as irritable bowel syndrome and pelvic inflammatory disease, are more common in women with endometriosis.

On laparoscopy, endometriosis lesions have a varied appearance: they may appear red, blue/brown, black, or clear/cystic. Black lesions are commonly described as "powder burn" lesions. Endometriosis may also result in peritoneal windows or increased vascularity. The degree or type of endometriosis seen at the time of surgery does not correlate well with patient symptoms. Women with minimal endometriosis seen at laparoscopy may have severe pain, yet women with extensive endometriosis may be asymptomatic. Endometriosis is classified from stage 1, which is minimal, to stage 4, which is severe. This staging system was developed by the American Society for Reproductive Medicine and incorporates the size, location, and number of endometriotic lesions, as well as the presence or absence of endometriomas and pelvic adhesions. In one series, there was no significant association between stage of endometriosis and pain symptoms.

Some evidence suggests that earlier, more active endometrial lesions are more commonly painful. In patients who underwent conscious sedation laparoscopy, 22% reported reproduction of pain when black endometriosis lesions were touched with a blunt probe. Clear or vesicular lesions were better correlated with pain symptoms, with patients describing pain up to 76% of the time these types of lesion were palpated. Furthermore, patients reported pain up to 86% of the time red lesions were palpated.

Endometriosis commonly is found on the ovaries, the anterior or posterior cul-de-sac, the posterior broad ligaments, or the uterosacral ligaments and less commonly on the uterus, fallopian tubes, sigmoid colon, appendix, or round ligaments. The location of endometriosis also does not always correlate well with pain symptoms. However, patients with posterior deep infiltrating endometriosis are more likely to describe noncyclic pain, deep dyspareunia, and painful defecation during menses.

Dyspareunia or painful intercourse with deep penetration occurs in approximately 50% of women with endometriosis. This pain is often most severe prior to menses and is usually positional in nature. It is commonly noted in association with deep endometriosis lesions on the uterosacral ligament or scarring of the uterosacral ligament due to endometriosis. Women with this type of endometriosis have impaired sexual functioning. They have intercourse less frequently and describe intercourse as less fulfilling.

The etiology of pain in endometriosis is not well understood. The number of nerve fibers in endometriosis lesions may be increased, and these fibers may have a different pattern of growth, which may explain the relationship between endometriosis lesions and pain. One theory is that the increased number of macrophages seen in endometriosis lesions interact with the nerve fibers to generate pain. Also, deep infiltrating endometriosis, which tends to be associated with more significant pain than peritoneal endometriosis, may be more richly innervated.

Another theory is that the pain experienced by women with endometriosis occurs due to bleeding of the endometriosis implants. Finally, pain in endometriosis may occur secondary to the production of growth factors or cytokines by the lesions.

EVIDENCE AT A GLANCE

One study examined the pain symptoms of 160 women who had endometriosis who underwent their first laparoscopy and staging. Of these women, 78% described dysmenorrhea, 39% described pelvic pain, and 32% described deep dyspareunia. After laparoscopy and staging had been performed, 25% of patients were found to have stage 1 endometriosis, 18% had stage 2, 36% had stage 3, and 21% had stage 4. Despite the wide variation in stage of endometriosis found at laparoscopy, the authors found no association between severity of disease and any of the pain symptoms. For example, 38% of women with stage 1 endometriosis had pelvic pain, as did 41% of women with stage 4 endometriosis. This study helped to establish the lack of correlation between pain symptoms and stage of endometriosis.

Treatment options

Endometriosis may be treated medically or surgically. If the clinical impression is that a patient has endometriosis without endometriomas, medical therapy is a good place to start. First-line medical therapy consists of oral contraceptive pills (OCPs) and nonsteroidal anti-inflammatory drugs (NSAIDs).

Medical treatment options

NSAIDs work by inhibiting cyclooxygenase and blocking prostaglandin production. In theory, they should be effective at treating endometriosis-related pain by preventing prostaglandin synthesis by the endometriosis implants. In observational studies of women with endometriosis, NSAIDs are effective at controlling mild pelvic pain. However, there are no randomized controlled trials of NSAIDs compared to placebo. A recent meta-analysis found no significant difference between NSAIDs and placebo at treating endometriosis-related pain, and NSAIDs do not prevent the growth of endometriosis implants.

NSAIDs have been proven effective at treating primary dysmenorrhea. Mefenamic acid may be more effective than ibuprofen or naproxen in the treatment of primary dysmenorrhea. Ibuprofen and naproxen, which have similar efficacy, are often chosen as first-line agents as they are readily available over the counter, are inexpensive, and have a favorable side effect profile. Their most common side effect is gastric irritation. Cyclooxygenase-2 inhibitors, which have a more serious side effect profile, are not frequently used. There is not strong evidence to support their use in treatment of endometriosis-related pain, but NSAIDs are frequently used, mainly due to their efficacy in treating primary dysmenorrhea.

EVIDENCE AT A GLANCE

Nonsteroidal anti-inflammatory drugs (NSAIDs) are a common first-line medical therapy for the treatment of pain in endometriosis and work by blocking prostaglandin synthesis. A Cochrane Database study reviewed all randomized controlled trials analyzing the use of NSAIDs in the treatment of endometriosis-related pain. Only one trial fitted their criteria. This study, which compared naproxen to placebo, included only 24 women. The authors concluded that there was inconclusive evidence on whether NSAIDs are more effective than placebo at controlling endometriosis-related pain.

OCPs are used and are effective in the treatment of endometriosis-related pain, particularly dysmenorrhea, and are generally well tolerated. The mechanism of action of OCPs is likely decidualization of endometrial tissue in both eutopic and ectopic endometrium, but they also decrease menstrual flow.

One study found OCPs to be more effective than placebo at reducing the degree of dysmenorrhea in patients with endometriosis. This study also demonstrated that 4 months of OCP therapy could decrease the size of endometriomas that were greater than 3 cm in size. One randomized trial comparing the use of cyclic OCPs to gonadotropin-releasing hormone (GnRH) agonists for the treatment of endometriosis-associated pain found that OCPs decreased dyspareunia and pelvic pain, although they were not as effective as GnRH agonists. Continuous oral contraceptive therapy may be preferable to cyclic therapy to control endometriosis-related dysmenorrhea. Side effects of continuous oral contraceptive use include amenorrhea, spotting, and breakthrough bleeding. There is no evidence to suggest that one formulation of OCP works significantly better than another at controlling endometriosis-related pain.

Danazol is another oral therapy used to treat pain due to endometriosis. It has been used in the treatment of endometriosis since the 1970s. Danazol is a 17-ethynyltestosterone derivative and works by creating a high androgen and low estrogen environment, or a pseudomenopause. Endometriosis implants as well as eutopic endometrium undergo atrophy during danazol therapy. Furthermore, gonadotropin secretion from the pituitary is inhibited, which can lead to anovulation, although not in all cases. Danazol is taken orally in doses ranging from 400 to 800 mg per day.

In a placebo-controlled study, 6 months of danazol significantly reduced endometriosis-associated pain including pelvic pain, lower back pain, and defecation pain. Endometriosis was diagnosed by laparoscopy, and a second laparoscopy 6 months after termination of the study found a total or partial resolution of the implants in 60% of patients receiving danazol. A meta-analysis confirmed the effectiveness of danazol at treating endometriosis-related pain and improving laparoscopic evidence of endometriosis post treatment. Overall, symptomatic improvement of endometriosis with danazol treatment ranges from 60% to 80% of patients, depending upon the dose and duration of treatment.

Despite its effectiveness, danazol therapy has largely fallen out of favor due to its side effects, most of which are androgenic in nature. Up to 80% of patients have a major side effect while taking danazol. The most common side effects are hot flashes, acne, and edema due to fluid retention or weight gain. Other side effects include amenorrhea or breakthrough bleeding, negative effects on lipid profile (increased low-density lipoprotein and decreased high-density lipoprotein), increased liver enzymes, and mood changes. Up to 8% of patients experience an irreversible deepening of the voice. With lower doses, there are decreased side effects but also lower efficacy of the treatment. Danazol is a known teratogen, and women taking danazol also need to be using contraception.

Progestins are also given as a single agent in the treatment of endometriosis, causing decidualization and atrophy of endometriosis lesions. Pituitary gonadotropins are inhibited during therapy with progestins, resulting in decreased estrogen production by the ovary secondary to a lack of follicular development and ovulation.

Progestins have efficacy rates that are similar to danazol. In one study, patients with moderate to severe endometriosis took 50 mg medroxyprogesterone acetate for 4 months, and 80% of patients reported symptom relief. A second-look laparoscopy during the last week of treatment demonstrated significant decreases in the mean stage score of disease using the American Society for Reproductive Medicine classification. Medroxyprogesterone acetate is given orally at doses of 30–100 mg per day in divided doses.

Another oral progestin, norethindrone acetate, can be started at 5 mg per day and titrated upward until symptom relief is achieved. The maximum dose per day is 15 mg, although doses of 5–10 mg per day are usually sufficient. Intramuscular depot medroxyprogesterone acetate at doses of 104–150 mg every 3 months has also been shown to be effective at treating endometriosis. However, prolonged use of this medication is associated with loss of bone mineral density.

The etonogestrel subdermal implant, or Implanon, is a newer formulation of progestin in which a single rod containing the progestin is inserted into the inner side of the upper nondominant arm. This implant may remain in place for up to 3 years. There is limited evidence that suggests this implant may be as effective depot medroxyprogesterone acetate at treating endometriosis-associated dysmenorrhea, pelvic pain, and dyspareunia after 4 months of treatment.

The most common side effects from progestin therapy include amenorrhea, breakthrough bleeding, fluid retention, and weight gain, which may be experienced by 40–80% of patients. Other side effects of this group of medications are acne, breast tenderness, and mood changes, and while less common, these symptoms are reported by 10–20% of women taking the medication. These side effects may limit the use and tolerability of progestins, especially at higher doses, in some patients.

The progestin intrauterine device or levonorgestrel-releasing intrauterine device (LNG-IUD) releases 20 μg levonorgestrel per day and can be kept in place for up to 5 years. The progesterone released is concentrated in the pelvis, with endometrial concentrations of levonorgestrel many times higher than those observed after oral progestin administration. However, plasma levels of levonorgestrel in LNG-IUD users are approximately half those seen in implant or oral progestin users. As a result, there are fewer systemic side effects from the LNG-IUD. This IUD does cause hypomenorrhea or amenorrhea, and the most common side effect is irregular bleeding. Six months of treatment with the LNG-IUD may be as effective as a GnRH agonist at decreasing endometriosis-associated chronic pelvic pain. Women who underwent laparoscopic treatment of their endometriosis and had a LNG-IUD placed postoperatively reported a decreased recurrence of dysmenorrhea compared to placebo. The LNG-IUD may also be effective at treating dysmenorrhea, pelvic pain, and deep dyspareunia related to rectovaginal endometriosis.

GnRH agonists are as effective as other available therapies to treat endometriosis, and when given with add-back therapy, they have minimal side effects. They have a longer half-life than endogenous GnRH and also bind for a longer period of time to the GnRH receptor. This results in an initial "flare" effect that stimulates the release of luteinizing hormone (LH) and follicle-stimulating hormone (FSH) from the pituitary. Ultimately, the GnRH agonists cause a down-regulation of the GnRH receptors and cause the pituitary to become desensitized to native GnRH. FSH and LH are not released in their normal fashion, and follicular development and ovulation are inhibited. This results in lower circulating estrogen and progesterone levels due to lack of production of these hormones by the ovaries, and induces a menopause-like state. The circulating levels of estradiol in treated patients are less than 30 pg/mL, similar to those seen in menopause. Up to 75% of patients achieve this level of hypoestrogenism in 4 weeks and up to 98% by 8 weeks of therapy with GnRH agonists.

GnRH agonists have been tested in randomized controlled trials and found to be superior to placebo at decreasing dysmenorrhea, pelvic pain, and dyspareunia. In addition, pre- and post-treatment laparoscopies have demonstrated decreases in endometriosis implants as measured by the American Society for Reproductive Medicine's scoring system. GnRH agonists are as effective as danazol at alleviating endometriosis-related pain symptoms.

GnRH agonists can be given as a nasal spray, nafarelin, at 400 μg per day in divided doses. More commonly, they are given as an intramuscular injection—depot leuprolide—at a dose of 3.75 mg each month or 11.25 mg every 3 months. Goserelin acetate is a formulation that is given subcutaneously 3.6 mg every 28 days.

Side effects of GnRH agonist therapy are mainly related to its hypoestrogenic effects. Hot flashes are experienced by 80–90% of patients. Other side effects include weight gain, bloating, acne, moodiness, headaches, vaginal dryness, and adverse lipid profile changes. Patients on GnRH agonist therapy also experience amenorrhea, but menstrual cycles generally return 60–90 days after stopping the medication. The main side effect that limits the duration of use of GnRH agonists is bone mineral density loss: up to a 4–6% decrease in bone mineral density is seen after 6 months of GnRH agonist use.

To avoid these side effects, GnRH agonists should be prescribed with add-back therapy, especially for patients who are treated for prolonged (>6 months) courses of therapy. The premise behind giving add-back treatment with progesterone and/or estrogen is that small amounts of these hormones will prevent some of the hypoestrogenic side effects such as hot flashes and bone loss, yet the small amount of hormone given back will not be great enough to stimulate the growth of the endometriosis implants.

A large trial has provided evidence for the following add-back therapy regimen: 5 mg norethindrone acetate daily with or without 0.625 mg conjugated equine estrogens daily. Both norethindrone alone and norethindrone plus low-dose estrogen were shown to preserve bone density after 1 year of continuous GnRH agonist use. Patients also took supplemental calcium. This add-back regimen did not reduce the efficacy of GnRH agonists in treating endometriosis-related pain. However, higher doses of estrogen add-back therapy, such as 1.25 mg conjugated equine estrogens daily with the norethindrone, did result in decreased suppression of pelvic pain symptoms. Upon discontinuation of GnRH agonists, endometriosis-related pain symptoms will usually return within 60–90 days, and up to 75% of patients will have recurrent symptoms.

No studies have been conducted on the safety of GnRH agonists with an add-back therapy regimen for periods longer than 12 months. For women who respond well to the treatment, some clinicians are choosing to continue them on this regimen for longer periods of time. Yearly bone mineral density evaluations and periodic assessments of lipid profile are advised in these cases.

★ TIPS & TRICKS

When starting a patient on a gonadotropin-releasing hormone (GnRH) agonist for the treatment of endometriosis, start the medication during the midluteal phase of the menstrual cycle. This could prevent some of the flare effect of GnRH agonists that would occur if the medication were given during the follicular phase of the menstrual cycle. Also, when GnRH agonists are given during the luteal phase, there is more rapid down-regulation of the pituitary. This may translate into more rapid relief of symptoms for patients with endometriosis-related pain.

✋ CAUTION

Treatment with a gonadotropin-releasing hormone (GnRH) agonist without add-back therapy is limited to a maximum of 6 months as continuing therapy for longer periods of time will result in a loss of bone mineral density. However, the addition of add-back therapy, such as low-dose estrogen or progesterone, prevents this unwanted side effect without reducing the efficacy of GnRH agonists in reducing pain symptoms. Patients taking GnRH agonists with add-back therapy may safely continue them for up to 1 year without compromising bone mineral density. Regimens for add-back therapy are:
- norethindrone acetate 5 mg orally daily;
- conjugated estrogen 0.625 mg plus norethindrone acetate 5 mg orally daily.

⬡ SCIENCE REVISITED

Aromatase is an enzyme in the estrogen biosynthetic pathway that catalyzes the conversion of the C19 steroids testosterone and androstenedione to the estrogens estradiol and estrone. In endometriosis implants, there is an overproduction of estrogen, which encourages the survival and proliferation of endometriosis in the peritoneal cavity. The increased estrogen in these lesions also up-regulates prostaglandin E2, which then induces aromatase activity, creating a positive feedback loop. By blocking a key step in the synthesis of estrogen, aromatase inhibitors, such as letrozole, decrease the production of estrogen by the endometriosis implants. This leads to atrophy of the endometriosis lesions. Patients with endometriosis taking these medications experience decreased pain.

Aromatase is also expressed in peripheral tissues such as fat. Aromatase inhibitors halt this peripheral production of estrogen, leading to lower plasma levels of estrogen and decreased estrogen feedback to the pituitary during the follicular phase of the menstrual cycle. This results in increased ovarian stimulation by follicle-stimulating hormone and the formation of ovarian cysts. For this reason, patients who are taking aromatase inhibitors should also be on a medication that prevents ovulation, such as a gonadotropin-releasing hormone agonist, a progestin, or an oral contraceptive.

A novel treatment option for patients with endometriosis is aromatase inhibitors. Endometriosis lesions and eutopic endometrium in patients with endometriosis express the aromatase enzyme and can produce estrogen. Aromatase inhibitors work by blocking local estrogen production in the endometriosis lesions, as well as in other parts of the body. See the "Science revisited" box for a more thorough explanation.

Small case series provide most of the limited clinical evidence for the use of aromatase inhibitors in the treatment of endometriosis. The aromatase inhibitors most commonly used are anastrozole 1 mg orally a day or letrozole 2.5 mg orally per day. Six months of treatment with aromatase inhibitors when used in conjunction with a GnRH agonist significantly decreased symptom recurrence after surgery in patients with severe endometriosis compared to treatment with a GnRH agonist alone. The combination therapy led to lower circulating estradiol levels than the

GnRH therapy alone but did not cause increased menopausal symptoms.

Side effects of aromatase inhibitors include some loss of bone mineral density. This is a concern in reproductive-aged women taking this medication, but studies thus far have not consistently shown significant losses in bone mineral density. By decreasing circulating estrogen levels, aromatase inhibitors increase FSH and ovarian stimulation, and cause the development of ovarian cysts. Aromatase inhibitors should be used with another medication that blocks follicular development such as a progestin or GnRH agonist to mitigate this side effect.

Progesterone antagonists and selective progesterone receptor modulators have some evidence for their use in the treatment of endometriosis. They may work by inhibiting endometriosis progression, preventing ovulation, and suppressing endometrial prostaglandin production. Patients using mifepristone at a dose of 50 mg per day for 6 months reported decreased pelvic pain and uterine cramping. Regression of endometriosis lesions was also noted. Amenorrhea occurred as a result of anovulation, although hypoestrogenism was not documented. Asoprisnil, a selective progesterone receptor modulator, used at doses of 5–25 mg per day over a 3-month period, decreased dysmenorrhea and pelvic pain. These medications are generally well tolerated and do not appear to cause bone mineral density loss.

Medical treatment of endometriosis may cause regression of lesions during therapy but does not destroy the implants. Once medical therapy is stopped, there is often a regrowth of endometriosis. While patients may be initially pain-free after termination of medical therapy, up to 30–70% will develop recurrent pain. The mean length of time to recurrence of pain is 6–18 months. If endometriosis-related symptoms are controlled with medical therapy, the regimen can be maintained, with continued success expected.

Medical suppression of endometriosis should not be attempted in women who desire to conceive. Up to 20–50% of women with infertility have endometriosis. The disease may affect fertility by impairing oocyte development and/or quality, sperm penetration or fertilization, tubal function, and implantation. For women with endometriosis who are attempting to conceive, spontaneous monthly fecundity rates are between 2% and 3%. Medical therapy suppresses endometriosis implants but does not improve fecundity rates. Hormonal therapies stop ovulation while in use, and they further delay fertility. Monthly fecundity rates of 4.7% are achieved after surgery for endometriosis-associated infertility. However, this does not represent a great improvement over no treatment. In patients with endometriosis-associated infertility, clomiphene ovulation induction with intrauterine insemination increases monthly fecundity rates to 9%, while gonadotropin-controlled ovarian hyperstimulation further increases monthly fecundity rates to 15%. Pregnancy rates of 30% per month may be achieved with in-vitro fertilization.

Surgical treatment options

Surgical management of endometriosis is considered when patients fail or do not tolerate medical therapy. Surgery allows for both definitive diagnosis and treatment of endometriosis. The laparoscopic approach is generally preferred as it can provide shorter operative times, quicker postoperative recovery, and better visualization of endometriosis lesions. Conservative surgery for endometriosis involves preservation of ovarian tissue. Ablation of endometriosis provides superior postoperative pain relief compared to diagnostic procedures.

A study looking at patients with minimal to moderate endometriosis who had either diagnostic laparoscopy or laparoscopy with laser ablation of endometriosis and uterine nerve ablation demonstrated symptom improvement in both groups 3 months postoperatively. However, by 6 months, some 77% of patients had a recurrence of their pelvic pain after diagnostic laparoscopy, compared to 37% of the patients after an operative laparoscopy. After 1 year, 44% of patients in the operative laparoscopy group reported recurrent pain. After 6 years of follow-up, the recurrence rate of pelvic pain was 74%, with the majority of this recurring in the first 1 or 2 years after the initial surgical procedure.

Another study looking at patients undergoing laparoscopy with full excision of their endometriosis compared to diagnostic surgery found that only 20% of patients in the operative group had recurrent pain at 6 months, compared to 68% of patients in the diagnostic group. In addition to pain recurrence, patients undergoing conservative surgery may have a 15–20% reoperation rate within 2 years of their initial surgery.

Aggressive surgical resection or ablation of visible disease, followed by postoperative medical therapy with a GnRH analogue, danazol, or a progestin, might offer increased duration of pain relief or decreased recurrence of disease. In one study, patients who underwent surgical resection of their endometriosis had a recurrence rate of approximately 40% at 2 years, whereas those who had ablation of the disease had a significantly higher recurrence rate—approximately 77% at 2 years. Postoperative GnRH agonist use after surgical ablation reduced the recurrence rate at 2 years from 77% to approximately 30%. However, a meta-analysis looking at postoperative medical therapies after surgery for endometriosis showed a benefit of therapy in decreasing disease recurrence rates but not in decreasing pain.

The addition of presacral neurectomy or laparoscopic uterine nerve ablation (LUNA) to surgery for endometriosis to provide additional pain relief has been evaluated. Presacral neurectomy at the time of conservative laparoscopic surgery for severe dysmenorrhea caused by endometriosis was compared to conservative surgery without nerve ablation. At 6 months after surgery, patients who underwent LUNA had significantly less dysmenorrhea. However, some studies have shown no difference in postoperative pain after presacral neurectomy. Presacral neurectomy is a technically difficult surgery that can result in severe hemorrhage from the sacral venous plexus. Additionally, up to 15% of patients report the development of constipation and 5% urinary urgency after the procedure. So while presacral neurectomy may prove to be effective at treating central pain related to endometriosis, the minority of patients have solely centrally located pain symptoms. The addition of LUNA to surgery for endometriosis implants compared to surgery alone does not add additional pain relief.

Surgery may be first-line treatment for patients with endometriomas. Endometriomas that are larger than 1 cm are not as likely to regress with medical therapy. Surgery provides relief for patients who are experiencing pain related to an endometrioma and also provides a histologic diagnosis of the ovarian cyst. The latter is important as endometriomas do have a small risk of developing into clear cell or endometrioid ovarian cancer. Laparoscopic excision of the endometrioma and the cyst wall is superior to aspiration and/or ablation of the cyst. Cystectomy compared to aspiration results in decreased rates of cyst recurrence, fewer recurrent symptoms of dysmenorrhea, dyspareunia, and pelvic pain, as well as decreased rates of reoperation. Long-term effects on fertility and ovarian reserve after surgical excision of endometriomas are not clear. However, cystectomy may result in loss of follicles adjacent to the cyst wall and potentially lead to earlier decreased ovarian reserve.

Definitive surgery for endometriosis consists of hysterectomy with or without single or bilateral salpingo-oophorectomy. This treatment approach is only acceptable for women who do not wish to preserve their fertility and most often reserved for patients who have failed medical therapy and conservative surgery. Women under the age of 30 years who undergo definitive surgery may be more likely to experience a sense of loss, life disruption, and residual pain symptoms than women over the age of 30.

Evidence supporting that hysterectomy alone is effective at relieving endometriosis-related pain in patients who have failed other treatment measures is unclear. Whether or not to remove one or both ovaries at the time of definitive surgery remains controversial. One study examining the definitive surgery consisting of hysterectomy with or without ovarian preservation found that 62% of patients with ovarian preservation had recurrent pain and 31% required reoperation, compared to a 10% recurrent symptom rate and a 3.7% reoperation rate in patients who had their ovaries removed. Overall, reoperation rates for recurrent pain are lower if bilateral salpingo-oophorectomy is performed at the time of the original surgery.

Hormone replacement therapy after definitive surgery for endometriosis is also controversial as estrogen replacement could result in recurrence of disease and pain. Patients symptomatic from hypoestrogenism may require estrogen replacement. Some experts advocate replacement with both estrogen and progesterone, but the addition of progesterone may increase the risk of breast cancer. Others argue that estrogen replacement alone may stimulate residual endometriosis lesions and may increase the risk for malignant transformation of the remaining endometriosis lesions.

Selected bibliography

Abou-Setta AM, Al-Inany HG, Farquhar CM. Levonorgestrel-releasing intrauterine device (LNG-IUD) for symptomatic endometriosis following surgery. Cochrane Database Syst Rev 2006, Issue 4. Art. No.: CD005072.

Allen C, Hopewell S, Prentice A, Gregory D. Non-steroidal anti-inflammatory drugs for pain in women with endometriosis. Cochrane Database Syst Rev 2009, Issue 2. Art. No.: CD004753.

Bulun SE. Endometriosis. N Engl J Med 2009;360:268–79.

Demco L. Mapping the source and character of pain due to endometriosis by patient-assisted laparoscopy. J Am Assoc Gynecol Laparosc 1998;5:241–5.

Du H, Taylor HS. Contribution of bone marrow-derived stem cells to endometrium and endometriosis. Stem Cells 2007;25:2082–6.

Fedele L, Parazzini F, Bianchi S, Arcaini L, Candiani GB. Stage and localization of pelvic endometriosis and pain. Fertil Steril 1990;53:155–8.

Hart R, Hickey M, Maouris P, Buckett W, Garry R. Excisional surgery versus ablative surgery for ovarian endometriomata: a Cochrane Review. Hum Reprod 2005;20:3000–7.

Hornstein MD, Surrey ES, Weisberg GW, Casino LA. Leuprolide acetate depot and hormonal add-back in endometriosis: a 12-month study. Lupron Add-Back Study Group. Obstet Gynecol 1998;91:16–24.

Hughes E, Fedorkow D, Collins J, Vandekerckhove P. Ovulation suppression for endometriosis. Cochrane Database Syst Rev 2003, Issue 3. Art. No.: CD000155.

Kettel LM, Murphy AA, Morales AJ, Ulmann A, Baulieu EE, Yen SS. Treatment of endometriosis with the antiprogesterone mifepristone (RU486). Fertil Steril 1996;65:23–8.

Luciano AA, Turksoy RN, Carleo J. Evaluation of oral medroxyprogesterone acetate in the treatment of endometriosis. Obstet Gynecol 1988;72(3 Pt 1):323–7.

Marcoux S, Maheux R, Berube S. Laparoscopic surgery in infertile women with minimal or mild endometriosis. Canadian Collaborative Group on Endometriosis. N Engl J Med 1997;337:217–22.

Selak V, Farquhar C, Prentice A, Singla A. Danazol for pelvic pain associated with endometriosis. Cochrane Database Syst Rev 2007, Issue 4. Art. No.: CD000068.

Soysal S, Soysal ME, Ozer S, Gul N, Gezgin T. The effects of post-surgical administration of goserelin plus anastrozole compared to goserelin alone in patients with severe endometriosis: a prospective randomized trial. Hum Reprod 2004;19:160–7.

Sutton CJ, Pooley AS, Ewen SP, Haines P. Follow-up report on a randomized controlled trial of laser laparoscopy in the treatment of pelvic pain associated with minimal to moderate endometriosis. Fertil Steril 1997;68:1070–4.

Yap C, Furness S, Farquhar C. Pre and post operative medical therapy for endometriosis surgery. Cochrane Database Syst Rev 2004, Issue 3. Art. No.: CD003678.

Pelvic Infections and Chronic Pelvic Pain

Nicole Paterson and John Jarrell

University of Calgary, Calgary, Alberta, Canada

Introduction

Infections in the pelvis are a common spectrum of illness in women principally in the reproductive years. They generally but not exclusively arise from infections in the lower genital tract due to upward spread into the uterus, tubes, and pelvic and abdominal peritoneum. The upper genital tract infections are known as pelvic inflammatory disease or PID. This term is used for diverse infections such as endometritis, salpingitis, oophoritis, pelvic peritonitis and tubo-ovarian abscess. In some instances, the condition arises due to therapeutic or diagnostic instrumentation. The complications of PID include increased rates of ectopic pregnancy, infertility, and chronic pelvic pain (CPP), which account for the significant costs to the healthcare system resulting from PID. This chapter is specifically directed to a presentation of the clinical, pathologic, and therapeutic considerations of PID and the specific complication of CPP.

Epidemiology and risk factors

PID is a disease that is due either to sexually transmitted infections (STIs), usually gonorrhea (*Neisseria gonorrhoeae*) or increasingly more commonly chlamydia (*Chlamydia trachomatis*), or to infections associated with organisms in the lower genital tract. It can be due to the upward spread of organisms into the normally sterile environment of the upper genital tract, and it may also be facilitated by manipulations of a diagnostic and therapeutic manner involving penetration of the uterine cervix.

A review of the patterns of hospitalization-based care from the early 1990s provides a good summary of the outcomes of PID in which a comparison was made between the outcomes of 1,355 women with a history of PID and those of 10,507 women controls discharged with other diagnoses. Although such comparison studies are limited, it did show that the women with PID were 10 times more likely to be readmitted for abdominal pain, 4 times more likely to be admitted for pelvic pain, 6 times more likely for endometriosis, 8 times more for a hysterectomy, and 10 times more for an ectopic pregnancy. The incidence and prevalence of PID are difficult to ascertain because of the difficulties associated with diagnosis. Better information is available from the prevalence and incidence of STIs, which are highly variable around the globe. Dallabetta has reported the annual incidence of acquiring a curable STI as follows: Western Europe 1–2%, North America 2–3%, Latin America 7–14%, South East Asia 9–17% and sub-Saharan Africa 11–35%.

The Centers for Disease Control (CDC) has estimated there are approximately 1 million cases in the United States annually, for which the annual costs are in the range of US$4.2 billion. However, the rates of hospitalization have declined 16% since 1988, and there has also been a reduction in the diagnosis in ambulatory clinics up to 2007. There has also been a parallel reduction in hospitalization rates in Canada from 364 per 100,000 to 125 per 100,000 women of reproductive age between 1984 and 1994. The reasons for these declines in utilization rate are unknown.

Chronic Pelvic Pain, First Edition. Edited by Paolo Vercellini.
© 2011 Blackwell Publishing Ltd. Published 2011 by Blackwell Publishing Ltd.

It is difficult to assume that this means a reduction in the rate of PID, given the increasing rates of chlamydia infection, so it may be that the condition has changed its pathophysiology to represent a more subclinical appearance. It should be noted that the effectiveness of ambulatory treatment has been reported in a randomized controlled trial.

The disease carries significant alterations in years lost due to disability and disability-adjusted life years. While CPP is a large part of the measures of disability, other aspects include infertility and increased rates of mortality years of life lost, depending on the community. Additional approaches to the condition involve the measure of costs associated with delayed complications, and of illnesses, which are substantial and support the processes of preventative care.

The prevalence and incidence of STIs in general vary greatly both by country and within a country. The factors that affect the spread of STI in a population are biologic, behavioral, medical, and socioeconomic. Spread at a population level will be affected by the efficiency of transmission, the mean rate of sexual partner change, and the average duration of infectivity. Therefore efforts to reduce disease burden include reducing unsafe practices, encouraging monogamous relationships, and ensuring public health programs to aid tracing and treating contacts.

Risk factors for the development of PID

PID is a complex disease that can be associated with multiple organisms and can spontaneously develop or be associated with a variety of clinical circumstances that can initiate the condition (Table 5.1).

The most important risk factor is the presence of a lower genital infection with chlamydia or gonorrhea. Bacterial vaginosis (BV) as a risk factor has been viewed as controversial. However, a large study looked at two clusters of vaginal cultures. The first cluster was microorganisms associated with BV (an absence of peroxidase-producing *Lactobacillus* and the presence of *Gardnerella*, *Mycoplasma hominis*, and Gram-negative rods). The second cluster was unrelated to BV and included enteroccocus and *Escherichia coli*. The authors found that being in the highest tertile for BV-related microorganisms increased

Table 5.1 Risk factors for the development of pelvic inflammatory disease

The bacterial flora of the vagina
- *Chlamydia trachomatis*
- *Neisseria gonorrhoeae*
- Bacterial vaginosis

Ethnicity, socioeconomy, and geography

Prior infections

Sexual behavior
- Multiple partners
- Lack of barrier contraception

Instrumentation
- Insertion of an intrauterine contraceptive device
- Dilatation and curettage
- Pregnancy termination
- Hysterosalpingography
- Dye transit studies

the risk for PID, whereas the presence of vaginosis with unrelated BV microorganisms did not.

Demographic markers of risk include a young age, lower socioeconomic status, being single, separated, or divorced, and involvement in the sex trade. There is evidence from the CDC that there are much higher rates of STI infection among men and women of African-American background. This is further translated into higher rates of PID among the same population. Reasons for these increased rates may reflect reduced access to healthcare, increased attendance at public health clinics with greater testing frequency, and more frequent exposure to infected black men (who have higher rates of STIs) than occurs for white women. A previous episode of PID is a risk factor in the development of recurrent infections. Sexual behavior, particularly activity involving multiple sexual partners, is a most prominent risk factor.

Procedures that can be associated with a pelvic infection include dilatation and curettage, pregnancy termination, hysterosalpingography, laparoscopically associated dye transit procedures, and insertion of an intrauterine device (IUD). The practice of illegal abortion is the most common instrumental cause of pelvic infections.

The IUD has important relationships with PID. A recent summary showed that the incidence of

PID associated with IUD use is dependent on the definition used for the diagnosis and the means available for diagnosis. The frequency varied from 1 in 100 to 1 to 1,000 woman–years in different studies. The rate is sixfold higher in the first month of use, with rates also varying according to other risk factors such as multiple sexual partners, community prevalence of STIs, and age. Recent systematic reviews based on multiple randomized controlled trials have shown that universal prophylactic antibiotics do not decrease the rate of PID after IUD insertion. However, if a patient is at risk, swabs testing for chlamydia and gonorrhea should be performed and insertion of the IUD delayed.

Women having induced abortions with insertion of an IUD at the time of the procedure have increased rates of pain and bleeding, but there are no reported increases in the incidence of PID. Although classical teaching has indicated that tubal ligation is protective, there have been reports suggesting that the conditions should be considered in any woman with abdominal and pelvic pain independent of tubal ligation status.

Pathology

Culture of the lower genital tract provides a good assessment of the cause of infections associated with the upper genital tract. The common organisms include *Chlamydia, N. gonorrhoeae*, and a variety or aerobic and anaerobic bacteria (*Mycoplasma, Bacteroides, E. coli, Haemophilus influenzae, Gardnerella vaginalis*). It has been estimated that 10% of women with chlamydia will develop PID, but the reasons for this low rate are not apparent.

Although STIs are associated with younger women, older women tend to have more severe infections associated with endogenous bacteria in association with IUD use and with the development of tubo-ovarian abscesses.

The upward ascent of the organisms is thought to be associated with passage along the endothelial lining, and this may occur in association with spermatozoon activity. Infections with chlamydia or gonorrhea develop further with the recruitment of additional organisms, particularly anaerobic bacteria. The infections with chlamydia and gonorrhea result in rapid destruction of the ciliated cells of the fallopian tube, the generation of pelvic adhesions, and later the development of abscesses involving the tubo-ovarian complex.

Clinical presentation and diagnosis

The hallmark of PID is its inherent variability. The differential diagnosis includes ectopic pregnancy, ovarian cyst rupture, torsion, infection, appendicitis, endometriosis, urinary sepsis, septic abortion, and inflammatory bowel disease. Many cases appear to be subclinical and are only appreciated when the woman is being investigated for other reasons, such as by laparoscopy for infertility. In terms of the initial infections, 50% and 30% respectively of individuals with *N. gonorrhoeae* and *C. trachomatis* infection develop nonspecific signs of infection, although these are generally mild, such as discharge and or abnormal bleeding shortly after infection.

When clinically apparent, the most common symptom of PID is lower abdominal pain. Other symptoms may include vaginal discharge, abnormal vaginal bleeding, and dyspareunia. In the event that the infection is severe, nausea, vomiting, and fever can develop. It should be noted, however, that fever is apparent in less than half of patients with PID. In some individuals with more widespread illness, there is tenderness in the upper abdomen from involvement of the hepatic capsule, which is known as Fitz-Hugh–Curtis syndrome.

The criteria for diagnosis of PID are imprecise, and the condition is often mistaken for other conditions such as endometriosis (Table 5.2). No single variable from the history, physical examination, or laboratory tests has been found to have high sensitivity and specificity, so the approach to diagnosis is to incorporate a number of findings. The CDC have provided minimal criteria for the diagnosis. These include lower abdominal tenderness, adnexal tenderness, and cervical motion tenderness. However, it is argued by some that these criteria will miss a substantial number of cases and that a minimal criterion of only adnexal tenderness provides more sensitivity. The incorporation of other laboratory markers then may be used to increase specificity.

Laboratory investigations may aid diagnosis and be valuable in ruling out other potential

Table 5.2 Criteria for the diagnosis of pelvic inflammatory disease (PID) from the Centers for Disease Control

Minimum criteria

Lower abdominal tenderness *or*

Bilateral adnexal tenderness *or*

Cervical motion tenderness

Additional criteria that support the diagnosis

Temperature >38.3 °C (100.9 °F)

Abnormal cervical or vaginal discharge

Elevated erythrocyte sedimentation rate

Elevated C-reactive protein level

Documented infection with *Neisseria gonorrhoeae* or *Chlamydia trachomatis*

Definitive criteria—warranted in selected cases

Laparoscopic abnormalities consistent with PID

Histological evidence of endometritis on endometrial biopsy

Imaging technique showing thickened, fluid-filled tubes with or without free pelvic fluid or tubo-ovarian complex

diagnoses; however, no single test or combination of tests can reliably predict PID. Laboratory tests that are often performed in the work-up for PID include beta-human chorionic gonadotropin, urinalysis, complete blood count, inflammatory markers, and endocervical and vaginal swabs for *N. gonorrhoeae*, *C. trachomatis*, and culture.

Erythrocyte sedimentation rate and C-reactive protein level have been shown to have sensitivities ranging from 65% to 85% but are also associated with a low specificity. Positive test results for *N. gonorrhoreae* and *C. trachomatis* are one of the most predictive criteria, but it is important to note that negative swabs do not rule out a diagnosis of PID given the polymicrobial nature of the condition.

The value of endometrial biopsy for diagnostic purposes remains to be elucidated. Multiple criteria for diagnosis have been proposed. The CDC use a count of five or more neutrophils per high-power field and one or more plasma cells per low-power field, which has been shown to have a sensitivity and specificity of approximately 90%. An endometrial biopsy might be used in women who are undergoing laparoscopy in which there is no evidence of salpingitis as some women have endometritis alone.

Ultrasound can be of value both to rule out other pelvic pathology and in addition to indicate markers of PID. Findings on transvaginal ultrasound may demonstrate thickened, fluid-filled tubes or a complex mass indicative of a tubo-ovarian abscess.

The use of laparoscopy should, because of its low sensitivity in making the diagnosis, be reserved for individual management when severity of disease or failure to respond to therapy dictates that more aggressive management may be required. In these situations, fallopian tube erythema, edema, and purulent exudates are indicators of PID. In addition, thin filmy adhesions on the anterior aspect of the liver capsule indicate Fitz-Hugh–Curtis syndrome.

Treatment and prevention

The management of PID should be initiated as soon as possible to avoid the sequelae of the condition as a consequence of injury to the fallopian tubes. PID can be managed on an outpatient basis, but admission is recommended in the presence of immunodeficiency states, diagnostic uncertainty, failure to respond to oral medications, suspected tubo-ovarian abscess, pregnancy, and where compliance may be a concern (Table 5.3). Admission to hospital provides options that include parenteral pain management, fluid rehydration, and observation

Table 5.3 Centers for Disease Control criteria for hospitalization

Surgical emergencies such as appendicitis cannot be excluded

Pregnancy

Failure to respond to oral antimicrobial agents

Inability to tolerate an outpatient regimen

Severe illness, nausea, vomiting, and high fever

Tubo-ovarian abscess

for the course of the illness. If there is an IUD in place, consideration should be given to its removal.

Centers for Disease Control treatment recommendations

Parenteral treatment

Parenteral and oral therapy appear to have similar clinical efficacy when treating women with PID of mild or moderate severity. Clinical experience should guide decisions regarding the transition to oral therapy, which usually can be initiated within 24 hours of clinical improvement. The CDC recommends the following parenteral regimes:

Recommended parenteral regimen A:
Cefotetan 2 g intravenously every 12 hours
  OR
Cefoxitin 2 g intravenously every 6 hours
  PLUS
Doxycycline 100 mg orally or intravenously every 12 hours.

Recommended parenteral regimen B:
Clindamycin 900 mg intravenously every 8 hours
  PLUS
Gentamicin loading dose intravenously or intramuscularly (2 mg/kg body weight), followed by a maintenance dose (1.5 mg/kg) every 8 hours. Single daily dosing may be substituted.

Alternative parenteral regimens:
Ampicillin/sulbactam 3 g intravenously every 6 hours
  PLUS
Doxycycline 100 mg orally or intravenously every 12 hours.

Oral treatment

Oral therapy can be considered for women with mild to moderately severe acute PID, as the clinical outcomes among women treated with oral therapy are similar to those treated with parenteral therapy. Women who do not respond to oral therapy within 72 hours should be re-evaluated to confirm the diagnosis and should be administered parenteral therapy on either an outpatient or an inpatient basis. The CDC's recommended oral regimen is:

Ceftriaxone 250 mg intramuscularly in a single dose
  PLUS
Doxycycline 100 mg orally twice a day for 14 days
  WITH OR WITHOUT
Metronidazole 500 mg orally twice a day for 14 days

OR

Cefoxitin 2 g intramuscularly in a single dose, and probenecid 1 g orally administered concurrently in a single dose
  PLUS
Doxycycline 100 mg orally twice a day for 14 days
  WITH OR WITHOUT
Metronidazole 500 mg orally twice a day for 14 days

OR

Other parenteral third-generation cephalosporin (e.g., ceftizoxime or cefotaxime)
  PLUS
Doxycycline 100 mg orally twice a day for 14 days
  WITH OR WITHOUT
Metronidazole 500 mg orally twice a day for 14 days.

Alternative oral regimens are also available. If parenteral cephalosporin therapy is not feasible, use fluoroquinolones (levofloxacin 500 mg orally once daily or ofloxacin 400 mg twice daily for 14 days) with or without metronidazole (500 mg orally twice daily for 14 days). However, rapid increases in quinolone-resistant *N. gonorrhoeae* have occurred, and therefore quinolones should only be used in select areas and where susceptibility testing is available; if antimicrobial testing is not available, a test of cure is essential. Therefore, if patient allergy to cephalosporin is an issue in a quinolone-resistance area, axithromycin (250 mg orally daily for 7 days) with or without metronidazole has been shown to be an effective treatment.

Although information regarding other outpatient regimens is limited, amoxicillin/clavulanic acid with metronidazole and either doxycycline or azithromycin has demonstrated short-term clinical cure. No data have been published regarding the use of oral cephalosporins for the treatment of PID.

Tests of cure should be performed when compliance is known to be suboptimal, in pregnant women, prepubertally or when there is re-exposure to an untreated partner. If a test of cure is performed, it is done 3–4 weeks after the treatment. Due to a high recurrence risk, repeat testing should be performed 6 months later if there have been positive results for chlamydia or gonorrhea.

Prevention

Correct approaches to the prevention of PID are extremely important because of the severity of the sequelae. Primary prevention involves community education regarding sexual activity and barrier contraception, as well as the use of prophylactic measures during pelvic instrumentation. Either the use of prophylactic antibiotics or screening for STIs should be performed in high-risk patients prior to termination of pregnancy, IUD insertion, or hysterosalpingography.

Screening for chlamydia in the community among women at risk has been shown to reduce the incidence of PID, and the relative cost-effectiveness of this measure will be associated with the underlying rates of infection in the community.

Complications

The complications of PID include tube-related infertility, the rate of which has been estimated at 8–20% depending on the number of PID episodes. Ectopic pregnancy is much more common after PID, and having a first pregnancy as an ectopic has been shown in a Swedish study to occur in approximately 9% of women with PID compared to 1% of women without PID. CPP occurs in 15–20% of women with PID.

Relationship to chronic pelvic pain

Pain is classified into nociceptive pain (which includes somatic and visceral) and neuropathic pain. In the case of PID, the overwhelming pattern of pain initially is visceral nociceptive pain, due to inflammation caused by the infectious processes. However, this can become a somatic type of pain with time. Somatic pain is characterized by its continuous nature, the presence of abdominal wall and perineal allodynia, and reduced pain thresholds in the accompanying musculature. When this pattern becomes fully developed, the intensity and impact of the somatic pain may not be related directly to the underlying pathology. Some women may have severe degrees of disability despite relatively minor anatomic abnormalities identified at surgery, whereas others may have minimal incapacity despite widespread intestinal and pelvic injury from chronic inflammation.

Evaluation of the patient with chronic pelvic pain

History

In some instances, there is a clear history of a preceding infection that has resulted in a chronic pain state. Previous acute pelvic infectious disease from confirmed *Chlamydia* infections or gonorrhea are not uncommon, but the women may also give a history of a postabortion infection, postpartum endometritis, or a ruptured appendix. In many cases, however, there are no indications of prior infections. This is due to the many instances of subclinical infection.

The quality and characteristics of the patient's pain can help guide the identification of potential etiologies contributing to CPP. It has be shown that bleeding, premenstrual exacerbation of pain, and cervical tenderness are more consistent with CPP after endometriosis or PID, whereas colicky pain, upper pelvis pain, abdominal dissention, nausea, bowel changes, and worsening with food are all more in keeping with CPP related to inflammatory bowel disease. A systematic review of patients with CPP found that previous PID infection was significantly associated with symptoms of noncyclic pelvic pain of longer than 3 months, duration and dyspareunia.

Diagnostic factors that may predict the development of CPP after PID have been explored, but no significant short-term markers have been found. It was found that cervical tenderness at 5 and 30 days after treatment was associated with the development of CPP, albeit with a weak positive predictive value.

Physical examination

The spectrum of CPP is large and in general poorly understood. PID, adhesions, and endometriosis occur in a large proportion of women who receive a diagnosis of CPP. In an evaluation of the predictors of those women with PID who go on to develop CPP, an increased risk for the condition with racial origin other than black, being married, a low SF-36 mental health composite score, two or more episodes of PID, and smoking all independently predicted a higher rate of CPP associated with PID. Notably, pelvic pain and recurrent episodes of PID have been shown to be reduced by a self-reported persistent use of condoms.

The examination of a woman with chronic pain has important differences from the general pelvic examination. In the first instance, women with chronic pain are usually hyperalgesic, meaning that painful stimuli are appreciated to a much greater degree than normal.

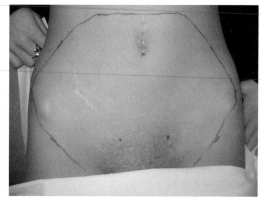

Figure 5.1 A demonstration of cutaneous allodynia that has developed from viscerosomatic pain referral on the abdomen and involves the dermatome segments T9–L1. Gentle pressure with a cotton-tipped applicator will generate a sudden change in sensation to sharp or painful in the presence of such neuroplasticity. The two dots indicate areas of myofascial dysfunction (trigger points)—areas of abdominal wall tenderness.

⚗ SCIENCE REVISITED

The referral of visceral pain to the somatic dermatomes has been established by Giamberardino. The number of episodes of visceral pain reflects the severity of somatic hyperalgesia.

In many instances, these women also have allodynia, in which a normal stimulus that is not normally associated with pain can be severely painful (Figure 5.1). As a result, palpation for somatic referral of pain from the abdomen should be very gentle. Pressure algometry has shown that, in women with CPP, a pressure of as low as 25 g with a von Frey anesthesiometer can effect severe pain in all four quadrants of the abdomen. A further examination with a cotton-tipped applicator can also demonstrate important clinical findings. There is commonly a sharply demarcated area of cutaneous allodynia that can be identified with the applicator if it is drawn gently down the abdomen. The woman will sense a change in the character of the touch to a sharpness or pain that is commonly identified in the T10–L1 dermatome area on the abdomen and in the S3 segment of the vulva. This is a marker for the presence of viscerosomatic pain referral. This sign is very common among women with visceral conditions that have led to the presence of chronic pain, including PID, endometriosis, and ovarian cysts.

★ TIPS & TRICKS

A cotton-tipped culture stick drawn gently down the abdomen in the midclavicular line becomes sharply painful in a woman with cutaneous allodynia due to neuroplasticity. This usually occurs in the T10–L1 dermatomes and is associated with the viscerosomatic referral of pain.

These areas are almost always associated with a significant degree of muscle tenderness, as indicated by the algometers. This tenderness is due in large part to the presence of myofascial dysfunction, another clinical finding associated with chronic pain. Such trigger points (Figure 5.1) can be located in the lower abdomen within the areas of cutaneous allodynia, or lie in the perineal body of the vulva. These represent the nervous innervations supplying the visceral organs of the pelvis, and when the pain becomes severe, referral occurs to the somatic aspects of the body in the same dermatome regions. In some cases of PID, the degree of inflammation extends to the upper abdomen, and hence the areas of cutaneous allodynia may extend into the upper abdomen as well.

The pelvic examination has to be modified for women with severe CPP. Essentially, it is directed most importantly to determine whether the pain is associated with ongoing muscle pain alone, as is commonly the case, or is also associated with ongoing recurrent or persistent visceral disease. As the woman is usually severely hyperalgesic, the pelvic examination should be undertaken with a single digit rather than as the traditional two-handed bimanual examination. The single digit can inform the clinician whether the pain being experienced can be reproduced by gentle pressure on the muscles of the pelvis. The examiner may also determine whether the pain may be reproduced by gentle pressure on the cervix and lower uterine area.

Medical management of chronic pelvic pain

The principles underlying medical management can be categorized into pain management (opioid and nonopioid), menstrual suppression, and surgical intervention. As in all aspects of the management of CPP, the objectives of care should be reducing the pain and improving the quality of life. Medical management alone is not sufficient to achieve these ends, and ancillary care is required through the availability of multidisciplinary teams.

Nonopioid pain management involves the use of nonsteroidal anti-inflammatory drugs and acetaminophen for inflammatory nociceptive pain, particularly in the treatment of dysmenorrhea. Increasing the potency and dose of medication may be required because of the severity of the condition or because of increasing pain during active physiotherapy. In selected cases, the use of opioid medication may be considered. Usage may be temporary during physiotherapy, or prolonged in severe cases of CPP. Although previously controversial, the management of chronic nonmalignant pain with opioids is recommended by the International Association for the Study of Pain (Tables 5.4–5.6). The medications should be used judiciously, and a formal contract that outlines the processes of management is recommended. Such contracts

Table 5.4 International Association for the Study of Pain: potential issues during the use of opioids in chronic noncancer pain

Tolerance

Physical dependence (patient or newborn)

Psychological dependence/addiction

Organ dysfunction (gastrointestinal, reproductive, genitourinary, ventilatory)

Neuropsychological and cognitive impairment

Diversion

Questionable efficacy for non-nociceptive pain

Hyperalgesia

Externalization of locus of control

Unproven effect on patient functional status

Table 5.5 International Association for the Study of Pain: therapeutic opioid trial for chronic noncancer pain: proposed entry criteria

A failure of reasonable pain management alternatives such as physical therapy, cognitive-behavioral techniques, and medical techniques

Physical and psychosocial assessment, preferably by two specialists

A history of substance abuse (a relative but not an absolute contraindication) requires consultation with drug abuse and drug control services

A final decision by a team of two or more medical practitioners

Informed, written, witnessed consent by the patient

Proposed practical guidelines

A preference for mu agonists with a long duration of action, such as slow-release morphine or methadone

Drug dosing by the oral route with scheduled administration

A 4-week trial period of planned therapy with frequent reviews to titrate dosage and assess clinical efficacy

Demonstration of a sustained improvement in pain control and/or function

Table 5.6 International Association for the Study of Pain: proposed guidelines for long-term

management after a successful therapeutic opioid trial for chronic noncancer pain
Prescriptions from a single medical practitioner (with deputy prescribers to cover absences)
Initially frequent and then at least monthly reviews and documentation of pain relief, functional status, appropriate medication use, and side effects
Review and discussion of concomitant education
An ongoing effort to gain an improvement in social and physical function as a result of pain relief
Contract between patient and practitioner explicitly detailing termination of supply (with appropriate tapering of the dose) and notification to drug control services if there is evidence of misuse such as diversion, loss, or theft of medication, unexplained escalation of dosage, or request for opioids from other sources
Use of drug assays and/or supervised inpatient treatment in case of problems (especially unexplained exacerbation of pain or escalation of dosage)
Continuing review of the overall situation with regard to nonopioid means of pain control

★ **TIPS & TRICKS**

Menstrual suppression with an oral contraceptive will initially produce some breakthrough bleeding in the first 2–3 months. If the woman stops the pill for 4 days and then restarts continuous medication, amenorrhea generally will ensue.

state that there should only be one prescribing physician.

Menstrual suppression is becoming a standard of management because recurrent menstrual bleeding is seen as a pain generator among women with CPP. Techniques for suppression include continuous oral contraception use (see the "Tips & tricks" box) and long term gonadotropin-releasing hormone administration with estrogen progesterone add-back therapy. The levonorgestrel-releasing IUD can be used for menstrual suppression in other CPP situations, but if there is a past history of PID, great caution is advised. In the setting of acute or recent PID or if a patient is high risk for STIs, an IUD should not be used.

Surgery in the presence of CPP should be reserved to treat conditions that may reduce the pain generation, but one should not anticipate a cure of the condition from surgical intervention unless there is a specific lesion. One such case is the persistent pain associated with an ovary bound in pelvic adhesions. During ovulation, the ovary can increase in volume considerably, so its removal is can result in a reduction in overall pain and an improvement in quality of life. Other similar cases that may benefit from a surgical procedure include hysterectomy and removal of the tubes and ovaries in the presence of a severe chronic tubo-ovarian abscess.

Multidisciplinary management

Determining that the pain is not due to contemporaneous active visceral disease is very important. If such a condition is present, it will be an active illness that will require active management and possible surgery and hospitalization. If the clinician has some assurance that the pain is due to muscle tenderness and reduced pain thresholds, the approach to management can be focused on a more rehabilitative approach, using multidisciplinary pain management approaches.

Multidisciplinary management involves physicians (neurologists, anesthetists, gynecologists, psychiatrists), nurses, physiotherapists, kinesiologists, psychologists, and dietitians, all of whom are involved in a woman's care. Much of the activity associated with such care is in group formats, although individual management is also used heavily in most multidisciplinary clinics. The overall effectiveness of such clinics has been reported. At the Calgary Chronic Pain Centre, subjects entering the clinic had an SF-36 rating that was equivalent to those with chronic congestive heart failure, but 1 year after discharge their

SF-36 ratings had increased to levels approaching Canadian norms. These approaches are directed therefore to improving the woman's quality of life and potentially reducing her reported pain levels.

It is important to note that a "cure" from CPP is unusual at best, but one can reasonably expect some measurable improvement in pain levels. Important areas that have been shown to give an improvement in pain have included cognitive-behavioral therapy.

Adhesions and the role of laparoscopy

Adhesions are among the most common abnormalities identified with CPP. They occur at a greater frequency following surgical procedures in the pelvis, in addition to being associated with inflammatory conditions such as PID. The relationship of adhesions to the pelvic pain and the basis for the surgical resection of such adhesions is controversial. Women with a history of pelvic pain have been found to have more frequent adhesions in the pelvis than women who did not have pelvic pain and were undergoing a tubal ligation. It should be noted that adhesions were found in 12% of 50 women who did not have pain, and it is possible that pericolic adhesions may simply reflect a congenital developmental variability in anatomy. Some have advocated for a laparoscopic approach early in the development of the chronic pain state to establish a diagnosis should one be available.

The clinical diagnosis of adhesions has been attempted using ultrasound and with magnetic resonance techniques; in general, magnetic resonance imaging appears to be more effective. The most common method remains laparoscopy with direct vision of the pelvis. Awake laparoscopy has been reported to demonstrate that there were greater increases in pain associated with filmy adhesions with attachment of the peritoneum or to ovarian tissues than with adhesions in which the tissues were relatively immobile. This procedure, however, remains experimental.

It is controversial whether intra-abdominal surgery for adhesions is a procedure with strong evidence of long-term benefit. In a review of the therapies effective for CPP, those which were found to be effective were progesterone (medroxyprogesterone acetate), gonadotropin-releasing hormone agonists, counseling supported by ultrasound scanning, and a multidisciplinary approach to care. Specifically, no benefit was noted from adhesiolysis (except where adhesions were severe), uterine nerve ablation, or photographic reinforcement after laparoscopy. Systematic reviews of the available literature have shown the same findings.

There are significant complications associated with surgical resection of adhesions, such as injury of organs during trochar insertion, inadvertent enterotomy, conversion from laparoscopy to laparotomy, and prolonged hospital stay. Delayed presentation of inadvertent enterotomy is associated with severe morbidity, and an unrecognized and delayed presentation of enterotomy carries with it a mortality rate of 7.7%.

Recently, adhesions have been recognized as the most common complication of pelvic surgery, causing bowel obstruction, infertility, and CPP, with a directive to explore new methods of prevention. One procedure of benefit has been fixation of the ovary to avoid persistent adhesion to the peritoneum of the ovarian fossa. A variety of agents, including low molecular weight heparin, aprotinin, and sodium hyaluronate/carboxymethylcellulose, to reduce adhesions have been evaluated in animal studies, with positive benefits noted over controls. The use of polypropylene mesh with and without Seprafilm (Genzyme Corporation; Cambridge, MA, United States), an absorbable adhesion barrier, and Composix (Bard Nordic Inc.; Helsingborg, Sweden) mesh application also did not prevent adhesions in experimental animals. In rabbits, Sepracoat (Genzyme Corporation) was found to be beneficial in the prevention of adhesions.

There have been several Cochrane Reviews on the benefits of various agents. In general, the results have been either limited in the scope of the recommendations or relatively negative. One review found that hyaluronic acid/carboxymethyl cellulose reduced the incidence severity and extent of adhesions but did not prevent subsequent intestinal obstruction. The use of barrier agents (oxidized regenerated cellulose, polytetraflouroethylene of fibrin sheets) showed that Interceed (Ethicon Inc., Johnson & Johnson, New Jersey USA) did reduce adhesions, but the data were insufficient to support its use in improving pregnancy rates. There was no benefit from Seprafilm and fibrin sheet. A Cochrane Review of the use of adhesion prevention strategies evaluated 15 randomized studies and showed there was no evidence for the use of steroids, icodextrin, SprayGel (Covidien, Waltham, MA, USA), or dextran, although there was some benefit from fluids that contained hyaluronic acid. A non-randomized study of the use of Seprafilm indicated potential benefits.

Outcomes of management

There have been no long-term studies of the outcomes of CPP associated specifically with PID, but the use of multidisciplinary care has been shown to be an effective management strategy overall. One must be cautious in this complex condition not to oversell treatment and promise cures as they are rare. The most effective strategy lies in reducing the woman's stress levels, improving her understanding that chronic pain is not a sign of tissue injury, reducing catastrophic thinking, and generating active management on the part of the women to pace her activities. These approaches differ significantly from the acute care management model and, in some women, take a long time to be achieved.

Conclusion

PID in the acute setting can cause significant morbidity, and in addition it is associated with significant long-term complications of ectopic pregnancy, infertility, and CPP. The impact of these diseases at a population and a patient level make prevention, diagnosis, and treatment of the disease important. No single non-invasive investigation can diagnose PID, so a combination of clinical symptoms, signs, and investigations must be used to prevent undertreatment of PID while minimizing false diagnosis.

Treatment primarily involves broad-spectrum antibiotics that cover the most common etiologic organisms of *Chlamydia* and *N. gonorrhoeae* as well as other Gram-negative bacteria and possibly anaerobes in complicated or severe cases. Inpatient versus outpatient treatment must be considered based on concerns such as severity and treatment compliance. In cases of unresolving tubo-ovarian abscess, surgical drainage may become necessary.

The development of CPP can be secondary to numerous initiating events but the condition may occur in up to 20% of those diagnosed with PID. The evaluation of CPP involves unique examination techniques to guide optimal treatment options. Optimal treatment involves multidisciplinary management with medication, physiotherapy, cognitive-behavioral therapy, and judicious use of surgery. The realistic goal of treatment is reduction in pain and improved quality of life rather than complete resolution.

Dyspareunia

Painful intercourse is a common problem in the complex array of symptoms of CPP. There are many causes of dyspareunia, as indicated in Table 5.7.

History

The history is critically important in attempting to make a diagnosis that will allow an appropriate course of management. The relationship of the pain to sexual function is important. It is important to determine whether the pain is on penetration, deep in the pelvis, both, or occurring with orgasm. Initiation of pain with penetration is associated with myofascial dysfunction of the perineal body. Pain with deep penetration may be secondary to endometriosis, PID, or a retroverted uterus. Pain that comes with orgasm or lasts for several days is an indication of obturator internus-related myofascial dysfunction.

It should be noted there are many reports that prior sexual abuse may cause CPP. Such an approach has suggested that once the individual

Table 5.7 Causes of dyspareunia

Physiological: atrophic vaginitis
Phobic: vaginismus
Inflammatory: vestibulitis
Viscerosomatic: visceral disease related
• Pelvic inflammatory disease • Endometriosis
Traumatic: postinjury
• Straddle injuries • Postpartum muscle injury • Motor vehicle accident • Pudendal nerve injury

reports a previous experience of sexual abuse, the diagnosis is complete and the focus of management is directed to psychological support alone. New evidence is casting doubt on this specific causal relationship. For example, in the Calgary Chronic Pain Centre, the self-reported rates of child and adult sexual abuse are exactly the same for patients in the headache, back pain, and pelvic pain programs—50%. Focus is now being directed to recognizing such prior experiences as adding to the multitude of stresses that can augment chronic pain, rather than singling this out as the only entity.

Other factors of importance relate to the issues surrounding the initiation of the pain. Primary dyspareunia may reflect vaginismus, which is an involuntary withdrawal from vaginal touch or penetrative attempt and is often associated with pain during tampon insertion. Atrophic vaginitis will accompany the development of a hypoestrogenic state. Viscerosomatic pain is associated with a previous or ongoing association with endometriosis or PID, so the history should inquire about symptoms or previous therapy for these conditions. A history of a previous motor vehicle accident is often not recalled because the pain of dyspareunia often occurs 2 years following the accident, after the management of whiplash and lower back pain. This delay may reflect a delay in reinitiation of intercourse or a delay in myofascial changes associated with paraspinal trauma.

Vestibulitis is a poorly understood condition that can be focal or generalized on the vulva. It begins spontaneously without any clear association with other causes but often is reported to begin as a urinary tract infection in which there are negative urinary cultures. Pain from involvement of the pudendal nerve is often, although not necessarily, associated with childbirth or pelvic surgery, and the woman will give a strong history of having increasing pain while sitting. The pain in this case is neuropathic and usually described as a burning sensation in the vulvar region.

Examination

The examination is critical to determining the cause of the pain. The woman should be informed that the examination is intended to identify the source and cause of the pain and may be uncomfortable, but that it can stop at any time if pain is too much. It is important for the examination to be gentle, using one finger. The traditional bimanual examination has virtually no place in this situation.

Examination begins with inspection of the tissues for atrophy, inflammatory or infectious changes, or traumatic injury. Redness of the introitus has been associated with vestibulitis. A cotton-tipped applicator can be used to isolate areas of the introitus that reproduce the pain associated with vestibulitis. The cotton-tipped applicator should also be used to delineate whether any cutaneous allodynia is present in the S3 dermatome (Figure 5.2). If present it is an indication of neuroplasticity and viscerosomatic pain.

With the pulp of the first digit, the perineum is examined for the presence of a band or nodule on the perineal body. This is present in cases of viscerosomatic neuroplasticity and trauma from long-previous motor vehicle accidents. Similar bands can be noted in the levator muscles and obturator muscles. In the levator muscles, the

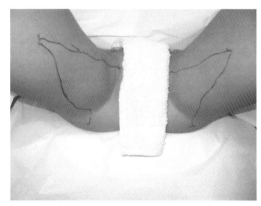

Figure 5.2 A demonstration of cutaneous allodynia that has developed from viscerosomatic pain referral on the abdomen and involves the dermatome segments S3. Gentle pressure with a cotton-tipped applicator will generate a sudden change in sensation to sharp or painful in the presence of such neuroplasticity. Not shown is an area of myofascial tenderness (a trigger point) located on the perineal body that was associated with severe pain on intercourse.

bands can have the feel of a cello's strings. In all of these cases, it is important to identify clearly whether the pressure being placed on the muscle is reproducing the pain. Pressure in the region of the ischial spines can at times increase the pain associated with pudendal nerve involvement.

> ⭐ **TIPS & TRICKS**
>
> A cotton-tipped applicator drawn across the buttocks from the left to the right side of the patient will suddenly produce a sharp sensation in the presence of cutaneous allodynia and neuroplasticity from visceral referral of pain.

Finally, a gentle examination should be made of the upper genital tract to determine, if possible, whether there is ongoing active disease present, usually endometriosis or PID. This can be extremely difficult and may not be possible to determine on one single assessment.

In the case of posthysterectomy deep pelvic pain, a small speculum should be inserted to expose the upper vault. A cotton-tipped applicator is then gently pushed against the upper vault to determine if the pain is reproduced in a focal area amenable to injection.

Management

Dyspareunia is a symptom with many causes and is not a diagnosis. Ideally, because of the frequent need for psychological support and physiotherapists trained to deal with the pelvis, it is best to undertake this therapy in a multidisciplinary program. It is also important to make a specific clinical diagnosis if possible. Some approaches that have promise are described below.

Vaginismus does not traditionally lie in the sphere of chronic pain management and is increasingly being seen as a phobic disorder. Approaches with physiotherapy and psychological support hold promise. Topical anesthetics, such as lidocaine gel, are often irritating but if tolerable can be used with cotton balls directly placed on the areas of pain. Medications of potential benefit include tricyclic antidepressants in low dosage, gabapentin, and pregabalin. Vaginal dilators can be very helpful in alleviating some of the difficulties associated with vaginismus.

In relation to vestibulitis, similar approaches to vaginismus can be used. Surgical excision of localized areas of pain and tenderness has been advocated but may be associated with a worsening of pain. Caution should therefore be exercised when contemplating this procedure.

Myofascial dysfunction, even as severe as to lead to unconsummated marriages, can be treated effectively by physiotherapy combined with self-directed exercise, vibrators, and dilators. In refractory cases, the use of myofascial injections with 1% xylocaine with or without botulinum toxin can be very helpful. Involvement of the partner in the discussions can be very helpful. This applies both to myofascial dysfunction associated with viscerosomatic pain and to traumatic myofascial dysfunction. Injections into the pelvis can be made into the levator ani and obturator internus muscles. These injections seem to provide relief for weeks to months but, to be successful, must include physiotherapy with a trained physiotherapist in the pelvis and self-exercise.

> ⭐ **TIPS & TRICKS**
>
> Xylocaine and botulinum toxin can be used to treat myofascial dysfunction in chronic pain states. Botulinum toxin for injection is made up in 1% xylocaine solution and injected into the affected muscles with about 1 cm^3 of solution being injected into each area of pain.

Myofascial dysfunction associated with ongoing active viscerosomatic disease should encompass other approaches to management appropriate to the initiating cause.

Posthysterectomy pain can be managed by direct injections of 1% xylocaine into the areas of the vaginal vault that show pinpoint tenderness with a cotton-tipped applicator. Apical vaginectomy can be undertaken if these injections fail, but it is less successful.

Women with pudendal nerve involvement as a cause of pain can benefit from injection of local anesthetic (1% xylocaine) as a nerve block. The addition of triamcinolone for one or two injections may assist in the reduction in nerve inflammation.

Conclusions

Dyspareunia may present as pain on initial or deep penetration. The etiology may be physiologic, psychological, inflammatory, post-traumatic injury, or a result of visceral disease. Delicate examination for skin health, trigger points and cutaneous allodynia, along with a limited bimanual examination, will aid in the diagnosis of common causes such as atrophic vaginitis, vestibulitis, vaginismus, myofascial or pudendal nerve damage, endometriosis, or PID. Treatment methods will vary depending on the type of dyspareunia, but options for treatment may include pelvic physiotherapy, vaginal dilators, tricyclic antidepressant or gabapentin medication, nerve block or trigger point injections, and possibly surgery.

Selected bibliography

Ahmad G, Duffy J, Farquar C et al. Barrier agents for adhesion prevention after gynecological surgery. Cochrane Database Syst Rev 2007, Issue 2. Art. No.: CD000475.

Buchan H, Vessey M, Goldacre M, Fairweather J. Morbidity following pelvic inflammatory disease. Br J Obstet Gynaecol 1993;100: 558–62.

Center for Disease Control and Prevention. Updated recommended treatment regimens for gonococcal infections and related conditions – United States April, 2007. Washington, DC: CDC; 2007.

Cheong Y, William SR. Chronic pelvic pain: aetiology and therapy. Best Pract Res Clin Obstet Gynaecol 2006;20:695–711.

Farquhar C, Vandekerckhove P, Watson A, Vail A, Wiseman D. Barrier agents for preventing adhesions after surgery for subfertility. Cochrane Database Syst Rev 2000, Issue 2. Art. No.: CD000475.

Gambone JC, Reiter RC. Nonsurgical management of chronic pelvic pain: a multidisciplinary approach. Clin Obstet Gynecol 1990;33: 205–11.

Giamberardino MA, Affaitati G, Lerza R, Lapenna D, Costantini R, Vecchiet L. Relationship between pain symptoms and referred sensory and trophic changes in patients with gallbladder pathology. Pain 2005;114(1–2): 239–49.

Haggerty CL, Peipert JF, Weitzen S et al. Predictors of chronic pelvic pain in an urban population of women with symptoms and signs of pelvic inflammatory disease. Sex Transm Dis 2005;32:293–9.

International Association for the Study of Pain. Opioids for chronic noncancer pain. Pain Clin Updates 1995;III(3).

Jarrell JF, Documentation of cutaneous allodynia among women with chronic pelvic pain. JoVE. 2009, 28, doi: 10.3791/1232. Available from http://www.jove.com/index/Details. stp?ID=1232.

Jarrell JF, Vilos GA, Allaire C et al. Consensus guidelines for the management of chronic pelvic pain. J Obstet Gynaecol Can 2005;27: 781–826.

Jarrell JF, Vilos GA, Allaire C et al. Consensus guidelines for the management of chronic pelvic pain. J Obstet Gynaecol Can 2005;27: 869–910.

Khaitan L, Scholz S, Houston HL, Richards WO. Results after laparoscopic lysis of adhesions and placement of Seprafilm for intractable abdominal pain. Surg Endosc 2003;17: 247–53.

Kresch AJ, Seifer DB, Sachs LB, Barrese I. Laparoscopy in 100 women with chronic pelvic pain. Obstet Gynecol 1984;64:672–4.

Kumar S, Wong P, Leaper D. Intra-peritoneal prophylactic agents for preventing adhesions and adhesive intestinal obstruction after nongynecological abdominal surgery. Cochrane Database Syst Rev 2009, Issue 1. Art. No.: CD005080.

Metwally M, Watson A. Fluid and pharmacological agents for adhesion prevention after gynecological surgery. Cochrane Database Syst Rev 2006, Issue 2. Art. No.: CD001298.

Ness RB, Randall H, Richter HE et al. Condom use and the risk of recurrent pelvic inflammatory disease, chronic pelvic pain, or infertility following an episode of pelvic inflammatory disease. Am J Public Health 2004;94:1327–9.

Ness RB, Kip KE, Hillier SL et al. A cluster analysis of bacterial vaginosis-associated microflora and pelvic inflammatory disease. Am J Epidemiol 2005;162:585–90.

Stones W, Cheong Y, Howard F. Interventions for treating chronic pelvic pain in women. Cochrane Database Syst Rev 2005, Issue 4. Art. No.: CD000387.

Vercellini P, Pisacreta A, Pesole A, Vinentini S, Crosignani P. Surgical management of endometriosis. Clin Obstet Gynecol 2000;14:501–23.

Vercellini P, Crosignani G, Abbiati A, Somigliana E, Vigano P, Fedele L. The effect of surgery for symptomatic endometriosis: the other side of the story. Hum Reprod Update 2009;15: 177–88.

Pelvic Congestion Syndrome

Aarti Umranikar[1] and Ying Cheong[2]

[1]Southampton University Hospitals NHS Trust, Southampton, UK
[2]University of Southampton, Southampton, UK

Introduction

Pelvic congestion syndrome takes its name from the vascular hypothesis that dilated pelvic veins are associated with chronic pelvic pain. The condition is in itself an enigma; much has been written in the literature about the syndrome, although its treatment, and indeed for many the acknowledgement of its actual existence as a gynecologic diagnosis, is still somewhat controversial. This chapter attempts to draw on the current literature to help provide evidence-based guidance on the treatment and management of this condition.

Pelvic congestion syndrome

This is a clinical syndrome associated with dilatation of the pelvic veins and reduced venous drainage in the pelvis. The characteristic symptom complex was first described by Gooch in 1831, and in the 1940s Taylor described the concept of venous congestion as dilatation associated with sluggish flow in the utero-ovarian veins that resulted in pelvic pain. The nature and very existence of this syndrome was a subject of much debate until the 1980s, when Beard and colleagues described the clinical syndrome based on the characteristic symptom complex. They put forward the hypothesis that pelvic pain can be caused by pelvic congestion. Much work has been done in the last 20 years that has enabled a better understanding of the basic mechanisms of vascular control and pelvic pain. With the advent of laparoscopy, ultrasound scanning, and pelvic venography, the etiology of the condition has now become clearer.

Symptoms

Pelvic congestion syndrome is a clinical syndrome typically seen in women of reproductive age. It is equally prevalent among nulliparous and multiparous women. Predominant symptoms include menorrhagia, congestive dysmenorrhea, deep dyspareunia, postcoital ache, and pelvic pain with exacerbations on prolonged standing.

Pathophysiology

It was Beard and colleagues who proposed an objective method of diagnosing pelvic varicosities using venography to measure vessel diameter, tortuosity, and dye transit time, thus demonstrating the anatomic changes associated with pelvic congestion syndrome. They also postulated that pain from vascular congestion is caused by the release of vasoactive peptides such as substance P and bradykinins.

Their study included 45 women who had a history of lower abdominal pain lasting more than 6 months. Transuterine pelvic venography was carried out on these patients. For comparison, venography was carried out on eight women admitted for laparoscopic sterilization who had no gynecologic symptoms and a normal pelvis. Venography was carried out on conscious patients in the lithotomy position. A long cannula with a 19-gauge needle was passed through the

Chronic Pelvic Pain, First Edition. Edited by Paolo Vercellini.
© 2011 Blackwell Publishing Ltd. Published 2011 by Blackwell Publishing Ltd.

cervix up to the uterine cavity. The tip of the needle was advanced into the myometrium, and a small amount of contrast medium and hyaluronidase was injected. The spread of contrast medium into the myometrial veins and upper vaginal, uterine, and ovarian venous plexuses was observed by fluoroscopic screening.

A pelvic venogram score was used to quantify ovarian vein dilatation, dye disappearance, and severity of pelvic congestion. A score of 3 indicated a normal venogram, and a score of 9 an abnormal one. The diagnostic potential of pelvic venography was shown by a venogram score of over 5 distinguishing patients with pelvic pain syndrome due to congestion from those with other causes of pelvic pain. A venogram score of 5 gave a diagnostic sensitivity of 91% with a specificity of 89%, confirming that pelvic varicosities with concomitant vascular stasis were found in women with pelvic pain syndrome due to pelvic venous congestion.

Anatomic changes

Pelvic vascular congestion predominantly affects the venous system as opposed to the arterial or lymphatic system. This is a feature similar to the changes noted in the pelvic vasculature in pregnancy. These characteristic changes enable pelvic veins to increase their capacity 60-fold to accommodate the increase in the volume of blood during late pregnancy. Another feature noted is a 2.5 times increase in the tension of these veins in pregnancy compared to the nonpregnant state. Furthermore, the network of pelvic veins is thin walled and relatively unsupported, with fewer valves compared to the veins in the legs, which makes them vulnerable to chronic dilatation and stasis, resulting in vascular congestion.

Vascular physiology

The ovarian circulation undergoes changes at menarche, during a menstrual cycle, in pregnancy, and at menopause both in the large vessels and in the capillary network. The different phases of reproductive life are associated with changes in size and volume flow in the uterine and ovarian arteries and veins.

Some of these changes are a consequence of fluctuating levels of ovarian steroid hormones. In a menstrual cycle, the ovarian veins are exposed to a 100-fold increase in estrone and estradiol concentrations. Studies from oophorectomized mice have shown an increased response of uterine and ovarian veins to estradiol or testosterone administration, but this response was not observed in the femoral or iliac veins or the inferior vena cava. This may suggest an increased sensitivity of uterine or ovarian vessels to steroid hormones. Evidence also indicates that estrogen may be responsible for the circulatory dysfunction of pelvic congestion by stimulating the release of nitric oxide or by interfering with the autoregulation of the pelvic circulation.

Anatomic studies in humans have shown that ovarian veins have both longitudinal and circular muscle coats, with nerve endings situated in the outer longitudinal layer of muscle. Autonomic nervous system instability may thus contribute to venous distension as seen in pelvic congestion syndrome. This layer also contains vasoactive endothelial substances such as substance P and bradykinin that contributes to the autoregulation of the ovarian circulation. Many of these agents are mediators of inflammation and pain sensation, which provides an explanation for the link between vascular changes and associated pain.

Ovarian dysfunction

Ovarian morphology is characterized by predominantly atretic follicles scattered throughout the stroma. The ovarian volume remains normal, in contrast to the increased volume noted in polycystic ovaries. Adams et al. have reported a prevalence of cystic ovaries in 56% of women with pelvic congestion, but these cystic ovaries were morphologically different from classical polycystic ovaries. Ultrasound studies have also demonstrated morphologic differences between polycystic ovaries and cystic ovaries noted in pelvic congestion. Pelvic congestion cystic ovaries (PCCO) have multiple atretic follicles with a random distribution and a normal ovarian volume. The stroma appears spongy and reduced. Classical polycystic ovaries have multiple small follicles with a peripheral distribution associated with an increased stromal tissue component along with an increase in ovarian volume.

There are clear differences in the steroid response of granulosa and theca cells between the two groups of ovaries too. An ovular polycystic ovary demonstrates a significant increase in estradiol secretion in response to follicle-stimulating hormone stimulation, whereas the granulosa cells of the PCCO showed a reduced response. Theca cell secretion of androstenedione in response to a luteinizing hormone stimulus is increased in both groups of ovaries. Thus, there are not only morphologic differences between polycystic ovaries and PCCO—functionally, the two groups of ovaries also behave differently. The cysts of polycystic ovaries are fully functional, whereas those of PCCO group have a large proportion of atretic follicles.

Menstrual dysfunction

One study provides evidence on the endometrial and myometrial response to circulating estrogen in women with pelvic congestion resulting in enlargement of the uterus and endometrial thickening. Menstrual dysfunction (menorrhagia, congestive dysmenorrhea) has been seen in 65% of women with pelvic congestion. If the myometrium and endometrium are increased in women with pelvic congestion, it may be possible that the effect of estrogen is similarly responsible for the chronic venous dilatation found in these women.

Psychological dysfunction

The prevalence of psychological abnormalities is higher in women with chronic pelvic pain compared to the control population with no pain, regardless of whether or not pelvic pathology has been found. Studies have shown an increased prevalence of anxiety neuroticism, hostility, and sexual dysfunction in these women. It may be a somatic response to chronic pelvic pain and a state of chronic stress.

Investigations

Ultrasound imaging

Transabdominal ultrasound (TAUS) or transvaginal ultrasound (TVUS) imaging has been used to visualize the dilated pelvic veins. One study prospectively evaluated TAUS and TVUS findings in patients with pelvic congestion syndrome and compared them to those of healthy volunteers. It was found that women with pelvic congestion showed the presence of a varicocele—dilated pelvic veins with reversed caudal flow in the left

ovarian vein. Transvaginal power Doppler imaging has improved the sensitivity for detection of low flow rates in the pelvic veins. Combined TAUS and TVUS is a useful, noninvasive screening tool for determining which patients with chronic pelvic pain may benefit from selective venography and embolization.

Pelvic venography

The transuterine injection of water-soluble radio-opaque contrast can be used to outline the pelvic veins. The ovarian vein diameter, evidence of pelvic congestion, and time taken for disappearance of the radio-opaque dye on the venogram can be used to score the severity of the syndrome. Beard and colleagues have devised a scoring system to grade the severity of pelvic venous congestion, a score of 6 being diagnostic of pelvic congestion. The scoring system for grading abnormalities on the venogram has a diagnostic sensitivity of 91% and a specificity of 89%. The procedure can, however, only be undertaken in specialized centres.

Use of dihydroergotamine in pelvic congestion

Dihydroergotamine (DHE) is a venoconstrictor that acts selectively on the capacitance vessels. It increases the venous tone by 150–250% and can mobilize up to 350 mL of blood by causing contraction of these vessels. DHE has been shown to have a vasoconstrictive effect on the pelvic veins and to reduce pelvic congestion, and one study has demonstrated that DHE might have diagnostic value and therapeutic value in patients with acute pain due to pelvic congestion.

This study demonstrated that, in women with venographic evidence of pelvic congestion with no other cause of pelvic pain, administration of DHE during an attack of acute pain produced pain relief, thus providing evidence that pelvic congestion is likely to be responsible for pain in these patients. Their study included 12 women who had chronic pelvic pain of over 6 months' duration with evidence of pelvic venous congestion. Transuterine pelvic venography was performed in six women before and after the injection of 1 mg DHE. The remaining six women were given an intravenous injection of 10 mL normal saline (placebo). The vasoconstricting effect of DHE on the pelvic veins was studied, and its effects on pain relief were assessed. The vasoconstrictor response was noted to start 1 minute after injection of the drug, with its maximum effect in 8–20 minutes. Pain was found to be considerably lower 4 hours after injection of DHE in the treatment group. The effect lasted for 2 days.

Treatment

Medical treatment

As pelvic congestion is related to ovarian activity and possibly mediated through estradiol, suppression of ovarian activity has been shown to reduce pelvic congestion and pain by reducing the calibre of the dilated pelvic veins and improving blood flow. Ovarian down-regulation with a progestogen or gonadotropin-releasing hormone (GnRH) agonist in combination with "add-back hormone replacement therapy (HRT)" is effective in the treatment of chronic pelvic pain. Psychotherapy combined with medical treatment is effective in the management of chronic pelvic pain: studies have showed that psychotherapy is effective in reducing the frequency and severity of pain in women with chronic pelvic pain.

Medroxyprogesterone acetate (MPA) is a well-tolerated medication without antiestrogenic side effects. Studies conducted have tried using 30 mg per day MPA in women with proven pelvic congestion on venography. The study by Reginald and colleagues included 22 women with lower abdominal pain caused by pelvic congestion. Findings on venogram before and after treatment were compared, as were pain scores. A 75% reduction in pelvic pain score was reported among women who showed a reduction in the venogram score after treatment compared to 29% among those who showed no reduction in venogram score. The significant association between reduction in pelvic congestion and pain indicated that treatment with MPA was effective in reducing symptoms.

A double-blind, randomized controlled trial investigated with MPA with or without psychotherapy. Psychotherapy for pain and stress management included relaxation exercises and alternative therapies such as yoga, reflexology, or aromatherapy. A total of 102 women were included in the study, all of whom had a history of pelvic pain of more than 6 months, with no obvious pathology on laparoscopy and a venogram score of over 5, indicative of pelvic congestion. The women were randomized into four groups: MPA only, MPA and psychotherapy, placebo only, and placebo plus psychotherapy. MPA treatment was given for 4 months, and the women were followed up at 9 months with pain assessments. At the end of therapy, 71% of women receiving MPA and psychotherapy showed over 50% reduction in their pain scores. Thus, therapy with MPA was a useful first-line therapy for women with pain associated with pelvic congestion.

Another study compared the efficacy of MPA 30 mg per day with that of a GnRH agonist (goserelin acetate 3.6 mg per month) over a period of 6 months. Both agents were associated with a significant improvement in pelvic pain at the end of the 6 months, but goserelin had longer lasting improvements at 12 months.

A recent randomized controlled study has been piloted on 25 women to study the efficacy of the subdermal implant Implanon for the treatment of chronic pelvic pain associated with pelvic congestion. The effects of Implanon on pelvic pain scores, menstrual scores, and changes on venography were recorded. At the end of 12 months, the objective venography score was reduced in the treatment group compared to the control group, and reduced pain scores and menstrual scores were also observed in the Implanon-treated group. Thus, Implanon seems to be an effective hormonal alternative for patients with pelvic pain related to pelvic congestion.

Surgical treatment

Since functioning ovaries are the cause of pelvic pain due to congestion, any surgical procedure that diminishes or ablates the functioning ovary will be effective.

Bilateral oophorectomy with hysterectomy relieves pain in the majority of cases (85%). This option is only suitable for a small proportion of women who have obtained no relief on medical treatment. Women need to be aware of the risks involved in undertaking a major surgical procedure and the need for HRT. In one study, only 4.6% (36 of 775 women) who attended for chronic pelvic pain were eventually treated with hysterectomy and oophorectomy. Studies have shown that a short period of nondirective counselling resulted in a substantial increase in the number of pain-free days 1 year after the start of treatment.

Embolization of ovarian veins under radiologic control is an alternate treatment modality and has a 50–80% success rate, but more studies are needed to verify the benefits.

EVIDENCE AT A GLANCE

Evidence from literature supports the use of progesterone treatment (medroxyprogesterone acetate) or gonadotropin-releasing hormone agonists for the treatment of pelvic pain secondary to pelvic congestion. In addition, randomized controlled trials have shown the efficacy of the subdermal implant Implanon in reducing pain scores and menstrual scores. Hysterectomy with bilateral oophorectomy is an option for women who do not respond to medical treatment.

---

more holistic and multidisciplinary management approach.

☆ TIPS & TRICKS

Pelvic congestion syndrome is a complex clinical syndrome that is the subject of much controversy, even though much has been written about it in the literature. It is a syndrome seen in women of reproductive age, with symptoms including menorrhagia, dysmenorrhea, deep dyspareunia, postcoital ache, and pelvic pain with exacerbations on prolonged standing.

Medical treatment includes the use of medroxyprogesterone acetate, Implanon, or gonadotropin-releasing hormone agonists. Hysterectomy with bilateral salpingo-oophorectomy is an option for women who do not respond to medical treatment. Appropriate counselling using a multidisciplinary team approach is needed.

Conclusions

The investigations available for the diagnosis of pelvic congestion are currently not often used by practicing gynecologists. This is mainly due to the invasiveness of the investigations, and many physicians institute empiric treatment for women presenting with this condition in any case. Current studies suggest that there is evidence of benefit for the use of MPA or a GnRH agonist (goserelin) along with a multidisciplinary team approach in the assessment and treatment of women presenting with pelvic pain secondary to pelvic congestion syndrome. Although the more radical surgical treatments have been shown to be partly effective, they will continue to be secondary treatment options due to their radical nature and the potential need for long-term HRT.

Pelvic congestion syndrome remains a gynecologic enigma. Although many medical and surgical approaches to this clinical entity are in part effective, the management of women presenting with chronic pelvic pain continues to be challenging and, in many respects, will require a

Selected bibliography

Adams JM, Tan SL, Wheeler MJ. Uterine growth in the follicular phase of spontaneous ovulatory cycles and during luteinizing hormone-releasing hormone- induced cycles in women with normal or polycystic ovaries. Fertil Steril 1988;49:52–5.

Adams J, Reginald PW, Franks S, Wadsworth J, Beard RW. Uterine size and endometrial thickness and the significance of cystic ovaries in women with pelvic pain due to congestion. Br J Obstet Gynecol 1990;97:583–7.

Beard RW, Reginald PW, Wadsworth J. Clinical features of women with chronic lower abdominal pain and pelvic congestion. Br J Obstet Gynecol 1988;95:153–61.

Farquhar CM, Rogers V, Franks S. A randomized controlled trial of medroxyprogesterone acetate and psychotherapy for the treatment of pelvic congestion. Br J Obstet Gynaecol 1989;96:1153–62.

Foong LC, Gamble J, Sutherland LA, Beard RW. Altered peripheral vascular response of women with and without pelvic pain due to congestion. Br J Obstet Gynecol 2000;107:157–64.

Luciano AA, Turksey RN, Dlugi AM, Carleo JL. Endocrine consequences of oral medroxyprogesterone acetate (MPA) in the treatment of endometriosis. Presented at the Annual Meeting of the endocrine society, Anaheim, California, USA, 1986.

Park SJ, Lim JW, Ko YT et al. Diagnosis of pelvic congestion using transabdominal and transvaginal sonography. AJR Am Roentgenol 2004;182:683–8.

Pearce S, Beard RW. Chronic pelvic pain in women. In: Somatization: physical symptoms and psychological illness. London: Blackwell Scientific; 1990. pp. 259–75.

Pearce S, Knight C, Beard RW. Pelvic pain—a common gynaecological problem. J Psychosom Obstet Gynecol 1982;1:12–17.

Reginald PW, Beard RW, Kooner JS. Intravenous dihydroergotamine to relieve pelvic congestion with pain in young women. Lancet 1987;2:352–3.

Reginald PW, Adams J, Franks S. Medroxyprogesterone acetate in the treatment of pelvic pain due to venous congestion. Br J Obstet Gynecol 1989;96:1148–52.

Shokeir T, Amr M, Abdelshaheed M. The efficacy of Implanon for the treatment of chronic pelvic pain associated with pelvic congestion: 1-year randomized controlled pilot study. Arch Gynecol Obstet 2009;280:437–43.

Soysal ME, Soysal S, Vicdan K, Ozer SA. Randomised controlled trial of goserelin and medroxyprogesterone acetate in the treatment of pelvic congestion. Human Reprod 2001;16:931–9.

Taylor HC. Vascular congestion and hyperaemia: physiologic basis and history of concept. Am J Obstet Gynecol 1949;57:211–30.

Van Buren GA, Yong D, Clarke KE. Oestrogen induced vasodilatation is antagonised by L-nitroarginine methyl ester, an inhibitor of nitric oxide synthesis. Am J Obstet Gynecol 1992;167:828–33.

Chronic Pelvic Pain and Adhesions

Michael P. Diamond, Manvinder Singh, and Elizabeth E. Puscheck

Wayne State University School of Medicine/Detroit Medical Center, Detroit, Michigan, USA

Introduction

The relationship of adhesions to pelvic pain remains an enigmatic dilemma. Controversy abounds both about the crucial questions of whether adhesions cause pain, as well as about whether adhesiolysis is successful in reducing or curing pain.

For purposes of consideration of the clinically significant syndrome of pelvic pain, an "adhesion" will be defined as a nonanatomic attachment of parietal and/or visceral peritoneal surfaces at locations where such attachments should not exist. As such, adhesions are distinguished from fibrosis within organs and the abdominal wall. Nonetheless, both represent deposits or collections of extracellular matrix material (e.g., collagen, fibronectin) that are often initially vascularly deficient and thus manifest tissue that is relatively hypoxic.

Adhesions have been classified in multiple ways. A common classification system uses the phenotypic appearance, such as filmy or dense (opaque), whether they are avascular or vascular, and their ease of separation (division), as well as the extent (or surface area) of the organs or sites involved in adhesions. Additionally, while filmy/dense and avascular/vascular adhesions represent bands connecting adjoining surfaces, an additional categorization is that of cohesive adhesions, in which tissue (organ) surfaces are intimately attached without intervening bands. The latter may be of particular clinical relevance because of both the difficulty in separating the adjoining organ surfaces without surgical injury to the underlying tissue, and the larger resultant "raw" surface area after surgical separation, which becomes a future potential adhesiogenic site.

Classification systems for adhesion development should also consider the presence or absence of pre-existing adhesions, as well as any additional pathology existing (and treated) at each site. These classifications are important to be able to assess both the advantages and disadvantages of surgical approaches and techniques (e.g., conduct of procedures at laparotomy or laparoscopy, approach utilized to lyze the adhesions, methods of treatment of the pathology), and the choice of and efficacy of antiadhesion adjuvants.

In order to have a systematic approach to such categorizations, we proposed a classification system nearly two decades ago (Table 7.1). This system distinguishes de novo adhesion formation from adhesion reformation, the former being defined as the development of adhesions as assessed at second-look laparoscopy at sites that did not have adhesions at the time of a preceding surgical procedure. This was contrasted with adhesion reformation, which was defined as the redevelopment of adhesions at sites at which adhesiolysis had been performed at the initial procedure.

Both de novo adhesion formation and adhesion reformation were subdivided based on whether a surgical procedure was performed at

Chronic Pelvic Pain, First Edition. Edited by Paolo Vercellini.

© 2011 Blackwell Publishing Ltd. Published 2011 by Blackwell Publishing Ltd.

Table 7.1 Categorization of adhesion development as assessed at second-look surgical procedures

Type 1: De novo adhesions
Adhesions occurring at sites/locations with no prior adhesion
1a Adhesion development at sites/locations at which no surgical procedure was performed at the initial procedure, such as adhesions that occur as a result of indirect trauma or tissue drying—so-called "incidental adhesions"   1b Adhesion development at sites/locations of surgical procedures (e.g., myomectomy, ovarian cystectomy) other than adhesiolysis at the initial procedure, thus representing adhesions caused by direct tissue trauma
Type 2: Reformed adhesions
Adhesions reforming at sites of adhesiolysis during the initial procedure
2a Adhesion reformation at sites/locations with adhesiolysis only at an initial surgical procedure   2b Adhesion reformation at sites/locations with both adhesiolysis and treatment of tissue pathology (such as an ovarian endometrioma with adhesions to adjacent organs)

Adapted from Diamond and Nezhat, 1993.

that site (other than adhesiolysis at that site to deal with reformation). Thus, de novo adhesion formation was subcategorized into type 1a and 1b. Type 1a represents sites with no surgical procedures at all that were identified to have developed adhesions at second-look laparoscopy; such adhesions may be due to peritoneal drying, injury from laparotomy pad abrasion, and/or tissue grasping. Other investigators have called adhesions at such sites incidental adhesions. Type 1b de novo adhesion formation represents adhesions that develop at sites of surgical procedures when have been no pre-existing adhesions at the site. Examples include adhesions identified as forming at the site of uterine incisions for myomectomy or cesarean section, ovarian adhesions after removal of an ovarian dermoid cyst, and adhesions after treatment of peritoneal endometriotic implants.

Adhesion reformation at sites at which adhesiolysis was conducted at the initial procedure would be classified as type 2a adhesion reformation; this might occur, for example, after lysis of adhesions between the uterus and sigmoid colon. In contrast, type 2b adhesion reformation represents identification of adhesions at the time of second-look laparoscopy at sites that, at the initial procedure, underwent both adhesiolysis and treatment of the underlying pathology. An example of type 2b would be adhesions to the ovary developing following ovarian adhesiolysis and excision of an ovarian endometrioma.

Thus, progression from type 1a to 1b to 2a to 2b would be expected to show an increasing frequency of the likelihood of developing adhesions, as has been demonstrated from a meta-analysis of clinical trials examining the frequency of adhesion development. Furthermore, a corollary would be that the ability of an antiadhesion adjuvant to minimize or eliminate adhesions would be inversely related to the stage, with 1a de novo adhesions being the easiest to prevent, and the greatest difficulty in manifesting efficacy occurring at type 2b adhesion sites. Such a classification system is important to allow a comparison of outcomes in different clinical trials with different modes of entry into the abdominal cavity and the use of varying instruments during the surgical procedure, as well as to compare the relative efficacy of different antiadhesion adjuvants.

Incidence of de novo adhesion formation and adhesion reformation

Adhesions develop in the vast majority of patients after gynecologic surgical procedures among women undergoing microsurgical procedures at laparotomy. Adhesions were identified in 86% of women at the time of a second-look procedure. Additionally, when examining individuals who developed de novo adhesion formation, such adhesions were identified at approximately one third of available sites. Similarly, among women

Table 7.2 Incidence of de novo adhesion formation and adhesion reformation following gynecologic surgery

Adhesion type	Mode of entry into abdominal cavity	
	Laparoscopy	Laparotomy
De novo 1a	18%	28%
De novo 1b	63%	55%
Adhesion reformation	86%	74%

Adapted from Wiseman et al., 1998.

undergoing laparoscopic adhesiolysis, although the average adhesion score was reduced by approximately 50%, postoperative adhesions developed in 66 of 68 women, or 97% of subjects. These findings of a very high incidence of adhesion development after procedures conducted at both laparotomy and laparoscopy is consistent with other reports, as well as with a meta-analysis. The percentage of patients with adhesions after laparotomy and laparoscopy in this latter report are depicted in Table 7.2.

⚠ CAUTION

Adhesion reformation after adhesiolysis occurs in approximately 85% of women, with worsening of adhesion scores after approximately 10% of procedures, despite the use of high-quality surgical techniques. Such adhesion reformation occurs with similar frequency after both open and laparoscopic surgical procedures and may limit the benefit currently achievable from adhesiolysis. Surgical procedures may also commonly be associated with de novo adhesion reformation, and repeat procedures may lead to injury of the abdominopelvic tissues during entry into the abdominal cavity and/or during adhesiolysis.

Relationship of adhesion to pelvic pain

The relationship of adhesions to pelvic pain has been difficult to assess for multiple reasons. First,

although some investigators have reported the ability to identify adhesions at specific locations such as the anterior abdominal wall using imaging modalities, it is generally recognized that surgical procedures are required to identify the existence and location of adhesions. Second, pelvic pain can also be caused by other gynecologic pathology in the pelvis such as endometriosis, or be due to gastrointestinal or urinary tract disorders. Additionally, musculoskeletal etiologies as well as abdominal wall etiologies such as entrapped nerves can be a cause of pain perceived to be within the pelvis. Such conditions can co-exist with adhesions, making determination of the etiology difficult.

Third, pain thresholds vary between individuals, as does the degree of pain tolerable before seeking clinical care and the willingness to undergo invasive procedures for their diagnosis and/or management. Fourth, pain is primarily subjectively reported, and individuals can describe a prolonged duration or extensive severity of their pain for ulterior motives, such as drug-seeking, attention and/or sympathy-seeking, or a desire for prolonged convalescence before returning to work.

An unresolved question is, why, if adhesions cause pelvic pain, do patients with extensive adhesions sometimes not have pain? The answer may lie in the position and attachments of the pelvic tissues. One hypothesis is that adhesions of tissues that are positioned in their normal anatomic locations will not cause pain, while adhesions that cause pain either stretch the parietal peritoneum or serosal surfaces of the organs (either at rest or with activity such as walking, running, and/or sexual intercourse) or hold tissues in nonanatomic locations. An anecdotal example of the latter is three patients that had an ovary adherent to the anterior abdominal wall, who were cured by lysis of this adhesion.

The contribution of adhesions to pain has also been pathophysiologically explained by some authors by the identification of nerve fibers within some adhesions. The variable presence of these fibers in adhesions could also partly explain the clinical observation that some, but not all, adhesions are associated with pain. However, others have questioned whether the reported finding of nerves within adhesions might actually represent a tissue sampling artifact. The latter could arise if adhesions were grasped and elevated, thereby "tenting" up normal peritoneum (containing nerve fibers), which the surgeon might consider to be part of the adhesion per se.

A third possibility is that adhesions may be associated with the etiology causing the pain, but not be the cause per se. This may in fact be the case in some women such as those with coexisting endometriosis and adhesions. In this case, the inflammation from the endometriotic implant or the cytokines and other products released into surrounding tissue and the peritoneal cavity may be an etiologic cause of pain. However, several series reporting laparoscopic evaluation of the pelvis of women with pelvic pain have identified varying percentages with adhesions, endometriosis, or a normal-appearing pelvis (without identified pathologic processes). Thus, the etiology of pelvic pain is often difficult to identify.

Multiple authors have reported descriptive evaluations of the contribution of laparoscopic adhesiolysis in women with pelvic pain to the reduction (or resolution) of the pelvic pain. Initial outcomes at short intervals (approximately 1 month) have often appeared promising and in some studies have continued for 6–18 months, lasting in one report for up to 60 months. However, these studies are limited by lack of a placebo arm. In one study with serial observations at later times, a return of pain to near pre-surgery levels has been demonstrated, thus obviating the benefit of laparoscopic adhesiolysis for reducing pelvic pain in these patient populations as a group (although individual patients, of course, may have a reduction or resolution of their pain). It remains unclear whether the return of the pain in these patients represents the loss of a "placebo effect" from the surgery. Alternatively, return of the pain could occur due to remodeling of adhesions that developed after the surgical procedure, with resultant repositioning of the tissues that have adhered together.

⚗ SCIENCE REVISITED

Well-designed studies have to date failed to identify long-term reductions in chronic pelvic pain attributable to adhesiolysis. However, the lack of efficacy of such procedures may reflect not that adhesiolysis per se is without benefit, but rather that the high incidence of adhesion reformation (often with worsening extent and/or severity) may limit eliminate the potential benefit of adhesiolysis procedures.

Clinical trials examining efficacy of adhesiolysis

When considering clinical trials of adhesiolysis for the resolution of pelvic pain, a major confounding factor also exists that has often gone unrecognized and not considered in evaluations of the efficacy of adhesiolysis for reduction of pelvic pain. Virtually all reports that have examined the efficacy of adhesiolysis for pelvic pain have failed to assess, and factor in, the very high likelihood of postoperative adhesion development. Thus, does persisting pain in women who have undergone adhesiolysis represent failure of treatment of the true underlying etiology, or does it represent adhesion reformation with ongoing causation of pain because of ongoing presence of the adhesions? Such a hypothesis is consistent with the observation from multiple reports that (1) adhesiolysis was associated with an immediate reduction in pelvic pain at initial postoperative evaluation points, but (2) the incidence and/or severity of pain had returned to preoperative levels at subsequent, more long-term postoperative evaluation time points.

Additionally, such a hypothesis could lead to a major reinterpretation of the findings of what are probably the two best clinical trials examining efficacy of adhesiolysis as a means of treating pelvic pain. Those two trials are to be commended for their study design and ability to convince women to be randomized to surgical treatment for pelvic pain, particularly since one arm was limited to observation without surgical treatment of the adhesions identified at the surgical procedure.

In the first report, randomization to laparotomy for adhesiolysis was not associated with an alteration in ongoing pelvic pain compared to the control subjects 9–12 months later. The exception was the women with the worst pelvic adhesions (dense and vascular adhesions that involved fixation of the small or large colon to the parietal peritoneum), in whom lysis of adhesions was associated with a reduction in pain.

Similarly, in the second report, women who were identified to have adhesions were randomized to undergo or not undergo laparoscopic adhesiolysis. In this report, after 1 year follow-up, there was a trend for improvement among the 100 women who underwent adhesiolysis, but this failed to reach statistical significance. However, if the high frequency of adhesion reformation is also considered, any benefit that might be achieved by adhesiolysis would be greatly minimized, leaving the possibly incorrect impression that adhesiolysis per se is not of benefit. What would be advantageous would be a repeat of the prior studies examining the efficacy of adhesiolysis for reduction of pelvic pain in association with the use of an antiadhesion adjuvant and a second-look procedure to assess adhesion reformation. Such a design would allow an examination of whether an actual reduction in adhesions is in fact associated with a reduction in pelvic pain.

★ TIPS & TRICKS

- Chronic pelvic pain treatments may benefit from a multidisciplinary approach.
- Attention to surgical technique, especially minimization of tissue damage, to the extent possible in the procedure being undertaken is probably the most important approach a surgeon can utilize to limit postoperative adhesion development. The use of antiadhesion adjuvants, in combination with meticulous attention to surgical techniques, may provide the best opportunity to limit both de novo adhesion formation and adhesion reformation.

Conclusions

Associations between chronic pelvic pain and adhesions have been described by many investigators, although the mechanism(s) by which adhesions cause pain in some patients but not others remains unclear. While well-designed studies examining adhesiolysis as a method to reduce pelvic pain have failed to demonstrate conclusive benefits, interpretation of such studies is difficult because of the high incidence of adhesion reformation and logistical considerations, which limit the ability to ascertain timely and accurate information on postoperative adhesion development.

Selected bibliography

Bremers AJ, Ringers J, Vijn A, Janss RAJ, Bemelman WA. Laparoscopic adhesiolysis for chronic abdominal pain: an objective assessment. J Laparoendosc Adv Surg Tech A 2000;10:199–202.

Chan CLK, Wood C. Pelvic adhesiolysis—the assessment of symptom relief by 100 patients. Aust NZ J Obstet Gynecol 1985;25:295–8.

Daniell JF. Laparoscopic enterolysis for chronic abdominal pain. J Gynecol Surg 1989;5:61–6.

Demco LA. Effect on negative laparoscopy rate in chronic pelvic pain patients using patient assisted laparoscopy. JSLS 1997;1:319–21.

Diamond MP, Nezhat F. Letter to the editor: adhesions after resection of ovarian endometriomas. Fertil Steril 1993;59:934–5.

Diamond MP, Daniell JF, Feste J et al. Adhesion reformation and de novo adhesion formation after reproductive pelvic surgery. Fertil Steril 1987;47:864–6.

Diamond MP, Daniell JF, Johns DA et al. Postoperative adhesion development after operative laparoscopy: evaluation of early second-look laparoscopy. Fertil Steril 1991;55:700–4.

Diamond MP, Bachus K, Bieber E et al. Improvement of interobserver reproducibility of adhesion scoring systems. Fertil Steril 1994;62:984–8.

Fayez JA, Clark RR. Operative laparoscopy for the treatment of localized chronic pelvic abdominal pain caused by postoperative adhesions. J Gynecol Surg 1994;10:79–83.

Herrick SE, Mutsaers SE, Ozua P et al. Human peritoneal adhesions are highly cellular, innervated and vascularized. J Pathol 2000;192:67–72.

Howard FM. The role of laparoscopy as a diagnostic tool in chronic pelvic pain. Baillieres Best Pract Res Clin Obstet Gynecol 2000;14:467–94.

Kligman I, Drachenberg C, Papadimitriou J, Katz E. Immunohistochemical demonstration of nerve fibers in pelvic adhesions. Obstet Gynecol 1993;82:566–8.

Kresch AJ, Seifer DB, Sachs LB, Barrese I. Laparoscopy in 100 women with chronic pelvic pain. Obstet Gynecol 1984;64:672–4.

Malik E, Berg C, Meyhofer-Malik A, Haider S, Rossmanith WG. Subjective evaluation of the therapeutic value of laparoscopic adhesiolysis. Surg Endosc 2000;14:79-81.

Peters AAW, Trimbos-Kemper GCM, Admiral C, Trimbos JB. A randomized clinical trial on the benefit of adhesiolysis in patients with intraperitoneal adhesions and chronic Pelvic pain. Br J Obstet Gynecol 1992;99:59–62.

Rapkin AJ. Adhesions and pelvic pain: a retrospective study. Obstet Gynecol 1986;68:13–15.

Saravelos HG, Tin-Chiu L, Cooke ID. An analysis of the outcome of microsurgical and laparoscopic adhesiolysis for chronic pelvic pain. Hum Reprod 1995;10:2895–901.

Steege JF, Stout AL. Resolution of chronic pain after laparoscopic lysis of adhesions. Am J Obstet Gynecol 1991;165:278–83.

Stout Al, Steege JF, Dodson WC et al. Relationship of laparoscopic findings to self-report of pelvic pain. Am J Obstet Gynecol 1991;164:73–9.

Suleiman H, Gabella G, Davis C et al. Growth of nerve fibers into murine peritoneal adhesions. J Pathol 2000;192:396–403.

Sutton C, MacDonal R. Laer laparoscopic adhesiolysis. J Gynecol Surg 1990;6:155–9.

Swank DJ, Swank-Bordewijk SC, Hop WC et al. Laparoscopic adhesiolysis in patients with chronic abdominal pain: a blinded randomized controlled multi-center trial [published correction appears in Lancet 2003;361:2250]. Lancet 2003;361:1247–51.

Wiseman DM, Trout R, Diamond MP. The rates of adhesion development and the effects of crystalloid solutions on adhesion development in pelvic surgery. Fertil Steril 1998;70:702–11.

Fibroids, Adenomyosis, and Chronic Pelvic Pain

David L. Olive

Wisconsin Fertility Institute, Middleton, Wisconsin, USA

Introduction

Chronic pelvic pain can have a variety of sources, and each anatomic structure residing within the pelvis has been implicated in some form of this entity. The uterus, the central organ in the pelvic cavity, is no exception. In many women, pain emanating from the uterus is a regular feature of the menstrual process; excessive pain may result from normal anatomy associated with locally abnormal neural/biochemical processes, or even pathologic central pain transmission or interpretation.

Uterine pain may, however, be a result of disease processes originating within the uterus. Two such disorders—adenomyosis and uterine leiomyomas—have long been linked to pain symptoms in the reproductive-aged female. This chapter will examine these diseases, the evidence for implicating them as a source of chronic pelvic pain, and the treatments available when women with pelvic pain present with these diseases.

Adenomyosis

Adenomyosis stands as perhaps the most poorly and infrequently investigated of all gynecologic disorders. It is defined as endometrial glands and stroma displaced within the uterine musculature. The endometrial tissue may be localized to a discrete mass, termed an adenomyoma, or be seen as diffusely scattered islands of abnormal tissue throughout the myometrium (diffuse adenomyosis). The endometrial tissue is frequently (but not invariably) surrounded by myo-

metrium that has undergone hypertrophy and hyperplasia.

Epidemiology and risk factors

The incidence and prevalence of adenomyosis have not been accurately determined, since definitive diagnosis can only be made with microscopic analysis of the uterus, usually following hysterectomy or other uterine excisional procedures. In such biased populations, the prevalence is found to be in the 20–30% range in most studies. However, the presence of adenomyosis has been found to be dependent upon the compulsivity of the examining pathologist and the number of cuts in the anatomic specimen per institutional protocol. This is best seen in a study by Bird et al., in which, when three routine sections of myometrium were examined in each specimen, the rate of adenomyosis in hysterectomy specimens was 31%; however, when nine blocks were examined, the rate among the same specimens rose to 61.5%. It may well be that if excised uteri are meticulously examined in a very large number of sections, the prevalence would approach 100%!

Necropsy studies have also been performed, although they contain the reverse selection bias (that women with hysterectomy are eliminated from analysis). In two such published studies, the prevalence of adenomyosis was 50% and 53%, respectively. These data suggest that the true prevalence is higher than generally anticipated by most authors and at the high end of the above-mentioned range.

Chronic Pelvic Pain, First Edition. Edited by Paolo Vercellini.

© 2011 Blackwell Publishing Ltd. Published 2011 by Blackwell Publishing Ltd.

Traditional dogma holds that adenomyosis is a disease of older, parous women. However, these findings may be the result of selection bias due to diagnosis by hysterectomy. Indeed, when radiologic criteria are used for diagnosis, the disease can be found in women of all ages, including adolescents. Moreover, studies have been unable to show increasing adenomyosis risk with increasing parity. Thus, the relationship between age, parity, and adenomyosis remains questionable.

Other risk factors that have been associated with adenomyosis include prior uterine surgery, endometriosis, and uterine fibroids. However, data supporting each are difficult to come by. In fact, although most authors write of the common coexistence of adenomyosis with other pelvic diseases, at least one study exists to refute that notion.

☆ TIPS & TRICKS

If a patient undergoes surgical excision of endometriosis and fails to respond, consider performing a magnetic resonance imaging scan to check for adenomyosis.

Pathogenesis

Two major theories exist for the origination of adenomyosis. The first is de novo development from müllerian rests. This theory is nearly purely theoretical, with the best available evidence consisting of case reports of adenomyosis in müllerian remnants lacking a developed endometrium.

The more highly investigated theory is that adenomyosis is derived from endometrium. One such mechanism by which this might occur is invagination of the endometrial basalis into the underlying myometrium. This has support from an existing mouse model of the disease. Of interest is the fact that all organs in the human body that contain cavities also possess a submucosal region, with the exception of the uterus. It is thought that one of the main functions of this submucosa is to prevent the inward growth of glands that line these cavities. A second proposed mechanism is via a disruption of continuity between the basalis and myometrium, as might occur during surgery or delivery.

Both pituitary and gonadal hormones have been implicated in the development of adenomyosis. Prolactin and follicle-stimulating hormone have both been identified in the mouse model as capable inducers of the disease. Early exposure to estrogen has also been implicated in the murine model as increasing the risk for adenomyosis.

Pathology

As stated previously, adenomyosis may be localized or diffuse. When diffusely located throughout the myometrium, the uterus on gross inspection appears uniformly enlarged and feels boggy to the touch. Uterine size in this situation is generally less than 200 g, and the uterus will generally be confined to the pelvis. Upon sectioning, the uterine wall will appear thickened with multiple punctuate areas of hemorrhage or chocolate-colored tissue. Adenomyomas generally produce an irregular-appearing uterus, resembling a fibroid. However, upon incision there is no protrusion of the tumor, and it is difficult if not impossible to find a plane separating normal and abnormal tissue.

Microscopically, adenomyosis is defined as the presence of endometrial tissue within the myometrium at a distance of at least one low-power field (3 mm) from the endomyometrial junction. Care must be taken, however, to insure that sectioning is performed perpendicular to the junction to avoid misdiagnosis due to distorted tissue relationships from skewed sections.

Ectopic endometrium may cycle along with eutopic endometrium, or it can fail to show a functional response to either estrogen or progesterone. Receptor studies show a wide range of findings in various lesions, from normal amounts of estrogen and progesterone receptors to reduced or absent steroid receptors. There also appears frequently to be a local dysregulation of immune function, with inflammation characterized by increased expression of cell surface antigens, heat shock proteins, and adhesion molecules on the endometrium. In addition, there is generally an increase in macrophages and other immune cells. Expression of numerous growth factors, including granulocyte–macrophage colony-stimulating factor, is increased in the glandular epithelial cells, possibly explaining the elevated macrophage content and activation level. The activated macrophages, in turn, release cytokines, prostaglandins, and matrix metallo-proteinases. The latter molecules may be responsible for destabilizing the extracellular matrix and provoking abnormal uterine bleeding (see below).

Adenomyosis and symptoms, including pelvic pain

The two primary symptoms of adenomyosis are abnormal uterine bleeding and pelvic pain. Bleeding, although frequently associated in the literature, may possibly represent selection bias due to the past requirement for diagnosis by hysterectomy. However, menorrhagia could be explained by the increased endometrial surface area secondary to uterine enlargement. Intermenstrual bleeding may be a result of the aforementioned immune dysregulation, with altered matrix metalloproteinase expression and function. Further research is needed to explore these issues.

Pelvic pain is quite frequently associated with adenomyosis, although the frequent coexistence of diseases such as endometriosis makes attribution of the symptoms somewhat difficult. For this reason, the scientific and lay literature is replete with claims of types of pain due to adenomyosis, with little scientific confirmation. Dogma suggests that adenomyosis can produce dysmenorrhea, dyspareunia, and even sporadic noncyclic pelvic pain. It is difficult to determine the rates of such symptoms due to problems associated with calculating their prevalence, but pain in some form seems to be present in approximately 25% of those diagnosed at hysterectomy. The use of alternative diagnostic techniques may greatly alter this rate in the future.

Diagnosis

A definitive diagnosis of adenomyosis can only be made by histologic examination of at least a portion of the uterus. Generally, that means a hysterectomy specimen, but more conservative procedures can occasionally provide sufficient tissue for the diagnosis.

Clinical examination can suggest the disease. Diffuse uterine enlargement with tenderness to palpation is highly suggestive of the condition, although the sensitivity and specificity of this have never been determined.

Radiologic evaluation provides a noninvasive opportunity to assess the uterine architecture and thus potentially diagnose adenomyosis. The most accurate method available is magnetic resonance imaging (MRI). T_2-weighted images are used to evaluate the thickness of the junctional zone (inner myometrium); by convention, a junctional zone of 12 mm or greater thickness is classified as adenomyosis, while 8–12 mm is the "gray zone," and less than 8 mm is considered normal. In addition, bright T_2-weighted foci within the myometrium often represent islands of endometrial tissue with cystic dilatation and/or hemorrhage. Occasionally, linear striations radiate from the endometrium to the myometrium, representing direct invasion of the endometrium to the ectopic location. Finally, an adenomyoma is a localized, low signal intensity mass within the myometrium on both T_2- and T_1-weighted images, with poorly defined margins. Using these criteria, MRI has a sensitivity and specificity in most studies of 80–100%.

Ultrasonography can also be used for diagnosing adenomyosis, although it is far more operator-dependent than MRI. Transabdominal ultrasound is of limited utility, but transvaginal sonography has proved highly accurate in experienced hands. The criteria used are heterogeneous (islands of heterotopic endometrium) and hypoechoic (smooth muscle hyperplasia) areas of myometrium. Small myometrial cysts represent dilated cystic glands. Doppler flow evaluation demonstrates a pulsatility index greater than that seen with leiomyomas. A meta-analysis of 14 studies calculated a sensitivity of 83% and a specificity of 85% for the diagnosis of adenomyosis.

Other methods used to diagnose adenomyosis include hysteroscopic punch or excisional biopsies, needle biopsies, serum CA125 levels, and hysterosalpingography (HSG). While all have ardent supporters, there are few or no data to suggest the clinical utility of each of these diagnostic tools.

Treatment of adenomyosis-associated pain

It would seem initially that determining the value of treatment modalities for adenomyosis-associated pain would be a relatively straightforward task. However, quite the opposite is true. First, adenomyosis, as stated above, is difficult to diagnose or exclude without a concerted effort. Unfortunately, most studies rely upon limited sectioning of uteri, poorly chosen or poorly analyzed controls, and a lack of preoperative diagnosis. Thus, most studies are retrospectively evaluating women with histologically demonstrated adenomyosis compared to either a control group that has been poorly investigated for evidence of the disease or no control group at all.

Second, pelvic pain relief is difficult to attribute to a single disease entity, as many frequently coexist and are treated simultaneously. Furthermore, randomization, properly chosen controls meticulously characterized, and a reasonable follow-up duration to insure decay of the placebo effect are essential components of a comprehensive, well-designed treatment trial. To date, none has been conducted for adenomyosis-associated pain.

Hysterectomy is the definitive treatment for adenomyosis, guaranteeing that the disease will be removed in its entirety. It has been the mainstay of treatment for decades. However, it is unclear what percentage of women with adenomyosis and pelvic pain actually improve with hysterectomy. This is critical information, in that we do not know how often adenomyosis is the *cause* of pain in women with coexistence of both pelvic pain and adenomyosis. In the past, when hysterectomy was the only reliable means of diagnosis, this could not be easily studied prospectively; now that MRI and ultrasonography (to a lesser extent) can be used for preoperative diagnosis, no study has determined the value of this procedure. It should be added that concomitant oophorectomy would be expected to have no additive effect upon pain relief if adenomyosis were indeed the culprit.

Multiple conservative procedures have been proposed for the treatment of adenomyosis-associated pain. When adenomyomas are identified, excision or electrocoagulation has been reported. Adenomyosis of the transition zone can on occasion be treated by hysteroscopic resection or endomyometrial ablation. Recently, MRI-guided focused ultrasound surgery has been employed. Each of these techniques can undoubtedly remove some or all of the adenomyosis present in patients with pain. However, their utility in producing pain relief is unknown.

Conservative nerve interruption procedures such as uterosacral nerve ablation and presacral neurectomy would be expected to provide significant pain relief in those women with adenomyosis/pain in whom the discomfort seemed limited to the uterus. However, there are no data evaluating these treatments for adenomyosis-associated pain. This would seem to be a fertile topic for future investigation.

Uterine artery occlusion, either surgically or by embolization, has also been suggested. Uncontrolled trials suggest there is utility in producing pain relief in the woman with pelvic pain, adenomyosis, and no other discernable cause. However, recommendations for use should only follow properly controlled treatment trials, which have not yet been conducted.

Medical treatments have been utilized sporadically in the treatment of adenomyosis-associated pain, with few organized forays into actual treatment trials. Oral contraceptives may be beneficial, particularly when given continuously. Additional medications that have been used with anecdotal success include bromocriptine, progestins, danazol, gonadotropin-releasing hormone analogs (GnRH) analogs, and aromatase inhibitors. However, quantification of benefits has not been established for these medications. Local delivery via intrauterine contraceptive devices has also been advocated for both progestins and danazol; again, however, only case reports and clinical opinions exist on the subject.

Numerous alternative and complementary medical treatments have been forwarded for adenomyosis-associated pelvic pain, including acupuncture, therapeutic Mayan massage, and reiki. Common herbal remedies include Indian gooseberry juice with sugar daily, Bael leaf paste once daily, coriander seed decoctions, and almond–honey paste with warm milk. Interestingly, these "home remedies" have as much scientific support as the above-mentioned surgical and medical approaches.

Conclusions regarding adenomyosis and pain

Pelvic pain is a relatively common disorder among reproductive-aged females. Adenomyosis may be even more common but is difficult to diagnose. The two frequently coexist, but whether or not a cause and effect relationship exists in most cases is completely unknown. In fact, it is unclear whether adenomyosis truly represents a "disease" in most cases, or is rather a normal variant that can become pathologic only in rare and extreme cases. Furthermore, where that line is drawn between normal variant and disease-producing pathology is completely unknown.

Although adenomyosis may indeed represent a handy diagnosis for the physician who performs a hysterectomy in the presence of no other apparent pathology, the scientific validity for specifically treating adenomyosis in the presence of pelvic pain is minimal. Fortunately, the aforementioned treatments are nearly uniformly beneficial in treating pelvic pain of other etiologies (e.g., endometriosis), and most have proven beneficial for undiagnosed/unexplained pelvic pain. While some portion of these unexplained cases may in fact be adenomyosis-induced pain, high-quality investigations are needed to determine the validity of this theory and help define optimal therapeutic approaches.

EVIDENCE AT A GLANCE

- The prevalence of adenomyosis on histologic examination is directly proportional to the number of sections examined.
- The two primary symptoms are abnormal uterine bleeding and pelvic pain.
- Imaging with magnetic resonance imaging is the optimal noninvasive method for diagnosis; ultrasonography is highly operator-dependent.
- Although numerous medical and surgical therapies exist for the treatment of adenomyosis-associated pain, few high-quality data have been generated to evaluate their efficacy.

Fibroids

Uterine leiomyomas, also known as myomas or fibroids, are highly prevalent benign tumors of the uterine myometrium. They may be present within the uterus or attached to adjacent structures (parasitic myomas). They may even be scattered throughout the body (disseminated leiomyomatosis and benign metastasizing leiomyomas).

Uterine fibroids are generally defined by their location. Those involving the endometrial cavity are termed submucous, and these must, by definition, displace the endometrium into the cavity. Intramural myomas are limited to the area within the uterine wall, and subserous myomas protrude into the peritoneal cavity. Obviously, many such tumors encompass several or all of these characteristics.

Epidemiology and risk factors

The prevalence of uterine fibroids varies with age, race, and diagnostic modality. In a random sample of women in the United States, the cumulative incidence by age 50 was over 80% for black women and approaching 70% for white women. African-American women have diagnosis at an earlier age, have larger and more abundant tumors, and have more symptoms and consequently more hysterectomies. European cohorts, by contrast, have a much lower prevalence. In Germany, 10.7% of women at a mean of age 40 report this diagnosis, while ultrasonography in Italy detected fibroids in 21.4% of those aged 30–60. Swedish women are far less amenable to the disorder: only 7.8% between 33 and 40 years of age had ultrasonographically detected fibroids.

Risk factors for fibroid development have been intensely investigated by epidemiologists and geneticists. There does seem to be a genetic predisposition, with an increased risk of 5.7-fold for patients with an affected first-degree relative less than 45 years old. There is an increased risk with earlier age of menarche, and postmenopausal women have a 70–90% reduction in risk. Risk reduction also occurs with childbirth, and the more children the lower the risk. Exogenous steroid hormones are controversial as a risk factor premenopausally but increase the risk two- to sixfold in postmenopausal women. Also controversial is an association with increased weight and red meat in the diet. Reduction in risk may be seen with cigarette smoking, physical activity, and the consumption of green vegetables.

However, all the above epidemiologic data should be viewed with caution. Many women never consult a physician for myoma-related symptoms, and many physicians do not perform radiologic evaluation. Only 30% or less will have their fibroids removed, and thus histologic confirmation is rare. There exists a strong need for a prospective, longitudinal study of a wide cross-section of women to adequately determine risk factors.

Pathogenesis

Fibroids are the proliferation of a single clone of smooth muscle cells, with each fibroid in a uterus with multiple tumors representing a distinct clone; 40% have demonstrable chromosomal abnormalities. The tumors grow under the influence of local growth factors, cytokines, and sex hormones (estrogen, progesterone). Estrogen in particular is believed to be a major growth stimulus due to the epidemiologic features of the tumors, but in vitro studies show progesterone also to be a powerful enhancer of growth.

Pathology

Fibroids can be of varying sizes and shapes, often taking on the outer contour of the structures adjacent to them. They may protrude from the uterine surface or out of the cervical os, or they may be confined to the uterus, causing it to appear large and smooth. They are most often harder and firmer than the surrounding myometrium, and when overlying tissue is incised to expose the fibroid, it will generally protrude from the opening.

On histologic examination, the fibroid is composed of well-differentiated, whorled bundles of smooth muscle cells that resemble normal myometrium. The cells are generally uniform in shape and size and have a long, slender, spindle-like cytoplasmic process. The nuclei are elongated with tapered ends. Mitotic figures are infrequent.

A variety of degenerative forms are the tumor can be seen microscopically, and such degenerative changes are more common the larger the tumor. Hyaline degeneration is the replacement of smooth muscle cells by collagen. Red degeneration is usually due to acute loss of blood flow and is commonly seen in pregnancy. Calcific degeneration can also occur, most commonly in long-standing fibroids after menopause.

A variety of variant forms of these tumors can also be seen by histologic examination. The cellular leiomyoma has an increased number of cells per unit area when compared to surrounding myometrium. Symplastic leiomyomas have variable numbers of smooth muscle cells with multiple, gigantic nuclei and abundant nuclear chromatin.

Fibroids and pelvic pain

Fibroids cause a variety of symptoms, including abnormal bleeding, bladder and bowel dysfunction, and infertility. They have also been related to pelvic pain. Pain is an unusual symptom, and when it occurs it is most commonly acute. Acute pelvic pain resulting from fibroids is generally associated with torsion of the pedicle of a pedunculated myoma, cervical dilatation and uterine contractions due to a prolapsing submucous myoma, or red degeneration resulting from ischemia, which is generally seen in pregnancy.

> ### ✋ CAUTION
>
> Avoid attributing chronic pelvic pain to uterine fibroids without first performing a complete search for other potential causes.

Chronic pelvic pain commonly coexists with uterine fibroids, but a cause and effect relationship is unlikely in most circumstances. In a study utilizing transvaginal sonography on a population-based cohort of 635 non-care-seeking women with an intact uterus, symptoms of dyspareunia, dysmenorrhea, or noncyclic pelvic pain were concurrently measured by visual analog scales. The women found to have myomas were only slightly more likely to report moderate or severe dyspareunia or noncyclic pelvic pain, and had no higher incidence of moderate or severe dysmenorrhea, than women without myomas. Neither the number nor the total volume of myomas was related to pain. A fibroid located in the broad ligament will cause unilateral lower abdominal/pelvic pain or pain along the sciatic nerve, but this is a very rare event.

Diagnosis

Clinically significant subserosal and intramural myomas can often be diagnosed by pelvic examination based on findings of an enlarged, irregularly shaped, firm, and nontender uterus. Uterine size, as assessed by bimanual examination, correlates well with uterine size and weight at pathologic examination, even in most obese women. However, submucous myomas and some fibroids that are small or difficult to palpate may require imaging studies for definitive diagnosis.

Imaging studies give an accurate portrayal of the size, number, and location of fibroids, information critical to the success of most therapies. Techniques available for confirming the diagnosis of myomas include sonography, sonohysterography, HSG, and MRI.

Transvaginal sonography is the most readily available and least costly technique and may be helpful for differentiating myomas from other pelvic conditions. Large myomas may be best imaged with a combination of transabdominal and transvaginal sonography. The sonographic appearance of myomas can be variable, but frequently they appear as symmetric, well-defined, hypoechoic, and heterogenous masses. However, areas of calcification or hemorrhage may appear hyperechoic, and cystic degeneration may appear anechoic. Sonography may be inadequate for determining the precise number and position of myomas, and their size is frequently overestimated due to misreading of the surrounding, compressed myometrium.

Sonohysterography uses saline inserted into the uterine cavity to provide contrast and better define submucous myomas, polyps, endometrial hyperplasia, or carcinoma. It allows evaluation of both the cavity and the surrounding myometrium simultaneously, providing excellent evaluation of the fibroid's position and size. HSG is a similar technique but uses radiographically apparent contrast and fluoroscopy to delineate the uterine cavity and the internal contour of the fallopian tubes. By not providing an assessment of the uterine musculature, HSG is inferior to sonohysterography when fibroids are the principal purpose of the study; however, by allowing observation of the tubes, this test provides an added dimension not available with ultrasonography.

MRI is an excellent method to evaluate the size, position, and number of uterine myomas and is the best modality for the exact evaluation of submucous myoma penetration into the myometrium. The advantages of MRI include a lack of dependence on operator techniques and the low interobserver variability in interpretation of the images for submucous myomas, intramural myomas, and adenomyosis when compared to transvaginal sonography, saline-infusion sonograms, and HSG.

Endoscopy is the definitive test for determining the presence of fibroids within the uterine cavity (hysteroscopy), and frequently will provide confirmatory evidence of fibroids in other locations (laparoscopy).

Treatment

Hysterectomy is the approach most often utilized to treat myomas, and the removal of the uterus and inclusive structures will undoubtedly remove any fibroid-induced symptoms. However, in the case of acute pain resulting from fibroids, there is generally no need to pursue such major surgery as the symptom is self-limited. Furthermore, complications resulting from hysterectomy may be as significant or as devastating as the pain that is being treated. Fortunately, if fibroid-associated chronic pelvic pain is in fact due to another cause such as primary dysmenorrhea, adenomyosis, or endometriosis, or if the pain is a result of compression of surrounding structures, hysterectomy will likely alleviate the symptoms.

In women with fibroid-associated symptoms who desire future pregnancy, or in those who simply do not want to undertake the expense and risks of major surgery, conservative surgical approaches are available. Fibroids can be removed while leaving the uterus in place, termed a myomectomy, and this can be performed by laparotomy, laparoscopy, or hysteroscopy depending upon the size, location, and number of tumors. The rate of morbidity is no greater and may be less than that seen with hysterectomy, but fibroid removal may be ineffective if the source of the pain is uterine but not emanating from the fibroid itself.

The fibroid may also be destroyed in situ in a procedure called myolysis. This can be accomplished by laser energy, electrosurgery, or cryosurgery; all have proven effective at reducing fibroid and uterine size, and thus decreasing bulk symptoms from pressure on surrounding structures. However, their utility in the treatment of chronic pelvic pain remains unproven.

Obstruction of the uterine arteries has recently been employed in the conservative treatment of uterine fibroids. This can be accomplished via laparoscopic occlusion, radiologic uterine artery embolization, or transvaginal uterine artery clamping. All produce ischemia and may induce considerable acute pain, but the long-term results include a reduction in size and symptomatic improvement, particularly in those whose symptoms are caused by uterine/fibroid volume. Current contraindications for radiologic embolization include coagulopathy, immunocompromise, previous pelvic irradiation, and a desire to maintain childbearing potential.

Several medical therapies have been utilized in an attempt to decrease myoma size, thus relieving many of the symptoms associated with the tumors. These include GnRH agonists, GnRH antagonists, aromatase inhibitors, selective estrogen receptor modulators, selective progesterone receptor modulators, and weak androgens such as danazol and gestrinone. Combinations of these drug classes have also been used. Raloxifene, a selective estrogen receptor modulator, is ineffective alone in premenopausal women at reducing fibroid volume or symptoms. However, when it is combined with GnRH agonists, the drug combination produces a profound effect upon fibroids. Limited data exist regarding most of these medications, particularly for long-term relief of symptoms and recurrence following discontinuation. Virtually no data are apparent for chronic pelvic pain when fibroids appear to be the exclusive cause.

Conclusions regarding fibroids and pain

Fibroids are a very common gynecologic pathology, and methods for treating these tumors are numerous and expanding daily. However, the preferred treatment of fibroids in the face of chronic pelvic pain remains obscure in that it is unlikely that fibroids are generally the source of such pain. Pressure symptoms from uterine/myoma bulk effect are more commonly seen in women with fibroids, and occasionally dyspareunia or noncyclic pain will be reported. If fibroid-associated pain exists, and the physician truly believes that treating the fibroids will improve this symptom, the decision on which treatment option to employ involves a consideration of cost, other health factors, desire for future fertility, and availability of resources.

EVIDENCE AT A GLANCE

- Fibroids have a very high prevalence in the United States but perhaps a lower one in Europe.
- Fibroids are a monoclonal disease, with each tumor representing a single cell that has escaped control.
- Pain is an unusual symptom of fibroids and is usually due to degeneration.
- Diagnosis can be made by a variety of radiologic modalities as well as endoscopy.
- Treatment of myoma-associated pain has not been adequately investigated, although numerous surgical, medical, and radiologic treatments are available.

Selected bibliography

ACOG practice bulletin. Surgical alternatives to hysterectomy in the management of leiomyomas. Number 16, May 2000 (replaces educational bulletin number 192, May 1994). Int J Gynaecol Obstet 2001;73:285–93.

Ascher S, Arnold LL, Patt RH et al. Adenomyosis: prospective comparison of MR imaging and transvaginal sonography. Radiology 1994;190:803–6.

Baird D, Dunson D, Hill M. High cumulative incidence of uterine leiomyoma in black and white women: ultrasound evidence. Am J Obstet Gynecol 2003;188:100–7.

Bird CC, McElin TW, Mandalo-Estrella P. The elusive adenomyosis of the uterus— revisited. Am J Obstet Gynecol 1972;112:583–93.

Dueholm M, Lundorf E, Hansen ES, Ledertoug S, Olesen F. Accuracy of magnetic resonance imaging and transvaginal ultrasonography in the diagnosis, mapping, and measurement of uterine myomas. Am J Obstet Gynecol 2002; 186:409–15.

Gordts S, Brosens JJ, Fusi L, Benagiano G, Brosens I. Uterine adenomyosis: a need for uniform terminology and consensus classification. Reprod Biomed Online 2008;17:244–8.

Lippman SA, Warner M, Samuels S, Olive D, Vercellini P, Eskenazi B. Uterine fibroids and gynecologic pain symptoms in a population-based study. Fertil Steril 2003;80:1488–94.

Meredith SM, Sanchez-Ramos L, Kaunitz AM. Diagnostic accuracy of transvaginal sonography for the diagnosis of adenomyosis: systematic review and meta-analysis. Am J Obstet Gynecol 2009;201:107 e1–6.

Olive DL, Lindheim SR, Pritts EA. Conservative surgical management of uterine myomas. Obstet Gynecol Clin N Am 2006;33:115–24.

Palomba S, Russo T, Orio F, Jr. et al. Effectiveness of combined GnRH analogue plus raloxifene administration in the treatment of uterine leiomyomas: a prospective, randomized, single-blind, placebo-controlled clinical trial. Hum Reprod 2002;17:3213–19.

Parker WH. Etiology, symptomatology, and diagnosis of uterine myomas. Fertil Steril 2007;87:725–36.

Payson M, Leppert P, Segars J. Epidemiology of myomas. Obstet Gynecol Clin N Am 2006; 33:1–11.

Pract Res Clin Obstet Gynaecol 2006;20:583–602.

Rackow BW, Arici AA. Options for medical treatment of myomas. Obstet Gynecol Clin N Am 2006;33:97–113.

Schwartz SM, Marshall LM, Baird DD. Epidemiologic contributions to understanding the etiology of uterine leiomyomata. Environ Health Perspect 2000;108(Suppl. 5):821–7.

Weiss G, Maseelall P, Schott LL et al. Adenomyosis a variant, not a disease? Evidence from hysterectomized menopausal women in the Study of Women's Health Across the Nation (SWAN). Fertil Steril 2009;91:201–6.

Wood C. Surgical and medical treatment of adenomyosis. Hum Reprod Update 1998;4: 323–36.

Bladder Pain Syndrome and Other Urological Causes of Chronic Pelvic Pain

Daniela Wittmann and J. Quentin Clemens

University of Michigan Medical Center, Ann Arbor, Michigan, USA

Introduction

Urologists are frequently consulted to assist with the management of chronic pelvic pain, especially when the pain appears to be associated with the bladder or urethra. A variety of specific disorders can cause pain in these areas, and some of these are readily identified and easily treatable. However, for the majority of patients with chronic urologic pain, effective treatment remains elusive. This chapter will review a number of specific urologic causes of pelvic pain, but will focus primarily on idiopathic bladder pain, typically termed "interstitial cystitis" or "bladder pain syndrome." The contribution of pelvic floor muscle dysfunction (PFMD) to these disorders will also be discussed. Finally, a brief review of dyspareunia will be presented.

Well-characterized urologic causes of pelvic pain

Urethral diverticula

Urethral diverticula are thought to be caused by infection and obstruction of the periurethral glands. The infected gland eventually ruptures into the lumen of the urethra, creating a communication between the urethra and the lumen of the diverticulum.

Common presenting symptoms include dysuria, postvoid dribbling, dyspareunia, and irritative voiding symptoms. Recurrent episodes of cystitis are also common. However, certain patients may have more subtle periurethral pain

or nonspecific symptoms, and a high index of suspicion may be warranted to identify these less obvious diverticula. In one series of 46 consecutive women who were diagnosed with a urethral diverticulum, the mean interval between the onset of symptoms to diagnosis was 5.2 years. On examination, most urethral diverticula are located ventrally over the middle and proximal portions of the urethra. Gentle compression of the diverticulum (if tolerated by the patient) may elicit purulent drainage from the urethral meatus.

If a diverticulum is suspected but not clearly evident on physical examination, additional diagnostic studies may be helpful. Cystoscopy may be used to visualize the ostium of the diverticulum from within the urethra, but this can be difficult to identify in some patients. Contrast urethrography using a specialized double-balloon catheter, or voiding cystourethrography, has traditionally been used to document urethral diverticula. More recently, magnetic resonance imaging has emerged as the "gold standard" for identifying these lesions and determining their size and location.

Treatment of urethral diverticula is surgical but may not be indicated if the lesion is an incidental finding and is asymptomatic. If a nonoperative approach is chosen, interval follow-up is warranted to ensure that the lesion does not enlarge with time. A variety of surgical techniques exist for treating urethral diverticula. The most common technique involves complete excision of the diverticular sac with closure of the urethra

Chronic Pelvic Pain, First Edition. Edited by Paolo Vercellini.
© 2011 Blackwell Publishing Ltd. Published 2011 by Blackwell Publishing Ltd.

over a catheter. Incomplete excision may result in recurrence of the diverticulum in the future. However, small diverticula may be successfully treated with simple marsupialization. In addition, in women presenting with a diverticulum during pregnancy, marsupialization and antibiotic therapy can treat the infection, alleviate the symptoms, and allow for a more definitive repair (if needed) following delivery.

Postsurgical pain

Postsurgical pain is often associated with the use of mesh, bone anchors, nonabsorbable sutures, or other synthetic materials as part of the surgical treatment of pelvic prolapse or stress urinary incontinence. These types of complication are frequently published as case series from referral centers, but the literature suggests that they are uncommon. For that reason, they may be unrecognized for an extended period of time following the initial surgery. The characteristic symptom is the new onset of urethral, vaginal, or suprapubic pain that was not present prior to the surgery. Other symptoms may include vaginal discharge, dyspareunia, or partner pain with intercourse ("hyspareunia").

On examination, there typically is focal tenderness at the site of the synthetic material that reproduces the symptoms. Visible mesh, granulation tissue, or a sinus tract may be visible on careful vaginal examination. Cystoscopy may identify foreign material such a suture or mesh within the urethra or bladder. Occasional patients with long-standing symptoms may develop pubic osteomyelitis, which can be identified on imaging studies. Effective treatment requires complete excision of the synthetic material. Certain patients may have long-standing pain and voiding dysfunction even after removal of all foreign materials.

Recurrent urinary tract infections

Recurrent urinary tract infections may cause repeated episodes of irritative voiding symptoms and pelvic pain. Approximately 30% of women who experience a single episode of bacterial cystitis will have a recurrence within the following year. The typical pattern is a series of separate symptomatic episodes that are interspersed by asymptomatic intervals. Common symptoms include dysuria, urinary frequency, urgency/urge incontinence, and gross hematuria. The symptoms typically respond after 1–3 days of antibiotic therapy. Rarely, a woman will demonstrate frequent recurrent infections with the same organism (bacterial persistence). In such cases, there is often a source of infection within the body, such as a kidney stone or urethral diverticulum.

Urinary tract infections in elderly individuals can be particularly challenging as the symptoms may be nonspecific (altered mental status, fatigue) and antibiotic side effects are more common. In addition, at least 20% of women over the age of 65 have asymptomatic bacteriuria. It is well documented that screening for and treating this condition confers no benefit to the patient. Furthermore, the presence of pyuria on urinalysis is not a good predictor of or indication for antimicrobial treatment in this population. This is important to understand because certain elderly patients may have other urologic conditions (idiopathic urge incontinence, bladder pain syndrome, etc.) in the presence of asymptomatic bacteriuria. These patients can be particularly complicated. Ideally, the bacteriuria can be eradicated for a period of time, and if the urologic symptoms do not resolve, this strongly suggests that the bacteria are not responsible for the symptoms. Often, it can be quite difficult to convince patients (and caregivers) of this fact after a pattern of ongoing treatment with antibiotics has been established.

Bladder carcinoma in situ

Bladder carcinoma in situ (CIS) refers to poorly differentiated transitional cell carcinoma that is confined to the urothelium. Over half of patients diagnosed with CIS present with irritative voiding symptoms (dysuria, frequency, urgency). Microscopic or gross hematuria is often, although not always, also present, and a high index of suspicion is needed to identify this condition, especially in individuals with risk factors (smoking, prior radiation therapy, exposure to aromatic amines). Between 40% and 80% of patients with CIS will develop muscle invasion if left untreated. On cystoscopy, the typical appearance is a velvety patch of erythematous mucosa, but the lesions may be subtle. Urine cytopathology is extremely important in diagnosis, as this test will be positive in 80–90% of patients with CIS. Treatment includes surgical resection and intravesical chemotherapy, particularly bacillus Calmette–Guérin (BCG). Recurrences are common, and frequent, long-term surveillance is required in all patients.

Idiopathic bladder pain—interstitial cystitis/bladder pain syndrome

The condition of interstitial cystitis (IC) refers to the presence of chronic pain that is perceived to be related to the bladder, and which is associated with other lower urinary tract symptoms such as urinary frequency or urgency, in the absence of infection or other identifiable causes. Some individuals will not use the term "pain" to describe their symptoms but instead will describe it as a sense of pressure, discomfort, burning, or urge to void. Common sites of pain include the suprapubic region, urethra, and genital region, but non-genitourinary sites (lower back, upper thighs, buttocks) may also be reported as associated symptoms. The association with the bladder is typically identified by a relationship with the voiding cycle, so that the symptoms worsen as the bladder fills or are at least partially relieved with voiding. Although a degree of symptom chronicity is implicit in the diagnosis, there is no consensus regarding the duration of symptoms that should present before the diagnosis is assigned. Traditionally, at least 6–9 months of symptoms were required to fulfill diagnostic criteria for IC, while some more recent research studies of IC have required only 6 weeks of symptoms for inclusion.

Nomenclature/definition

Although the term "interstitial cystitis" is widely recognized and is firmly embedded in the medical lexicon, it is somewhat of a misnomer. There is no clear evidence that IC is associated with pathology involving the bladder interstitium, nor is it associated with inflammation of the bladder wall. In fact, IC is a syndrome (collection of symptoms) with no objective diagnostic sign or test. In recent years, there is a growing consensus that IC actually represents a chronic pain condition of the bladder. With this recognition, nomenclature changes have occurred. The term "painful bladder syndrome" was coined by the Interna-

tional Continence Society to refer to the presence of "suprapubic pain related to bladder filling, accompanied by other symptoms such as increased daytime and nighttime frequency, in the absence of proven urinary infection or other obvious pathology." The condition IC was defined as the subset of individuals with PBS who also demonstrate the "typical cystoscopic and histologic features." Others have suggested that the term IC be dropped altogether, and that the term "bladder pain syndrome" should be used to describe the condition. This is currently an area of considerable controversy. The term "interstitial cystitis/bladder pain syndrome" (IC/BPS) will be used to describe the condition throughout this chapter.

⚠ CAUTION

In 1988, the National Institutes of Diabetes and Digestive and Kidney Diseases (NIDDK) published a research definition of interstitial cystitis/bladder pain syndrome (IC/BPS). This was an important landmark in IC/BPS research as it provided strict inclusion criteria for research studies so that a uniform group of individuals could be studied. To meet these criteria, patients were required to demonstrate:
- pain associated with the bladder or urinary urgency;
- symptom duration of 9 months or longer;
- glomerulations or a Hunner ulcer on cystoscopy under anesthesia;
- at least eight voids per day and one void at night;
- a cystometric bladder capacity of less than 350 cm^3.

This research definition was quickly adopted for clinical use by practising clinicians to define the condition. However, it has become quite clear that the NIDDK definition is too rigid for everyday clinical use as up to 60% of patients clinically diagnosed with IC/BPS by experienced clinicians were being missed when the NIDDK research criteria were used as the definition of the disease. Currently, less rigid criteria are used for clinical diagnosis and entry into clinical trials. For instance, cystometric capacity and the presence of glomerulations or ulcers are frequently not needed to make the clinical diagnosis of IC/BPS. Furthermore, clinical trials of IC/BPS patients with a symptom duration of as little as 6 weeks have been conducted.

IC/BPS versus overactive bladder

IC/BPS and overactive bladder (OAB) are considered to be separate clinical syndromes with unique defining characteristics. As mentioned above, IC/BPS is defined by bladder pain. In contrast, OAB is defined by the presence of urinary urgency (a sudden, compelling desire to pass urine, which is difficult to defer). In general, patients with IC/BPS will have fairly constant symptoms that worsen gradually as the bladder fills and then improve somewhat after voiding. In contrast, patients with OAB are usually completely asymptomatic between sudden urgency episodes. Most patients with IC/BPS do not have incontinence and do not have concerns about incontinence. Some individuals with IC/BPS will describe their symptoms as "urgency," but this urgency is typically due to pain rather than due to a fear of leakage. In contrast, many patients with OAB do experience urge-related incontinence ("OAB wet"), and their urgency is associated with impending incontinence if they are not able to reach a bathroom quickly.

Conceptually, IC/BPS and OAB are distinct, and indeed the symptoms are clear-cut along these lines in many patients. However, there are also a considerable number of patients with symptoms that span both conditions, and these patients are difficult to categorize.

Etiology

Despite extensive efforts to identify the pathophysiology responsible for the development of IC/BPS, the etiology remains unknown. It seems likely that the causes underlying the development of IC/BPS symptoms are multifactorial, with different factors responsible in different patients. A common belief is that IC/BPS results from a deficient urothelial protective lining that allows toxins from the urine to enter the subepithelium of the bladder and cause pain. Certain experimental studies have identified increased epithelial permeability in patients with IC/BPS, but other experiments do not support this theory, and it is clear that this is a nonspecific finding that is also observed with bacterial cystitis and radiation cystitis. Other investigators have identified increased numbers of mast cells in the detrusor muscle in women with IC/BPS, but it is not clear whether the mast cells represent an etiologic factor or a nonspecific response to injury or inflammation. Attempts to identify an infectious cause have been unsuccessful to date, but infection continues to be postulated as a possible etiologic factor. Other studies have suggested autoimmune or neurogenic etiologies.

⚙ SCIENCE REVISITED

Experimental evidence indicates that bladder epithelial cells from patients with interstitial cystitis/bladder pain syndrome (IC/BPS) patients produce a novel antiproliferative factor (APF), which is found in the urine of approximately 95% of patients with IC compared to only 5% of controls. APF is a low molecular weight glycosylated peptide related to the membrane receptor frizzled-8. APF has been found to profoundly inhibit urothelial cell proliferation, alter the production of several growth factors, increase transcellular urothelial permeability, and lower the expression of proteins that form intercellular junctional complexes. APF may therefore contribute to the pathogenesis of IC/BPS by altering the differentiation, tight junction formation, and proliferation of bladder epithelial cells, resulting in decreased epithelial barrier integrity. However, attempts to measure APF for use as a clinical marker for IC/BPS have not been successful to date, and additional research is needed to help understand the clinical utility of these findings.

Epidemiology of IC/BPS

Numerous studies have been performed to help quantify the prevalence of IC/BPS. Since there is no clear diagnostic test to identify the condition, and no uniform epidemiologic definition to use for research studies, it is not surprising that such studies have yielded disparate results.

It is clear that IC/BPS occurs more commonly in women than in men, with the typical ratio being between 5:1 and 10:1. On cross-sectional studies, approximately 0.5% of women report that they have been diagnosed with IC/BPS at some point in their lives, but these results are subject to recall bias. In particular, women may confuse the term "interstitial cystitis" with other forms of cystitis. Using administrative billing data, the prevalence of physician-diagnosed IC/BPS is approximately 200 per 100,000 women. However, the prevalence of symptoms suggestive of IC/BPS is much higher, ranging from 2% to 6%. The reason for the discrepancy is not clear, but it is increasingly being recognized that the condition is not nearly as rare as previously assumed. There does not appear to be substantial variability in IC/BPS prevalence across racial/ethnic minorities in the few studies that have examined this question.

Overlap with other conditions

It is well documented that women with IC/BPS are more likely to exhibit certain medical conditions than age-matched controls. Conditions that have been most strongly associated with IC/BPS include endometriosis, depression, anxiety/panic disorder, irritable bowel syndrome, vulvodynia, fibromyalgia, chronic headaches, allergies, chronic fatigue syndrome, back pain, and noncardiac chest pain. The relevance of these associations is not clear at this time, but the findings imply that certain patients with IC/BPS may have a systemic pain disorder rather than a disorder that is limited to the bladder. Whether this information can be exploited to improve treatment efficacy is an unanswered question at this time.

Diagnosis

History

A thorough and accurate history is probably the most important factor in making the diagnosis of IC/BPS. The character, duration, and severity of the symptoms must be accurately documented. It is important to understand that many patients will not describe their symptoms as pain but instead will use descriptors such as "pressure," "urgency," or "discomfort." Association of the pain with the voiding cycle is a cardinal feature of IC/BPS that is typically not present in other pelvic pain conditions.

It is often very informative to have the patient complete a voiding diary to better quantify the degree of urinary frequency and the amount of oral fluid intake, and to determine functional bladder capacity (the largest voided volume on the diary). Information about previous treatments (including self-care) should be obtained. In addition, a thorough past medical history should be obtained to identify specific conditions that could be responsible for the symptoms (e.g., previous pelvic surgery, pelvic malignancy, neurologic disease).

Standardized questionnaires

A number of standardized questionnaires for IC/BPS have been developed as both clinical and research tools. These instruments can be quite useful for quantifying the degree of symptoms in patients diagnosed with IC/BPS and for assessing response to therapy. However, these instruments are not intended for use as screening tools for IC/BPS, and they should not be used for diagnostic purposes.

Physical examination

The primary purpose of the physical examination is to identify conditions that could be contributing to the symptoms, such as a vaginal infection, a urethral mass, or a large pelvic prolapse. Transvaginal palpation of the bladder can be performed to see if this reproduces the patient's symptoms. Furthermore, identification of significant pelvic floor muscle tenderness can suggest that a trial of physical therapy may be helpful (see the section on "Pelvic floor muscle dysfunction" below).

Office testing

A urinalysis should be performed to evaluate for microscopic hematuria or possible infection. If the urinalysis is suspicious, a urine culture should be performed to document whether an infection is present. Certain patients may feel as though they are not completely emptying their bladder, and an assessment of postvoid residual (with a catheter or an ultrasound) can be performed to evaluate this.

★ TIPS & TRICKS

Interstitial cystitis/bladder pain syndrome is a strictly clinical diagnosis, with the inherent subjectivity that is present with all clinical syndromes. In general, the diagnosis should be suspected in a patient with suprapubic pain or discomfort, urinary frequency (over eight times in 24 hours), no evidence of a vaginal infection or urethral mass on examination, no hematuria on urinalysis, and a negative urine culture while symptomatic. In addition, there should be no history of neurologic problems, malignancy, pelvic radiation, or recent pelvic surgery that could cause the symptoms.

✋ CAUTION

There is no evidence that interstitial cystitis/bladder pain syndrome (IC/BPS) is a premalignant condition. However, it is possible for unrecognized bladder cancer to be mistakenly diagnosed as IC/BPS. Studies indicate that approximately 1% of women referred to a specialty IC/BPS clinic will ultimately be found to have bladder cancer. Women suspected of having IC/BPS who also have unevaluated hematuria (microscopic or gross) or a strong history of smoking should undergo a comprehensive urologic evaluation to exclude malignancy.

Provocative testing

The potassium chloride test is performed by infusing a supraphysiologic 0.4 M potassium chloride solution into the bladder through a catheter. A positive test (pain, provocation of symptoms) is considered to be diagnostic of IC/BPS, and treatment is then typically oriented toward reducing the bladder permeability defect. However, the sensitivity and specificity of this test have been questioned, and it is not clear if the results of the test can be used to predict any meaningful response to therapy. In addition, the test can be quite painful and unpleasant for both patient and clinician.

Using the opposite approach, an anesthetic bladder challenge can be performed by instilling a lidocaine solution into the bladder to assess symptomatic response. If the pain resolves or is significantly improved, this indicates a bladder source for the pain, while persistence of the symptoms implies a source of pain other than the bladder.

Cystoscopy

Office cystoscopy is frequently performed in patients with persistent bladder symptoms, primarily to exclude the presence of a bladder malignancy. This can be quite uncomfortable for many IC/BPS patients, and in such cases the procedure can be performed under an anesthetic in the operating room.

When the diagnosis of IC/BPS is suspected, hydrodistension is frequently performed, in which the bladder is filled to capacity while cystoscopy is performed. A Hunner's ulcer can be identified before hydrodistension, but it can become more apparent following distension, when the mucosa at the ulcer will often crack and bleed. Following hydrodistension, the presence of glomerulations (pinpoint bleeding sites in the bladder mucosa) is considered indicative of the presence of IC/BPS. However, it is important to understand that glomerulations are nonspecific findings that have been observed in asymptomatic individuals. Therefore, the presence of glomerulations as an isolated finding (in the absence of symptoms) is of no clinical significance.

★ TIPS & TRICKS

Although Hunner's ulcers are uncommon (approximately 10% of all patients with interstitial cystitis/bladder pain syndrome), their identification and treatment can result in a significant and durable symptom improvement in these patients. Using a cystoscope, the ulcers can be resected, fulgurated, or ablated with a laser. Repeat cystoscopy is indicated if symptoms recur, as new ulcers can form after years of quiescence. The pathophysiology responsible for ulcer formation is not understood. Histologic, microbiologic, and electronic micrographic studies have not identified an etiologic factor.

⚠ CAUTION

There is no standardized method to perform cystoscopy with hydrodistension for interstitial cystitis/bladder pain syndrome. However, a few principles can be used to guide clinicians who perform the procedure. The irrigant is typically placed no higher than 80–100 cm above the level of the bladder to avoid excessive intravesical pressures during filling. It is typically recommended to perform the procedure under a full general or spinal anesthetic as this allows the clinician to determine the bladder capacity without the abdominal straining that often occurs due to bladder pain. A capacity of less than 250 cm³ under anesthesia is associated with a poor prognosis.

The duration of hydrodistension is not standardized, but prolonged distension (>10 minutes) has been associated with bladder necrosis. In addition, the practice of manually "overdistending" the bladder with a syringe once capacity has been reached is to be discouraged as this has been associated with bladder perforation. Some clinicians performed multiple short-duration hydrodistensions, while others conduct a single hydrodistension. There are no data to indicate whether one practice is superior to the other in terms of safety or sensitivity in identifying pathology.

The need for bladder biopsy in the diagnosis of IC/BPS is somewhat controversial. It is quite clear that there are currently no histologic findings that are diagnostic of IC/BPS. Therefore, the primary clinical role for a bladder biopsy is to exclude bladder pathology (such as CIS) which could be responsible for the symptoms. As such, routine, random bladder biopsies in the absence of abnormal findings may not be warranted. However, others have argued that the presence of

histologic abnormalities may be important in identifying specific patient subtypes. For instance, the European Society for the Study of Bladder Pain Syndrome (ESSIC) classification system includes bladder biopsy data as an essential feature, so that patients with biopsy findings of inflammatory infiltrates, and/or detrusor mastocytosis, and/or granulation tissue, and/or intrafascicular fibrosis are separated from those with no histologic abnormalities. Of note, it is recommended that a bladder biopsy should be performed after hydrodistension in order to reduce the risk of bladder rupture.

Treatment

Nonpharmacologic

Studies have shown a median duration of 3-5 years between symptom onset and the diagnosis of IC/BPS. During this time, patients can feel isolated, anxious, confused and frustrated. Simply recognizing the diagnosis of IC/BPS and providing education about the condition can be a great relief to these patients. Patient support groups such as the Interstitial Cystitis Association (www.ichelp.org) can provide support and information that is extremely important for patients with newly diagnosed IC/BPS. Behavioral modification (voiding diary, fluid modification) and timed voiding may be helpful, especially in patients in whom urinary frequency is a more dominant symptom than pain. Dietary modification may improve symptoms in some patients. In particular, caffeinated beverages, citrus, alcoholic beverages, spicy foods, and vinegar are often reported as exacerbating IC/BPS symptoms. Various elaborate "IC diets" exist, but there is no systematic evidence to support their routine use.

Oral medications

Pentosan polysulfate (Elmiron) is the only oral agent that is approved for use for IC/BPS by the U.S. Food and Drug Administration (FDA) (see Table 9.1 for medications used to treat IC/BPS). This medication is a heparin analog that is designed to correct defects in the bladder glycosaminoglycan layer and thereby reduce the abnormal epithelial permeability associated with IC/BPS. Success with this agent has been modest, and it may require 3–6 months of therapy before improvement is seen.

Table 9.1 Common medications used to treat interstitial cystitis/bladder pain syndrome (IC/BPS)

Name	Dose	Common side effects
Oral medications		
Pentosan polysulfate (Elmiron)	100 mg three times a day	Gastrointestinal distress, hair loss (reversible), elevated liver function tests
Amitriptyline (Elavil)	10–75 mg at bedtime	Sedation, dry mouth, constipation, weight gain
Hydroxyzine (Vistaril)	10 mg at bedtime, up to 25 mg three times a day	Sedation
Gabapentin (Neurontin)	100 mg at bedtime, up to 300 mg three times a day	Dizziness, somnolence, peripheral edema, wieght gain
Pregabalin (Lyrica)	50–200 mg times a day	Dizziness, somnolence, peripheral edema, weight gain
Intravesical medications		
Dimethyl sulfoxide (DMSO; Rimso-50)	Supplied as 50 cm³ 50% DMSO solution—the entire 50 cm³ is instilled for 15 minutes weekly for 6 weeks	Garlic odor for several hours, symptoms of IC/BPS may initially worsen

The tricyclic antidepressant amitriptyline (Elavil) is also frequently utilized as initial therapy, and it too has demonstrated modest benefit when compared to placebo. Based on the increased number of detrusor mast cells that have been associated with IC/BPS, antihistamines such as hydroxyzine (Vistaril) have been studied as a possible therapy, but the results to date have been disappointing. Anticonvulsants that are useful for other pain conditions (gabapentin, pregabalin) have been utilized to treat IC/BPS, but the data are too few to determine efficacy at this time. A single research group has reported promising results with the use of low-dose cyclosporine, but these results need to be reproduced before treatment with this potentially toxic drug can be recommended for use outside clinical trials. For certain patients with severe and refractory pain, oral narcotics can provide some benefit. Many other therapies have been studied or described, but the evidence to support their use is scant.

EVIDENCE AT A GLANCE

A systematic review of the literature through 2007 assessed the efficacy of various pharmacologic approaches to interstitial cystitis/bladder pain syndrome (IC/BPS).

Pooled analysis suggested a modest benefit to oral pentosan polysulfate treatment compared with placebo, with a relative risk of 1.78 for patient-reported "global improvement" in symptoms (95% confidence interval 1.34–2.35). The evidence also suggested a benefit for intravesical dimethyl sulfoxide and oral amitriptyline therapy, but there were insufficient data for the effect of these agents to be conclusive.

Intravesical

A variety of agents have been utilized as intravesical instillation therapy for IC/BPS symptoms. One mainstay of therapy has been dimethyl sulfoxide (DMSO), which is the only FDA-approved intravesical agent for the treatment of IC/BPS. DMSO is a product of the wood pulp industry and is a solvent with anti-inflammatory, bacteriostatic, analgesic, and muscle relaxant activities. It is typically administered in the office setting as a course of six instillations each given a week apart. Intravesical DMSO administration is quite safe, with no adverse systemic affects. However, it can cause the IC/BPS symptoms to worsen transiently. Also, systemic absorption of the DMSO results in a garlic odor that persists for several days. Response rates of up to 70% have been reported.

Another approach is to combine a variety of agents with or without DMSO for intravesical instillation. Common ingredients in these intravesical "cocktails" include heparin, sodium bicarbonate, hyaluronic acid, and pentosan polysulfate. Although this management approach is quite common, evidence to support its efficacy is lacking. Intravesical BCG has also been studied for use to treat IC/BPS. Initial uncontrolled trials of this agent were promising, but a subsequent randomized controlled trial failed to demonstrate efficacy. Intravesical therapy with numerous other agents has been described, but the evidence to support their use is minimal.

Intravesical instillations of lidocaine are often utilized to treat IC/BPS "flares." These instillations are most commonly performed in the office setting, but certain patients may be instructed on how to perform the instillations at home as needed. The lidocaine is typically alkalinized based on in vitro evidence that alkalinization improves the absorption of the lidocaine and increases its duration of efficacy. Some patients utilize this therapy on a daily basis, but most use it only as salvage therapy for symptom exacerbations.

EVIDENCE AT A GLANCE

A systematic review of intravesical treatments for interstitial cystitis/bladder pain syndrome (IC/BPS) included studies published up until May 30, 2006. Nine eligible trials were identified, with a total of 616 subjects. These included trials of six different intravesical preparations (resiniferatoxin, dimethyl sulfoxide, bacillus Calmette–Guérin, pentosan polysulfate, oxybutynin, urinary pH alkalinization). Overall, the evidence base for treating IC/BPS using intravesical preparations was limited, and the quality of trial reports was mixed. Conclusive evidence to support any of the therapies was absent. Adverse events were commonly reported after instillation, irrespective of whether "active" or placebo treatments were administered.

Surgical

In addition to providing diagnostic information, hydrodistension may have therapeutic benefit in certain patients, although the duration of the improvement is typically short (months at most). In patients with Hunner ulcers, resection or fulguration of the ulcers can provide dramatic and long-term symptom resolution. Currently, this is the single instance where a true "cure" is reliably obtained in patients with IC/BPS. Sacral neuromodulation has been utilized for the treatment of IC/BPS, and it is clear that this therapy may benefit certain patients. While some reductions in pain have been observed, it appears that the urinary frequency component is more effectively treated with sacral neuromodulation than the pain component of the symptoms.

In certain end-stage IC/BPS patients with severe symptoms and reduced bladder capacity, more aggressive surgical approaches may be considered. Bladder augmentation utilizing bowel segments has been performed, but this treatment has been largely abandoned due to poor results (persistent pain). More commonly, urinary diversion is performed so that the urine is diverted away from the bladder into an incontinent urostomy or a continent catheterizable urinary pouch. These urinary diversion procedures can be effective for symptom control in carefully selected patients. However, they involve significant risks, and this approach eliminates the possibility of other less invasive treatment options. Furthermore, postoperative resolution of all IC/BPS symptoms is not guaranteed.

Pelvic floor muscle dysfunction

The primary support for the pelvic organs comes from the levator ani muscles and associated connective tissue, which form a horizontal plane under the bladder and urethra. It is well known that laxity of these structures is associated with the development of pelvic prolapse. Conversely, abnormal tension or abnormal sensory processing in these structures can be associated with pain and functional abnormalities. The term "pelvic floor muscle dysfunction" is used to describe these abnormalities. PFMD frequently coexists with other pelvic pathology, possibly due to the fact that the levator muscles and the pelvic organs share the same innervation (S2–S4). For instance, the reported prevalence of PFMD in patients with IC/BPS is 85%.

Common symptoms of PFMD include pelvic pain, constipation, dyspareunia, urinary hesitancy, increased residual urine volumes, and back pain. These are nonspecific symptoms, and the diagnosis of PFMD is largely based on the identification of muscle or connective tissue abnormalities (tenderness, trigger points, tight muscle bands, decreased mobility, increased tone, etc.). Relaxation techniques and skeletal muscle relaxants may improve the symptoms, but the mainstay of therapy is pelvic floor physical therapy. PFMD can exist as a secondary abnormality in patients with chronic pelvic pain due to other etiologies, and it is reasonable to assume that recognition and treatment of the PFMD in these patients is quite important for optimal outcomes.

Dyspareunia

Dyspareunia is a Greek expression for "ill mating" and is used in the medical literature to define pain with sexual intercourse or sexual pain. It is described as persistent or recurrent pain with attempted or complete vaginal entry and/or penile vaginal intercourse. It should be distinguished from *vaginismus*, which is characterized as difficulties of the woman to allow vaginal entry of the penis, a finger, and/or any object despite her expressed wish to do so. The World Health Organization estimates that dyspareunia is reported by 8–22% of women in the general population. In the context of urologic illnesses, dyspareunia may be experienced by patients suffering from recurrent urinary tract infections, lower urinary tract symptoms and IC/BPS: as many as 75% of women with IC/BPS report such difficulties.

Diagnosis

Since dyspareunia is present in a variety of medical conditions such as IC/BPS, vulvodynia, vestibulodynia, endometriosis, and others, a careful differential diagnosis is necessary to guide intervention. A diagnostic work-up should include a detailed history of the pain as well as the patient's response to it and its effect on the couple. Physical examination of the urinary structures and the vaginal vault can lead to a more precise location of the pain. In patients with IC/BPS, dyspareunia is diagnosed when pain, rather than the urge, can be provoked by palpating the urethra and the base of the bladder.

It is helpful to ask specifically about sexual pain because patients may not report it without prompting. Including a partner in the discussion during the diagnostic interview can facilitate information-gathering as well as legitimize the need to address sexual pain/dyspareunia as a part of the experience and management of the urologic disorder.

> ### ★ TRICKS & TIPS
> When doing an internal examination, it may be helpful for the patient to view the examination in a mirror. Many women are not well acquainted with their genitals and their function. Giving the patient a mirror and involving her in the examination provides education and involves the woman in the process of evaluation.

Psychosexual dysfunction

The experience of dyspareunia can have a significant effect on sexual functioning. Pain and/or fear of pain can diminish desire for sexual activity and impair the patient's orgasmic capacity. Associated anxiety and or depression can also complicate the picture.

> ### ⚠ CAUTION
> It is important to recognize that dyspareunia can lead to psychological and sexual difficulties and that the psychological difficulties may further potentiate the experience of sexual pain. Both the physiologic pain and the psychological and sexual distress must be addressed as bona fide components of the same problem and not blamed on one another.

Treatment

Since dyspareunia is a multidimensional disorder, its treatment requires a multidimensional, multidisciplinary approach. A team of clinicians with expertise in urology, physical therapy, and sex therapy can help the individual and the couple understand the condition and its management, with the aim of gradually regaining sexual functioning to the extent possible in each individual case. Patients and partners should be informed of the effects and limitations of available approaches to dyspareunia treatment so that they can participate fully in their care. Although evidence regarding the efficacy of treatment of dyspareunia is primarily based on clinical expertise and has been developed in the context of gynecologic disease, research in the management of dyspareunia in urologic disease is beginning to develop.

Medical

Antidepressants such as venlafaxine (Effexor) or amitriptyline have been used with some effect without eliminating pain completely. Their positive contribution to pain relief must be balanced by their effect on sexual functioning—loss of desire and diminished orgasmic capacity. More recently, a promising new approach has used an intravesical instillation of a mixture of lidocaine, bicarbonate, and heparin with moderate success. However, the researchers did not report the effect of using this mixture on their subjects' sexual arousal.

Physical

Pelvic floor rehabilitation and vaginal electromyographic biofeedback have been used with some success in combination with medical and psychological approaches in the treatment of dyspareunia.

Sex therapy

Patients are encouraged to empty their bladder prior to sexual activity so as to minimize pain. Learning about positions for intercourse that are most comfortable can help optimize the experience. Cognitive-behavioral approaches can be used to redirect thinking and distract the patient from pain. Patients can practise such thinking exercises with the use of a vibrator to stimulate pleasure before attempting partnered sex. Patients can learn to distinguish between discomfort and pain as a useful way to make decisions about whether to pursue penetrative sexual activity or decline it in favor of limited sexual intimacy or affection. Discomfort can be typically overcome during sexual activity, while pain can lead to sexual and emotional trauma. Gaining control over one's sexual experience through these techniques can prepare the individual for a positive experience with a partner.

Couple sex therapy

Patients and partners can learn together how to maximize sexual pleasure by learning to communicate effectively during sexual activity. When both parties recognize the legitimacy of the pain concern, they can work together on deciding when sexual intercourse might be initially uncomfortable but ultimately satisfying, or when they might resort to nonpenetrative sex to avoid pain and sexual trauma.

Conclusions

Chronic pain in the urethra or bladder may be due to a variety of sources, some of which are readily treatable. A systematic approach, including a thorough history, a focused physical examination, and basic laboratory tests can provide clues to the presence of specific, identifiable sources of the symptoms. Additional diagnostic tests such as cystoscopy, imaging studies, and bladder biopsies may be warranted in selected patients. The diagnosis of IC/BPS should be reserved for patients in whom this diagnostic approach fails to identify an alternative source for the symptoms. IC/BPS symptoms can be improved with treatment, although no single therapy is uniformly successful and therefore it is common for patients to receive multiple therapies. Dyspareunia is frequently reported in patients with IC/BPS and may have a major impact on their quality of life. It is important to identify and address this when present.

Selected bibliography

Abrams P, Cardozo L, Fall M et al. The standardization of terminology of lower urinary tract function: report from the standardization sub-committee of the International Conti-nence Society. Neurourol Urodyn 2002;21: 167–78.

Clemens JQ, Joyce GF, Wise M, Payne C. Intersti-tial cystitis and painful bladder syndrome. In: Litwin MS, Saigal CS, eds. Urologic diseases in America. US Department of Health and Human Services, Public Health Service, National Insti-tutes of Health, National Institute of Diabetes and Digestive and Kidney Diseases. Washing-ton, DC: US Government Publishing Office, 2007. pp.123–56.

Dawson TE, Jamison J. Intravesical treatments for painful bladder syndrome/interstitial cystitis. Cochrane Database Syst Rev 2007, Issue 4. Art. No.: CD006113.

Dimitrakov J, Kroenke K, Steers WD et al. Phar-macologic management of painful bladder syndrome/interstitial cystitis. Arch Intern Med 2007;167:1922–9.

FitzGerald MP, Anderson RU, Potts J et al. for the Urological Pelvic Pain Collaborative Research Network. Randomized multicenter feasibility trial of myofascial physical therapy for the treatment of urological chronic pelvic pain syndromes. J Urol 2009;182:570–80.

Hanno PM, Landis JR, Matthews-Cook Y, Kusek J, Nyberg L, Jr. The diagnosis of interstitial cystitis revisited: lessons learned from the National Institutes of Health Interstitial Cystitis Data-base study. J Urol 1999;161:553–7.

Heim LJ. Evaluation and differential diagnosis of dyspareunia. Am Fam Phys 2001;63: 1535–44.

Homma Y, Ueda T, Tomoe H et al. and the Inter-stitial Cystitis Guideline Committee. Clinical guidelines for interstitial cystitis and hypersen-sitive bladder syndrome. Int J Urol 2009;16: 597–615.

Keay SK, Szekely Z, Conrads TP et al. An antipro-liferative factor from interstitial cystitis patients is a frizzled 8 protein-related sialoglycopep-tide. Proc Natl Acad Sci U S A 2004;101: 11803–8.

Latthe P, Latthe M, Say I, Gulmezoglu M, Khan KS. WHO systematic review of prevalence of chronic pelvic pain: a neglected reproductive health morbidity. BMC Pub Health 2006; 6:177–83.

Peters KM, Carrico DJ, Kalinowski SE, Ibrahim IA, Diokno AC. Prevalence of pelvic floor dysfunc-tion in patients with interstitial cystitis. Urology 2007;70:16–18.

Peters KM, Killinger KA, Carrico DJ, Ibrahim IA, Kiokno AC, Graziottin A. Sexual function and sexual distress in women with interstitial cysti-tis: a case controlled study. Urology 2007; 70:543–7.

Romanzi LJ, Groutz A, Blaivas JG, Urethral diver-ticulum in women: diverse presentations resulting in diagnostic delay and mismanage-ment. J Urol 2000;164:428–33.

Schultz WW, Basson R, Binik Y, Eschenbach D, Wesselmann U, Van Lankveld J. Women's sexual pain and its management. J Sex Med 2005;2:301–16.

Steege JF, Zolnoun DA. Evaluation and treatment of dyspareunia. Obstet Gynecol 2009;113: 1124–36.

van de Merwe JP, Nordling J, Bouchelouche P et al. Diagnostic criteria, classification, and nomenclature for painful bladder syndrome/ interstitial cystitis: an ESSIC proposal. Eur Urol 2008;53:60–7.

Welk BK, Teichman MH. Dyspareunia response in patients with interstitial cystitis treated with intravesical lidocaine, bicarbonate and heparin. Urology 2008;71:67–70.

Chronic Pelvic Pain of Enterocolic Origin

Andrea J. Rapkin and Tevy Tith

Department of Obstetrics and Gynecology, University of California, Los Angeles, California, USA

Introduction

"Chronic pelvic pain" (CPP) refers to pelvic pain in the same location lasting 6 months or more. Dysfunction or pathology of the gastrointestinal tract commonly manifests as CPP. The most common enterocolic conditions presenting as CPP are the functional pain disorders irritable bowel syndrome (IBS), and functional abdominal pain and bloating. A thorough medical history and knowledge of the differential diagnosis of enterocolic pain and of the inclusion criteria for the functional abdominal pain disorders can help the clinician to distinguish when chronic pain derives from enterocolic pathology.

Up to 60% of women referred to a gynecologist for CPP are found to have IBS. These patients often seek the care of a gynecologist or may be referred to gynecologist as opposed to a gastroenterologist for a number of reasons:

- The functional pain disorders, especially IBS, have a female predominance, affecting twice as many women as men.
- Gastrointestinal pain is generally exacerbated by the premenstrual and menstrual phases of the cycle and can be confused with pain related to gynecologic pathology.
- Many gynecologic disorders such as endometriosis and dysmenorrhea are accompanied by gastrointestinal symptoms, including bloating, constipation, and pain in association with bowel movements.

- Women with IBS often have gynecologic symptoms such as dysmenorrhea and dyspareunia.
- The colon and reproductive organs share the same thoracolumbar and sacral autonomic and somatic innervations and thus have common regions of pain referral.
- Inflammation or infection in one organ can decrease the threshold for pain sensation in other pelvic organs and overlying muscle.

Epidemiology

Between 20% and 40% of the general female population suffer from CPP. A major proportion of these women also suffer from IBS. IBS prevalence rates of 50–79% are typical among women with CPP seen in gynecologic referral clinics. IBS and other gastrointestinal diagnoses, including diverticulitis and diverticulosis, accounted for almost 42% of all diagnoses in one study of a general practice database in Great Britain. Age over 40, a history of muscular back pain, fibromyalgia, or six or more pain sites, and physical abuse in adulthood were associated with the diagnosis of IBS in a multivariate model of women with CPP. The IBS diagnosis was missed 40% of the time, and IBS treatments were not initiated in 67% of CPP patients with IBS.

Reproductive and gastrointestinal system pain disorders often share common symptoms, and the presence of symptoms related to more than one pelvic organ system was associated with more severe pain and disability. Among

Chronic Pelvic Pain, First Edition. Edited by Paolo Vercellini.
© 2011 Blackwell Publishing Ltd. Published 2011 by Blackwell Publishing Ltd.

women with IBS, at least 43% reported dyspareunia. Fifty-five percent of women with suffering from both CPP and IBS (and who had urinary symptoms) refrained to some degree from intercourse due to pain, whereas only 22% of those with CPP alone had less sexual activity due to pain. Up to 43% of women with CPP alone, compared to 58% with both CPP and IBS, rated their pain as moderate to severe. Dysmenorrhea was also more severe if both CPP and IBS were present.

Twenty percent of hysterectomies in the United States are performed for CPP, and although abdominal hysterectomy does not appear to increase the risk of developing IBS, women with IBS are more three times more likely to have had a hysterectomy or other surgery for CPP. If operative laparoscopy or abdominal hysterectomy was performed for CPP, there was less improvement in pain in women with IBS.

There is significant comorbidity of IBS with other chronic visceral and somatic functional pain and mood disorders primarily affecting women, such as endometriosis-related pain syndrome, painful bladder syndrome/interstitial cystitis, fibromyalgia, migraine, anxiety, and depression. It is estimated that 42–59% of patients with some sort of functional bowel disorder have an associated psychiatric disorder, and stress is a major common denominator. Patients with panic disorder had the highest rate of unexplained gastrointestinal symptoms (7.2%), with a fivefold increased risk of having IBS-like symptoms compared to those without panic disorder. Substantial proportions of patients with refractory IBS symptoms suffered from coexisting depression (39%) and anxiety (10%).

Enterocolic and pelvic innervation

The pelvic organs (lower gastrointestinal tract, reproductive and genitourinary systems) derive innervation from the thoracolumbar (sympathetic) and sacral (parasympathetic) autonomic nervous system, as well as the lumbosacral somatic sensory nervous system. Innervation of the lower gastrointestinal tract and other pelvic viscera and surrounding somatic tissues is outlined in Table 10.1.

Projections from the thoracolumbar and sacral spinal cord converge into peripheral neuronal plexuses and then distribute fibers throughout the pelvis. Most of the visceral afferents converge on the dorsal root ganglia and enter the spinal cord through the dorsal roots. The important nervous plexuses in pelvis are the superior hypogastric plexus, hypogastric plexus, inferior hypogastric plexus (IHP), and pelvic splanchnic nerve. The IHP, located in the retroperitoneal tissues lateral to the rectum, is a major neuronal integrative center for most of the pelvic organs: urinary bladder, urethra, distal ureter, rectum, internal anal sphincter, upper vagina, cervix, uterus, and proximal fallopian tubes. In females, the anterior division of this IHP is referred to as the paracervical ganglia and provides innervation to the clitoris, vagina, and periurethral tissues.

Sympathetic autonomic input into the IHP arises from fibers originating in the thoracolumbar segments T10–L1 of the spinal cord, with nerve cell bodies in the dorsal root ganglia; nerve fibers then project and fuse distally before diverging into branches destined for the IHP, which condense into the superior hypogastric plexus. Parasympathetic autonomic nerves arise from cell bodies of the sacral nuclei located in the intermediolateral gray matter of the spinal cord at S2–S4. These nerves fuse as the pelvic splanchnic nerve and enter the IHP. Parasympathetic afferents also course through the splanchnic nerves and have cell bodies in the dorsal root ganglia of S2–S4. Parasympathetic fibers encode the full range of sensations from the lower gastrointestinal tract, including pain.

SCIENCE REVISITED

The vagina, cervix, uterus, and adnexa share the same visceral innervation as the large intestine, rectum, and lower small intestine. Therefore pain from both the reproductive organs and the gastrointestinal tract are referred to the same dermatomes.

True visceral pain is a diffuse, poorly localized sensation. Acutely visceral pain is associated often with autonomic changes such as pallor, diaphoresis, and alterations in blood pressure or heart rate, but these changes are absent in chronic visceral pain states. This nondescript pain results in part because of the relatively few sensory nerves from the viscera, the lack of second-order neurons in the dorsal horn of the spinal cord that respond solely to visceral sensation, and the extensive divergence of visceral afferent input.

Referred pain is thought to be caused by the convergence of somatic and visceral afferents onto the same second-order sensory neurons in the dorsal horn of the spinal cord, leading to sharper, well-localized pain. Referred visceral pan is not accompanied by neurovegetative signs.

Table 10.1 Nerves carrying nociceptive impulses from the pelvic organs and surrounding somatic tissues

Anatomic structure	Spinal segments	Nerves
Rectosigmoid, rectum, and internal anal sphincter, upper vagina, cervix, lower uterine segment, uterosacral, and cardinal ligaments, lower ureters, posterior urethra, bladder trigone	S2-4	Pelvic (sacral) autonomics (parasympathetics)
Terminal ileum, cecum, appendix, distal large bowel, upper bladder uterine fundus, broad ligament, proximal fallopian tubes	T11–12, L1	Thoracolumbar autonomics (sympathetic) through the inferior hypogastric plexus
Ascending colon Transverse colon Descending colon	S2–S4 L1–L2	Pelvic (sacral) autonomics (parasympathetics) through the inferior hypogastric plexus Lumbar autonomic (sympathetics) innervation through celiac, mesenteric, and superior hypogastric plexuses
Outer two-thirds of fallopian tubes, upper ureters	T9–10	Thoracic autonomics (sympathetics) through aortic and superior mesenteric plexuses
Ovaries	T9–10	Thoracic autonomics (sympathetics) through renal and aortic plexuses and celiac and mesenteric ganglia
Lower abdominal wall and inguinal region	T12–L1 T12–L1 L1–2	Iliohypogastric nerve Ilioinguinal nerve Genitofemoral nerve
External anal sphincter and puborectalis muscle	S2–4	Medial branches of the pudendal nerve
Perineum, vulva, lower vagina	S2–4 L1, L2	Pudendal, vaginal branch of S2, ilioinguinal, genital branch of genitofemoral, posterofemoral cutaneous
Pelvic floor muscles Levator ani muscles (puborectalis, iliococcygeus, piriformis) Obturator internus	S2-4	Pudendal nerve (S2-4) and division of sacral nerves (S2–3) mingle with fibers of the inferior hypogastric plexus

Viscerovisceral and viscerosomatic cross-sensitization

There is a high co-occurrence of IBS, painful bladder syndrome, endometriosis-related pain syndrome, and vulvodynia. It is not surprising that gastrointestinal and reproductive and genitourinary tract symptoms overlap with referred pain from the pelvic viscera.

The uterus and inner parts of the adnexa share the same visceral innervation with the distal ileum, ascending, transverse, and sigmoid colon (T10–L1), and the ovaries and the lower small bowel both derive innervation from the T9–T10 spinal segments. The cervix, upper vagina, descending colon, and rectum share innervation through nerves traveling with the sacral autonomics (S2–S4), and the somatic innervation of the lower vagina, vulva, and perineum and anus is via S2 and the pudendal nerve (S2–S4) (see Table 10.1). Within the central nervous system (CNS), there are neurons that receive convergent input from the uterus, colon, and bladder. This cross-system or cross-sensitization could potentially provide a mechanism whereby pathology in one organ would influence the functioning of another organ. Comorbidity of chronic medically unexplained pain and mood disorders can also be attributed to stress-mediated alterations in CNS processing in genetically predisposed individuals.

Studies have shown cross-organ interactions between the reproductive, gastrointestinal, and urinary tracts. Neural "crosstalk" in the pelvis occurs when afferent activation of one pelvic structure alters the neural output and input of another organ. Cross-sensitization results in a lowering of the threshold for sensation (painful and nonpainful, i.e., hyperalgesia and allodynia) in one organ or tissue due to inflammation of or neural up-regulation in different pelvic viscera, with resultant sensory interaction between two different internal organs. Thus, women with IBS have more severe dysmenorrhea, possibly because of shared neural pathways between the uterus and lower gastrointestinal tract.

Evaluation of chronic pelvic pain with enterocolic symptoms

In evaluating a patient with gastrointestinal complaints and CPP, it is important to rule out an acute surgical abdomen and an infectious, inflammatory, or neoplastic etiology before assuming the pain is of a benign functional nature. A functional disorder is one in which an organic cause cannot be found.

History

A thorough history delineates the pain intensity (quantified on a verbal analog scale from 0 = no pain to 10 = the most severe pain imaginable), events proximal to the onset of the pain (bacterial gastroenteritis, stress, major life events, lifestyle changes, etc.), change in the symptoms over time, duration of the pain when it occurs, whether the pain is persistent or intermittent, and its quality, location, and alleviating/aggravating factors.

It is important to query the relationship of pain to bowel movements and to changes in the form and/or frequency of bowel movements, change in the caliber of bowel movement, presence of mucous in the stool, straining, urgency, incomplete evacuation, abdominal distension or bloating, nausea, fecal soiling, and the effect of eating or stress. To rule out infectious and iatrogenic causes of gastrointestinal symptoms, dietary, travel, and medication histories are necessary. Since IBS is defined by symptoms within a criteria set called the Rome Criteria (see the "Evidence at a glance" box below), symptom questions regarding the relationship of the bowel movement to the pain must be asked. Symptoms of acute and/or potentially morbid conditions including red flag warning signs (see "Tips & tricks") should be solicited: rectal bleeding, anorexia, persistent watery stools, weight loss, emesis, a major change in symptoms, fever, syncope, or current pregnancy.

Although many CPP disorders (e.g., endometriosis, adenomyosis, pelvic congestion, painful bladder syndrome, IBS) are exacerbated by the perimenstrual phases of the menstrual cycle, making this connection is the key to a diagnosis of gynecologic pathology and may help with management by suppressing menses, etc. A general history for CPP also documents associated visceral and somatic symptoms such as abnormal vaginal bleeding, dysmenorrhea, dyspareunia, urinary symptoms (frequency, urgency, dysuria, hematuria), and myofascial or neuropathic pain symptoms and conditions.

The meaning of the pain for the patient (e.g., fear of cancer, fear of fecal soiling), the impact on activities of daily living, sex, personal relationships, and occupation, and disability or litigation related to the pain should be determined. A thorough psychosocial history should be taken, including current stressors, stressful past life events, substance use and abuse, and past and current psychiatric symptoms and diagnoses. It is very helpful to use validated questionnaires for the assessment of depression, anxiety, physical, and sexual and emotional (past and current) trauma.

Any prior evaluations, including diagnostic studies, operative and pathology reports, or past treatments for pain, should be included. The family history is particularly important in evaluating for inflammatory bowel disease (IBD), IBS, endometriosis, and colon cancer.

★ TIPS & TRICKS

Red flag warning signs for comorbid conditions:
- Age over 50 years
- Rectal bleeding or positive fecal occult blood
- Watery stool or refractory diarrhea
- Abrupt changes in bowel characteristics
- Weight loss
- Anorexia
- Abdominal mass
- Anemia
- Family history of colon cancer.

Physical examination

An acute abdomen, a palpable abdominal mass, ascites, or organomegaly should be ruled out first. A "pain mapping" examination is recommended for the evaluation of all women with CPP. Each somatic and visceral structure should be palpated separately when possible. Localized point tenderness (versus diffuse tenderness) of the abdominal wall, vulva, or pelvic floor suggests musculoskeletal or neuropathic sources rather than visceral one.

The Carnett test can be used for this: localize the painful point(s) on the abdominal wall, ask the patient to perform a bilateral straight leg raise or abdominal crunch, repalpate the tender point, and if the pain is increased and not diminished,

the test is considered positive and correlates well with an abdominal wall etiology or component, such as myofascial trigger point, iliohypogastric neuropathy, ilioinguinal neuropathy, or uncommonly a hernia. The presence of a mass alerts the clinician to order further diagnostic studies for elucidation.

A vulvar examination should include a cotton swab test of the vestibule if there is entry dyspareunia. A pelvic examination should sequentially evaluate the anterior vaginal wall for bladder or urethral tenderness, the cervix for motion tenderness, and the paracervical region for tenderness in the region of the IHP (suggesting neural up-regulation) and for nodularity (indicating possible endometriosis or cancer), and then uterine size, shape, and consistency, fixed position, and tenderness should be ascertained; this should if possible be done without palpating the bladder if there is bladder tenderness. The pelvic floor muscles should be tested for tenderness, tightness, and ability to contract and relax. Tenderness of the pudendal nerve area should be checked. A rectovaginal examination is particularly important for ruling out rectal masses, for examining the uterosacral ligaments for nodularity, and for performing a test for fecal occult blood.

Diagnostic studies

A fecal occult blood test is important, and a complete blood count is performed for signs of infection or anemia suggesting occult bleeding or chronic disease. A transvaginal ultrasound should be a part of the work-up for CPP. Other imaging studies such as computed tomography (CT) with contrast, magnetic resonance imaging (MRI), or abdominal ultrasound should be considered where appropriate or in patients with warning signs (see the "Tips & tricks" box above) or where the differential includes other organic causes. For those with the following warning signs— symptom onset over the age of 50, rectal bleeding, anemia of unknown etiology, positive fecal occult blood, family history of colon cancer, weight loss, or a major change in symptoms—a colonoscopy should be performed.

A pregnancy test, gonorrhea and chlamydia screen, Papanicolaou smear, and routine laboratory studies (blood chemistry, liver, kidney, and thyroid function) are performed as indicated. Special consideration must be made where celiac sprue is in the differential diagnosis, particularly in those with signs of malnutrition or anemia. If celiac disease is suspected, individuals can be empirically tested with a gluten-containing diet, or assays for antibodies to endomysium or tissue transglutaminase or antigliadin can be done.

Irritable bowel syndrome

IBS, often called "hypersensitive gut syndrome," is a functional pain disorder characterized by recurrent abdominal pain or discomfort and altered bowel habits. Because of the strong association between IBS and stress, and the altered CNS processing associated with the syndrome, it has recently been described as a "brain–gut" disorder. The epidemiology of IBS has been described above. The first time women usually present with IBS is between 30 and 50 years of age.

Pathophysiology

The lowered threshold for sensation, increased intensity of visceral pain, and enlarged viscerosomatic region of pain referral are the hallmark of IBS and constitute a visceral hypersensitivity that is thought to contribute to the discomfort and pain of IBS. The visceral hypersensitivity, demonstrated in both human and animal models, appears to be a consequence of CNS sensitization. Up to 95% of female subjects with IBS exhibit enhanced sensitivity to balloon distension of the rectum in experimental studies. Altered gastrointestinal motility and secretion, as well as abnormal immune activation of the gastrointestinal mucosa and alterations in gut microflora, may contribute to the altered frequency and form of stool and to abdominal bloating.

Perimenstrual exacerbation may be related to the release of prostaglandins, which can sensitize the nerves of the gut, to hormonal actions, or to the effect of hormones on mediators in the central or peripheral nervous system. Experimental subjects with IBS manifest increased rectal sensitivity to balloon distension at the time of menses.

Studies have identified that adverse early life events are significant risk factors for IBS and other functional pain syndromes. CPP, anxiety, depression, and somatization, post-traumatic stress disorder (PTSD), fibromyalgia, temporomandibular joint syndrome, migraines, burning mouth syndrome, and interstitial cystitis/painful bladder syndrome are present more often in women with IBS. Many patients with these chronic "medically unexplained" pain syndromes have been exposed to early stressful childhood events and exhibited excessive childhood shyness, anxieties, or phobias, which implicates excessive autonomic and hypothalamic–pituitary–adrenal system activation. This enhanced stress responsiveness—or hypervigilance—may be programmed into the central and peripheral nervous systems, potentiating stimulus perception.

In addition to behavioral changes in IBS patients, structural brain abnormalities and neural changes are evident. Functional MRI studies of women with IBS, fibromyalgia, migraine, or PTSD show a decrease in gray matter density or cortical thickness in the frontal cortex, cingulate cortex, hippocampus, and perihippocampal gyrus. Positron emission tomography scans to evaluate blood flow in specific areas of the brain during painful rectal balloon distension in females with IBS revealed increased cerebral blood flow in regions of the brain that are involved in anticipation of pain.

Clinical manifestations and diagnosis

IBS is characterized by abdominal pain and dysfunctional defecation. The diagnosis for IBS is one of exclusion, based on satisfying the Rome Criteria (see the "Evidence at a glance" box). The following symptoms must be present for at least 3 months: disturbed defecation and abdominal pain at least 3 days per month relieved by defecation and associated with changes in stool form or frequency. Patients should be subclassified as predominant diarrhea- or constipation-predominant IBS or mixed stool habits.

Once the Rome Criteria have been met, and in the absence of red flag warning signs, a diagnosis of IBS can be made. Other causes of altered bowel habits such as Crohn's disease, ulcerative colitis (UC), or celiac sprue should be ruled out if indicated. If the Rome Criteria are met and the warning signs are absent, a serologic test for celiac sprue is also indicated before initiating treatment for IBS in high-risk populations. If warning signs are positive, perform a complete blood count, thyroid-stimulating hormone test, and stool examination for ova, parasites, and, if indicated, specific bacteria; a gastrointestinal subspeciality consultation should be arranged.

EVIDENCE AT A GLANCE

The Rome III Criteria for the diagnosis of irritable bowel syndrome (IBS) are as follow:

Abdominal pain or discomfort occurring for 3 or more days per month for at least 3 months over the past year, and two or more of the following:
- Alleviation of symptoms with defecation
- Onset of pain is associated with a change in stool frequency
- Onset of pain is associated with a change in stool appearance or form.

Supportive symptoms that are not part of the diagnostic criteria:
- Three or fewer bowel movements per week
- More than three bowel movements per day
- Abnormal stool form, lumpy/hard stool
- Loose/watery stool
- Defecation straining
- Urgency
- A feeling of incomplete bowel movement
- Passing mucus
- Bloating.

Subtyping IBS by predominant stool pattern:
- IBS with constipation—hard or lumpy stools in 25% or more and loose or watery stools in fewer than 25% of bowel movements
- IBS with diarrhea—loose (mushy) or watery stools in 25% or more and hard or lumpy stool in fewer than 25% of bowel movements
- Mixed IBS—hard or lumpy stools in 25% or more and loose (mushy) or watery stools in 25% or more of bowel movements
- Unsubtyped IBS—insufficient abnormality of stool consistency to meet the criteria for any of the above subtypes.

Management

Therapy for IBS is multimodal. There must be an established physician–patient relationship as better outcomes have been seen in patients who had more contact with their physician. Edu-cation regarding the role of the brain (that it is a brain–gut disorder, triggering factors such as physical and emotional stress) should be provided, and realistic expectations must be set—i.e., patients must understand that this will likely be a chronic disorder and that there is no magic bullet. Dietary modifications can be tried. Lactose intolerance and food allergies can often present with similar symptoms so a trial of a lactose-free diet or a diet low in gas-forming foods may be therapeutic. The addition of fiber may help with diarrhea-predominant IBS. The various medications for alleviating diarrhea, constipation, and/or pain symptoms generally modulate the neurophysiology of the disorder (see the "Evidence at a glance" box below).

For diarrhea, anti-diarrheal medications decrease motility. Urgency can be managed with tricyclic antidepressants, which modulate the pain circuitry associated with IBS and help diarrhea by their anticholinergic effects. Aloset-ron (1 mg twice daily for 12 weeks) improved stool frequency, urgency, pain, and quality of life but has a limited U.S. FDA approval for women with severe diarrhea-predominant IBS of greater than 6 months' duration and carries a black box warning for rare complications such as ileus, bowel obstruction, fecal impaction, and perfora-tion and ischemic colitis.

For constipation-predominant IBS patients, laxatives and secretory stimulants (polyethylene glycol 3350, lactulose, lubiprostone) should be used. Tegaserod has modest efficacy in control-led trials and was approved by the FDA with restrictions, to be prescribed only to women under the age of 55 years with constipation-predominant IBS or chronic constipation without known ischemic cardiovascular risks or disease.

For IBS pain, antispasmodic drugs can help and antidepressants have salutary effects on the central and peripheral nervous systems for pain modulation, anxiety, and depression. A multi-disciplinary approach including pharmacologic and cognitive-behavioral psychological therapy, hypnotherapy, or yoga has the most potential for success; the number needed to treat for cognitive-behavioral therapy or hypnosis for one patient to be improved was 2.

EVIDENCE AT A GLANCE

Pharmacologic management of irritable bowel syndrome

Medication	Modes of action
Antidepressants • Tricyclic antidepressants (TCAs) • Selective serotonin reuptake inhibitors (SSRIs) • Selective norepinephrine reuptake inhibitors (SNRIs)	Central mechanisms: • Treat comorbid depression • Restore sleep • Analgesic • Antihyperalgesic Peripheral mechanisms: • Normalize gastrointestinal transit • Antineuropathic
TCAs • Amitriptyline (10–75 mg at night) • Nortriptyline (10–75 mg at night) • Desimipramine (50–150 mg)	Modulates descending serotonergic and noradrenergic (norepinephric) pain inhibition systems: • Decrease sensitivity to somatic painAnticholinergic: • Alter gastrointestinal motility
SSRIs • Paroxetine (10–60 mg/day) • Citalopram (5–20 mg/day) • Fluoxetine (20–40 mg/day)	5-HT$_2$ serotonin receptor agonist • Treat depression and anxiety • Decrease abdominal pain and bloating • Increase overall wellbeing
SNRIs • Duloxetine (30–60 mg/day) • Milnacipran (50–100 mg twice a day, titrated from 12.5 mg/day) • Venlafaxine (37.5–225 mg/day)	Affect descending serotonergic and noradrenergic pain inhibition systems
Antidiarrheals • Loperamide (2 mg/day)	Slow gut motility
Other, including antispasmodics • Alosetron (0.5–1 mg twice a day)	5-HT$_3$ receptor antagonist • Decreases stool frequency and bowel urgency • Relieves abdominal pain and discomfort
• Tegaserod (6 mg twice a day) • Hyoscyamine or mebeverine	Partial 5-HT$_4$ receptor agonist Antispasmodic

Postinfectious IBS

The development of IBS after an acute bacterial enteritis has been suspected based on the new occurrence of IBS symptoms in patients after a diarrheal illness that has been documented in 4–26% of women with IBS. The risk was increased in females who were younger, more anxious, and more depressed or who had prolonged fever.

Pathophysiology

Although the underlying mechanism is unclear, there is clearly a role for persistent inflammation in the pathogenesis of the condition. This process leads to an increased number of proinflammatory mediator cells and processes (enterochromaffin cells, T lymphocytes) and increased intestinal permeability. Several enteric pathogens lead to this phenomenon, including *Campylobacter* species, *Salmonella* species, and diarrheagenic strains of *Escherichia coli* and *Shigella*. It is possible that infection with these pathogens leads to more severe mucosal damage in the gastrointestinal tract.

Clinical manifestations and diagnosis

The diagnosis is made clinically when these patients meet the Rome Criteria for IBS after an episode of acute gastroenteritis. Most acute bacterial diarrheal illnesses are self-limited, with symptoms lasting less than 5 days. The onset of postinfectious IBS is usually insidious following an acute episode of enteritis. Acute gastroenteritis is diagnosed by at least two of the following: fever, vomiting, diarrhea, or a positive stool culture result. Traveler's diarrhea is defined as three or more loose stools with one or more symptom of infection (vomiting, abdominal pain, cramps) within a 24-hour period and at least 48 hours after arriving at a destination country.

Management

There are no widely accepted treatment options for postinfectious IBS. The management of symptoms is similar to that for IBS, focusing on symptom alleviation. Another arm of treatment is antibiotics, such as rifaximin (400 mg three times a day), which have reportedly benefited patients with documented intestinal bacterial overgrowth in the small intestine. Although there are many routes of therapy, only 14% of patients with IBS were completely satisfied with therapy, pointing to the need for primary prevention of the disease. Probiotics such as *Bifidobacterium infantus* 35624 (one capsule daily) may decrease bloating.

The remission rate for postinfectious IBS is generally better than that for IBS without an infectious onset (43% versus 32%). Complete remission rates are inversely related to the presence of coexisting psychiatric conditions.

Functional abdominal pain syndrome

Functional abdominal pain syndrome (FAPS) or "chronic functional abdominal pain" is prevalent in 1.7% of the general population. FAPS can significantly impair quality of life and is associated with significant absenteeism from work and many visits to the physician.

Clinical manifestations and diagnosis

The diagnosis is based on the following symptoms being present for at least 6 months: continuous or nearly continuous abdominal pain, pain not typically related to physiological events such as eating or menses, loss of daily function, absence of malingering, and lack of criteria for other enterocolic disorders that would cause abdominal pain. The patient often describes intense, diffuse, nonlocalized pain, often associated with other painful symptoms. Frequently, the pain is described in an emotional or bizarre fashion, and patients often request diagnostic studies or surgery and seek validation that the pain is secondary to an organic cause. They often deny a role for a psychosocial component of their pain and place high expectations on physicians to relieve the pain—requests for narcotics are common.

Management

As in IBS, there is a need for a good doctor–patient relationship that outlines pathophysiology, management plan, and goals, including concurrent psychological treatment. A multidisciplinary approach has the most potential for being efficacious. Analgesics are not effective, and narcotics should not be used in treatment. Anxiolytics should be used sparingly, if at all, but selective serotonin reuptake inhibitors or tricyclic antidepressants may be helpful. There are no good studies on psychotherapeutic approaches in this disorder. Overall, goals should be realistic, and there should be regular communication between the physician and the patient.

Functional bloating syndrome

"Bloating" refers to a sense of abdominal fullness, while "distension" refers to a visible or measurable increase in abdominal girth. This feeling of abdominal bloating is attributed to excessive gas production by patients and may or may not be associated with measurable distention. Up to 96% of IBS patients report symptoms of bloating. Community surveys reveal that 10–30% of individuals report bloating during the previous year. Like IBS, it is twice as common in women as men, and is exacerbated with menses.

Pathophysiology

Abdominal bloating may be secondary to delayed transit of gas in the small intestine, as compared to a healthy control population. A sensation of abdominal bloating sometimes is accompanied by increased girth (distension). It is a common and intrusive feature of functional bowel disorders. Bloating appears to be associated more frequently with visceral hypersensitivity, whereas distension is more often related to hyposensitivity and delayed transit. Many studies have shown that there is no single cause for bloating and distension. Food intolerance, abnormal gut bacterial flora, weak abdominal musculature, and fluid retention have been implicated but have not been proven in studies. Other hypotheses regarding the causes of bloating and distension include excess gas production, altered gas transit, abnormal perception of a normal amount of gas within the gastrointestinal tract, or dysfunctional somatic muscle activity in the abdominal wall.

Clinical manifestations and diagnosis

Diagnosis is based on the presence of two criteria: (1) a recurrent feeling of bloating or visible distension for at least 3 days per month over 3 months, and (2) insufficient criteria for a diagnosis of functional dyspepsia, IBS, FAPS, or other functional gastrointestinal disorder. There is typically a diurnal pattern of symptoms in which symptoms worsen after meals and throughout the day but improve or disappear overnight.

Management

Most research has been done on patients with IBS or other functional abdominal pain disorders. Treatment of bloating is symptom-based and is independent of whether it occurs in isolation or in association with another disorder. The goals of treatment are to reduce flatus, although data have not proven the importance of gut gas in bloating. Furthermore, symptoms of bloating may improve if associated gut syndromes, such as IBS or chronic constipation, are improved. Dietary exclusions may be worthwhile, especially if bloating is accompanied by diarrhea: avoid flatogenic foods or weight loss. The use of surfactants such as simethicone or antibiotics is also conflicting. The use of enzymes such as alpha-galactosidase—the active ingredient in Beano—may help decrease rectal passage of gas. Tegaserod may improve bloating in some IBS patients.

Diverticular disorders

Diverticulosis is one of the most common conditions in Western society. Approximately 5% of adults have diverticular disease by age 40, increasing to 30–40% in adults over 65 years of age. Of patients with diverticular disease, 20–30% have symptoms. There is some evidence to suggest that patients are developing diverticular disease at a younger age, and that the increasing prevalence of obesity is contributing to this. Between 20% and 60% of individuals will experience pain and inflammation/infection associated with their diverticulitis.

Pathophysiology

Diverticulosis is defined as small outpouchings in the colonic wall. These outpouchings tend to develop at specific sites where the vasa recta penetrate the bowel wall—weak points in the bowel wall. In Western countries, the disease often affects the sigmoid colon, whereas in Asian patients, it affects the proximal colon. The low-fiber Western diet may be one factor responsible for the development of diverticular disease; small-volume stools lead to alterations in colonic motility and a subsequent increase in intraluminal pressure, which leads to outpouchings in the colonic wall.

Clinical manifestations and diagnosis

Most patients with diverticulosis are asymptomatic. Patients can present with mild, intermittent attacks to severe, recurrent disease, separated by periods of mild colonic inflammation. Two-thirds of those with symptoms present with diverticulitis, while the other one third present with diverticular bleeding. Of those who are symptomatic, the most common symptom is abdominal pain, usually localized to the left lower quadrant. The pain often lasts hours to days, increases with eating, and decreases after passage of a bowel movement or flatus. Other less common symptoms include nausea, vomiting, crampy diarrhea, or constipation, flatulence, or dyspepsia. Morbid complications occur in 8% of patients with diverticulosis. One hallmark of diverticular disease is painless rectal bleeding; 5% of patients can present with massive hemorrhage or hypovolemia.

Diverticulitis occurs when there is inflammation of the diverticuli and can be associated with fever, generalized tenderness, or leukocytosis. Pain may be recurrent and chronic.

Potential complications include fistula formation, abscess, perforation, obstruction, or involvement of adjacent organs, referred to as complicated diverticulitis.

Abdominal examination may reveal tenderness in the region of the sigmoid colon. A mass is not usually palpable unless an abscess is present. The abdomen is usually soft and without rebound or guarding, unless diverticulitis is present. Diverticulitis is accompanied by fever and an elevated erythrocyte sedimentation rate, and diagnosis is confirmed by CT scanning with contrast or with barium enema.

Management of diverticulitis

Treatment of diverticulitis depends on multiple factors, such as the severity of illness, laboratory testing, the ability to tolerate oral antibiotics and hydration, and the presence of morbid complications. The mainstay of treatment of acute episodes of uncomplicated diverticulitis is broad-spectrum antibiotic therapy that covers Gram-negative organisms. Severe attacks with evidence of abscess, phlegmon, or obstruction require inpatient intravenous antibiotics, intravenous hydration, and pain control. Percutaneous drainage can be used for abscesses greater than 4 cm in size. In a select group of patients who suffer from chronic abdominal pain, there is some evidence that they may benefit from anti-inflammatory medications, such as 5-aminosalicyclic acid. Patients with recurrent attacks of acute diverticulitis who fail medical therapy may benefit from sigmoid resection, but this is controversial.

Inflammatory bowel disease

IBD is a complex of disorders that affects 1.5 million people in the United States and 2 million in Europe, and whose incidence is rising in Asia and other developing countries. IBD encompasses both Crohn's disease and UC. The incidence of UC is about three times that of Crohn's disease.

There appears to be a bimodal peak of IBD. The first peak occurs between the second and third decades, while the "late peak" occurs in the sixth to seventh decade. The incidence of Crohn's disease has increased over the years, while that of UC has remained the same. The risk factors are similar for both diseases: Ashkenazi Jewish descent, higher northern latitudes, especially Scandinavian regions, or having a family history of either disease. Crohn's disease is more common in smokers, whereas UC is less common in smokers.

In certain patients, symptoms are indistinguishable from those reported by patients with IBS, including bloating, abdominal distension, or a sensation of incomplete evacuation after a bowel movement. Symptoms may be chronic and intermittent in nature and may even be present during remission. The cancer risk in UC is increased by about 0.5% above baseline per year after diagnosis, and the risk of cancer is also increased with Crohn's disease.

Pathophysiology

IBD occurs when there is inappropriate or ongoing activation of the mucosal immune system secondary to normal bowel flora. Visceral pain can originate from a nonobstructed and inflamed bowel, from an inflamed bowel due to obstruction, or from an extension of the disease process beyond the bowel wall in the form of perforation, fistula, or abscess formations. Abdominal pain is more common in Crohn's than in UC, and probably results from stricture formation and an increased incidence of perirectal disease.

Differential diagnosis of inflammatory disease

Abdominal pain associated with diarrhea and rectal bleeding can present as a result of infectious gastroenteritis or colitis, antibiotic-related *Clostridium difficile* infections, or ischemic colitis. Ischemic colitis can present with nausea, vomiting, abdominal pain, fever, or signs of peritoneal irritation, and is more common in the elderly population. Other disorders included the differential diagnosis include tuberculosis, intestinal lymphoma, diverticulitis, colon cancer, and fungal infection. Colon cancer is something that must always be ruled out in elderly patients who present with anemia, weight loss, and chronic abdominal pain.

Crohn's disease

Crohn's disease is a chronic inflammatory condition, usually manifesting in the 15–30-year age range, that can affect the entire gastrointestinal tract, from mouth to anus. The inflammation is transmural, extending through all layers of the gut wall, leading to thickened bowel, which can become stenotic and lead to the development of adjacent thick fibrotic mesentery. Sinus tracts can develop and extend into the serosa and peritoneal cavity, retroperitoneal area, or perineum.

The most common symptoms reported in Crohn's disease are abdominal pain (82%), diarrhea (70%), weight loss (56%), and rectal bleeding (26%). Abdominal pain is reported in 80% of patients and is usually associated with diarrhea and fever. Symptoms often differ in severity, depending on the location in the gastrointestinal tract and the extent of disease. Disease that is localized to the small bowel is usually accompanied by moderate diarrhea (five or six soft stools per day). Colonic disease can present with urgency, incontinence, and rectal bleeding. Pain is often steady and localized tenderness to the periumbilical area of the right lower quadrant. A narrowed bowel lumen can lead to symptoms of a partial or complete bowel obstruction, with associated postprandial periumbilical pain, nausea, and vomiting. Colonic involvement can present as cramping in both lower quadrants, whereas disease in the distal colon may cause the pain to be referred to the lower back.

Ulcerative colitis

The inflammation in UC can be of variable severity; however, it is usually limited to the mucosa within the colon and/or rectum. In older patients, there is a predilection for the distal colon (proctitis, proctosigmoiditis, left-sided colitis). Pancolitis occurs more commonly in younger patients (26%) than in older ones (12%). Symptom onset can be insidious, with vague abdominal cramping and a gradual change in bowel habits and character of the stool. Constipation with rectal bleeding can be a presenting symptom in 3% of patients. Mild symptoms include intermittent rectal bleeding, mild diarrhea, pain, and occasional constipation. Frequent loose and bloody stools, anemia, and low-grade fevers are characteristic of moderate symptoms. In contrast, severe symptoms can cause bleeding requiring transfusion, high fevers, and severe crampy abdominal pain.

Diagnosis of inflammatory disease

Differentiating between UC and Crohn's disease can be difficult, as the symptoms can overlap. UC and Crohn's disease can be differentiated histologically (Table 10.2). Physical examination findings are usually nonspecific, unless there are extraintestinal manifestations. The physical examination is usually normal in patients with UC, although one may find pallor, weight loss, abdominal pain, and red blood on rectal examination.

Laboratory studies may reveal anemia, elevated erythrocyte sedimentation rate, and transaminases, but this is also nonspecific and would not distinguish between UC and Crohn's disease. Vitamin B_{12} level may be lower secondary to malabsorption. Stool studies for bacteria, ova, and parasites are indicated to rule out infectious colitis, but, ultimately, upper and lower endoscopy or upper gastrointestinal radiographs with small bowel follow-through and colonoscopy are necessary for pathologic diagnosis and to confirm disease location. Sigmoidoscopy with biopsy can be performed if there is a higher suspicion for UC. Barium enemas should be avoided as they can cause ileus and subsequent toxic megacolon.

Management of inflammatory bowel disease

Treatment in both UC and Crohn's disease necessitates decreasing the inflammation. First-line treatment is usually with oral sulfsalazine or mesalamine (which can be given orally, or as enemas, foams, or suppositories). Broad-spectrum antibiotics (metronidazole, ciprofloxacin) have been shown to be beneficial for mild to moderate IBD. For flares, corticosteroids are used, but they have no role in maintenance therapy due to the multiple adverse, long-term side effects. In patients with refractory symptoms, immunosuppressant therapies, such as 6-mercaptopurine, azathioprine, methotrexate, and cyclosporine can be considered. Surgical therapy can be considered for patients who ultimately fail medical therapy or present with morbid complications such as toxic megacolon, perforation, or sepsis.

Table 10.2 Clinical and pathologic comparison of ulcerative colitis and Crohn's disease

	Ulcerative colitis	Crohn's disease
Sites affected	Rectum Colon	Colon (20%) Ileum (80%) Skip lesions throughout gastrointestinal tract (mouth to anus)
Gastrointestinal complications	Fulminant colitis (15%) Hemorrhage Perforations (20%) Cancer Strictures (10%)	Strictures Fistulas Toxic megacolon Perforation Cancer
Extraintestinal manifestations	Uveitis Erythema nodosum Pyoderma gangrenosum Sclerosing cholangitis Autoimmune hemolytic anemia	Uveitis Erythema nodosum Pyoderma gangrenosum Peripheral arthritis Amyloidosis Thromboembolism
Pathologic and microscopic findings	Friable pseudopolyps Lesions are continuous from the rectum to the colon Superficial ulceration that involves the upper layers of the mucosa Crypt abscesses Loss of glands	Aphthous and linear ulcers Cobblestone appearance Thickened-appearing mucosa Skip lesions throughout gastrointestinal tract Transmural inflammation
Immunologic reaction	CD4+ cells Th2 cells predominance Transforming growth factor-beta Interleukin-5	CD4+ Th1 predominance Interferon-gamma Interleukin-2

Enterocolic endometriosis

Enterocolic endometriosis is almost always associated with genital organ and peritoneal endometriosis and can be a cause of severe pain. Between 3% and 37% of women with pelvic endometriosis have bowel endometriosis. Most cases of bowel endometriosis involve the sigmoid colon (65%); other sites include the rectum, ileum, cecum, appendix, and small bowel. Microscopically, there are endometriotic-like glands and stroma infiltrating the bowel wall through the subserosal fat. If the lesions involve only the serosa, it is considered peritoneal and not bowel endometriosis. In the muscularis layer, endometriotic nodules or foci can be surrounded by submucosal hyperplasia and fibrosis. Pain arises as a result of the neurovascular branches in the subserous plexus that are adjacent to these proinflammatory lesions. The rate of malignant transformation in unknown.

Clinical manifestations and diagnosis

Bowel endometriosis is often a difficult diagnosis to make. The differential diagnosis of bowel endometriosis is highly variable, depending on its presentation and location, and includes IBS, IBD, diverticulitis, functional bloating syndrome, or gastrointestinal or ovarian carcinoma. There are no clear recommendations for the diagnostic evaluation of patients with suspected endometriosis in the gastrointestinal tract.

The most common presenting symptoms for endometriosis are dysmenorrhea, pelvic pain, and dyspareunia. Rectovaginal endometriosis can present as dyschezia, nausea, or bloating. Gastrointestinal symptoms are widely variable.

Women with lesions may experience no pain or severe excruciating pain, with the severity of symptoms often depending on the size and location of the lesions. Symptoms overlap with those of IBS and endometriosis. Small nodules on serosal surfaces are usually asymptomatic; larger lesions in the lower colon can cause diarrhea, constipation, bloating, or pain. Nausea and bloating may be due to a sympathetic response from severe visceral pain, as seen in IBS. Unlike in IBS, defecation does not alleviate the symptoms. Cyclical rectal bleeding is rare as the mucosa is rarely infiltrated. Patients may also have dyschezia, tenesmus, and even acute bowel obstruction. Other nonspecific symptoms include back pain or a change in posture, associated with depression and bowel symptoms. Multifocal lesions make this disease process particularly difficult to diagnose and treat.

The patient's history and examination are typically consistent with endometriosis. Tender nodules reflecting indurations in the cul-de-sac are usually noted on rectovaginal examination. Definitive diagnosis can usually be made via laparoscopy. Bowel endometriosis may be visualized during routine laparoscopy performed by gynecologists to investigate pelvic endometriosis. Given that these findings are unexpected, many gynecologists are not equipped to intervene surgically, leaving lesions untreated or neglected. Furthermore, intraoperative consultation with a general surgeon may be frustrating due to the lack of experience of general surgeons in the management of colorectal endometriosis.

There is no "gold standard" for imaging procedures for visualizing bowel endometriosis. TVUS may allow visualization of bowel endometriosis as an irregular hypoechoic mass with hypoechoic or hyperechoic foci that infiltrates the mucosa, but it is difficult to see lesions above the rectosigmoid junction. Rectal endoscopic ultrasonography evaluates the involvement of the muscularis layer of the bowel and depth of infiltration of lesions, with a sensitivity and specificity of 97.1% and 89.4% respectively, but cannot evaluate the upper colon and requires anesthesia, rendering it impractical in the office setting.

Double-contrast barium enema has been used since the 1980s for diagnosing bowel endometriosis. Nodules may appear like extrinsic masses that impinge on the colonic lumen. The specificity of this test is low, and it cannot assess the full thickness of the bowel wall or the depth of infiltration of the lesions. Colonoscopy is not particularly useful, as most lesions do not penetrate the bowel mucosa.

The sensitivity and specificity of MRI are 76.5% and 97.9%, respectively. An endoluminal rectal coil is needed to visualize the lesions. Furthermore, it is not possible to visualize a nodule with MRI if it is more than 8 cm above the anal margin.

Management

The treatment of bowel endometriosis must take into account the severity of symptoms and its effect on the quality of life. Expectant management is an option, but little is known about the natural history of bowel endometriosis. Patients must be educated about the rare occurrence of bowel obstruction that might require emergent radical surgery for a benign process that can appear malignant. Medical therapies, such as gonadotropin-releasing hormone agonists, have been used with mixed results. Most lesions are unresponsive as they are fibrotic rather than glandular and lack hormone-responsive elements.

Surgery is recommended if there is evidence of obstruction. Most studies looking at postoperative outcomes are retrospective; complete relief (or near-complete relief) is estimated to be 72–86% after resection. There is an estimated 4% chance of recurrent disease. However, it is unclear just how much to resect and when to perform surgery if obstruction is absent. Most trials have shown a modest improvement in pain and quality of life.

Celiac sprue

Celiac sprue is a malabsorptive immune-mediated enteropathy characterized by damage to the small intestinal mucosa by the gliadin portion of the wheat protein secondary to an inappropriate T-cell-mediated response against gluten. Celiac disease is common in individuals of European ancestry, and the incidence was once thought to be 1 in 4,000. However, after the advent of specific serologic assays for antibodies to gliadin and endomysium, the prevalence was found to be as high as 1 in 300 to 1 in 500 (or 0.5–1%) of the general population. Specific predisposing immune genotypes (HLA-DR2, HLA-DQ8) are found in 95% of all affected individuals but exist in 9.9–15.6% of the population. Patients are at an increased risk of colorectal cancer (CRC) or lymphoma, infertility and short stature, and delayed puberty. Treatment can potentially prevent the sequelae of malabsorption.

Clinical manifestations and diagnosis

Symptoms vary depending on the age at presentation, duration of disease, and presence of extraintestinal manifestations. Classically, it is a young infant with failure to thrive and chronic foul-smelling floating stools or diarrhea due to malabsorption, but over 50% of patients with celiac disease present between the ages of 10 and 40. Patients can be asymptomatic or present with diarrhea, abdominal pain, mood changes, osteoarthritis, and depression. Other extraintestinal manifestations include anemia, dental enamel hypoplasia, and osteoporosis. There is often evidence of intestinal damage, despite the absence of symptoms. Furthermore, even though symptoms may be mild, micronutrient deficiencies can still persist, and women with celiac disease are at higher risk of having low birth weight neonates or preterm birth.

Testing should take place in those with risk factors or chronic diarrhea, evidence of weight loss or malabsorption, or iron-deficiency anemia of unknown origin. The list of individuals who should be tested includes those with a personal history or family history of immune thyroid disorders, celiac disease, type 1 diabetes, Sjögren disease, connective tissue disorders, Down syndrome, or Turner syndrome. Screening should start with serologic testing for IgA against endomysium and tissue transglutaminase. In those who screen positive, histologic studies should be performed with intestinal biopsies. There should then be an obvious clinical and serologic response to a gluten-free diet. Other causes of symptoms should be ruled out.

Management

The mainstay of treatment is lifelong avoidance of gluten-containing foods (wheat, barley, other related cereals). The presence of this protein is common, and education and avoidance involves major lifestyle changes, noncompliance being common. It was thought that patients could reintroduce foods after attaining remission of symptoms; however, reaction to foods is variable. Thus, after identification and diagnosis of the condition, patients must work with a dietitian and have long-term follow-up with a multidisciplinary team.

Colorectal cancer

CRC is the second most common cause of cancer death in the United States, the rate increasing exponentially after the age of 40. The risk increases in individuals with a family history or a familial CRC syndrome, those with IBD or diabetes, and those who smoke or drink alcohol. About 26% of lesions are found in the cecum and ascending colon, 18% in the transverse colon, 23% in the descending and sigmoid colon, and 52% in the rectosigmoid colon.

Clinical manifestations and diagnosis

Although there are advances due to screening, the majority of CRC will still be diagnosed clinically. Symptoms can overlap with benign conditions. Rectal bleeding occurs in 3–15% of the general population, and only 3% of those will be found to have cancer. Abdominal pain and changes in bowel habits are found in other benign conditions, especially IBS. The differential diagnosis includes villous tumors or adenomatous polyps of the gastrointestinal tract, peptic ulcer disease, and carcinoid syndrome. Patients with benign tumors beyond the ligament of Treitz may even present with intussusception or intermittent obstruction. Other malignancies to consider include gastrointestinal stromal tumors, ovarian cancer, lymphoma, and melanoma.

The three most common presenting symptoms in patients with CRC are rectal bleeding or hematochezia (43–58%), vague abdominal pain (22–65%) often increased with meals, often on the side of the disease, and a change in bowel habits (43–74%); 11% have anemia alone without other gastrointestinal complaints, weight loss occurs around 6% of the time, and 20% of patients will present with metastatic disease. Symptoms associated with proximal colon cancers include anemia with anorexia, nausea, vomiting, or abdominal pain. Distal CRC tends to be associated with rectal bleeding, altered stools, rectal pain, or tenesmus. Approximately 60% have had symptoms for over 6 weeks.

A positive fecal occult blood test is present only three-quarters of the time in asymptomatic individuals. A complete blood count can detect anemia. Suspected cases should undergo endoscopic examination with colonoscopy, as most lesions occur intraluminally and arise from the mucosa. Colonoscopy is the single best test to use as it can visualize the lesion, biopsies can be performed, and it can remove polyps detected. Barium enemas or CT colonography can be used in cases that cannot be reached with colonoscopy.

Management

Once a colorectal malignancy has been diagnosed, the next step is to evaluate the pathology to determine the extent of surgery or staging required. Further discussion of surgical management, chemotherapy, and radiation is beyond the scope of this chapter.

Conclusions

It can be difficult to distinguish between chronic enterocolic pain and CPP due to other visceral and somatic etiologies. Given the high prevalence of CPP in women that is unrelated to the reproductive organs, it is important to understand the innervation, differential diagnosis, comorbidities, and multidisciplinary approaches to treatment. The clinician must be adept at taking a thorough history, be vigilant for warning signs, and know the limitations of specific diagnostic tests. Functional abdominal pain disorders such as IBS and FAPS are very prevalent in women with CPP and are diagnosed by clinical criteria. IBS and FAPS are highly associated with other visceral and somatic pain disorders, anxiety, and depression, and treatment must involve extensive education and multimodal therapy.

Selected bibliography

Bailey HR, Ott MT, Hartendorp P. Aggressive surgical management for advanced colorectal endometriosis. Dis Colon Rectum 1994;37: 747–53.

Fasano A, Catassi C. Current approaches to diagnosis and treatment of celiac disease: an evolving spectrum. Gastroenterology 2001;120: 636–51.

Gurudu S, Fiocchi C, Katz JA. Inflammatory bowel disease. Best Pract Res Clin Gastroenterol 2002;16:77–90.

Hasler WL. Irritable bowel syndrome and bloating. Best Pract Res Clin Gastroenterol 2007;21:689–707.

Kavallaris A, Kohler C, Kuhne-Heid R, Schneider A. Histopathological extent of rectal invasion by rectovaginal endometriosis. Hum Reprod 2003;18:1323–7.

Lamvu G, Steege JF. The anatomy and neurophysiology of pelvic pain. J Minim Invasive Gynecol 2006;13:516–22.

Longstreth GF, Thompson WG, Chey WD, Houghton LA, Mearin F, Spiller RC. Functional bowel disorders. Gastroenterology 2006;130: 1480–91.

Majumdar SR, Fletcher RH, Evans AT. How does colorectal cancer present? Symptoms, duration, and clues to location. Am J Gastroenterol 1999;94:3039–45.

Matheis A, Martens U, Kruse J, Enck P. Irritable bowel syndrome and chronic pelvic pain: a singular or two different clinical syndrome? World J Gastroenterol 2007;13: 3446–55.

Mayer EA. Clinical practice. Irritable bowel syndrome. N Engl J Med 2008;358:1692–9.

Remorgida V, Ferrero S, Fulcheri E, Ragni N, Martin DC. Bowel endometriosis: presentation, diagnosis, and treatment. Obstet Gynecol Surv 2007;62:461–70.

Schwetz I, Bradesi S, Mayer EA. The pathophysiology of irritable bowel syndrome. Minerva Med 2004(5):419–26.

Sheth AA, Longo W, Floch MH. Diverticular disease and diverticulitis. Am J Gastroenterol 2008;103:1550–6.

Ustinova EE, Fraser MO, Pezzone MA. Colonic irritation in the rat sensitizes urinary bladder afferents to mechanical and chemical stimuli: an afferent origin of pelvic organ cross-sensitization. Am J Physiol Renal Physiol 2006;290:F1478–87.

Wesselmann U, Burnett AL, Heinberg LJ. The urogenital and rectal pain syndromes. Pain 1997;73:269–94.

Whitehead WE, Palsson O, Jones KR. Systematic review of the comorbidity of irritable bowel syndrome with other disorders: what are the causes and implications? Gastroenterology 2002;122:1140–56.

Winnard KP, Dmitrieva N, Berkley KJ. Cross-organ interactions between reproductive, gastrointestinal, and urinary tracts: modulation by estrous stage and involvement of the hypogastric nerve. Am J Physiol Regul Integr Comp Physiol 2006;291:R1592–601.

Zondervan KT, Yudkin PL, Vessey MP et al. The community prevalence of chronic pelvic pain in women and associated illness behaviour. Br J Gen Pract 2001;5:541–7.

Musculoskeletal Causes of Pelvic Pain

Frank Tu[1,3], Colleen Fitzgerald[2], Sangeeta Senapati[1,3], and Kristen Pozolo[1]

[1]Northshore University HealthSystem, Evanston, Illinois, USA
[2]Rehabilitation Institute of Chicago and Feinberg School of Medicine at North-western University, Chicago, Illinois, USA
[3]University of Chicago, Chicago, Illinois, United States

Introduction

The American College of Obstetricians and Gynecologists defines chronic pelvic pain (CPP) as "non-cyclic pain of 6 or more months' duration that localizes to the anatomic pelvis, anterior abdominal wall at or below the umbilicus, the lumbosacral back, or the buttocks and is of sufficient severity to cause functional disability or lead to medical care." Musculoskeletal etiologies are not well recognized by gynecologists in the initial evaluation of women and often are recognized only after primary treatment failure with surgery or hormonal suppression. This is not ideal, as only one in five women with pelvic pain have a condition that is primarily gynecologic.

Evaluation for musculoskeletal disorders in tertiary clinics is routinely part of the work-up for patients with pelvic pain, but is often not included in these population studies due to an absence of specific presenting symptoms. There are a variety of conditions that fall under the grouping of musculoskeletal dysfunction of the pelvis, such as levator ani syndrome, piriformis syndrome, sacroiliac joint dysfunction, coccygodynia, and pudendal neuralgia, to name but a few. Collectively, many of these disorders are often referred to as myofascial pain syndromes or described as conditions in which trigger points are present. In some circumstances, musculoskeletal pain may be secondarily referred from a primary visceral pain source, as in the rectus abdominis guarding seen with acute appendicitis. Clinically, this somatovisceral convergence can make identification of the primary pain generator difficult at times. More precise diagnosis and treatment of pelvic pain may reduce the impact of this disorder, which has a prevalence approaching that of low back pain and asthma.

Epidemiology

Musculoskeletal pain conditions in this area are classified into categories based upon the diagnosis and location of the pain, two common classifications being CPP and pelvic girdle pain (PGP). Tertiary clinics report the prevalence of nonpregnant pelvic musculoskeletal issues at anywhere between 20% and 90% but obviously are limited by selection bias. In contrast, the point prevalence of pregnant women in Europe suffering from PGP has been reported at 20%.

The use of varying definitions of pain conditions and inconsistent inclusion and exclusion criteria may explain the differences in prevalence rates. Many gynecologic clinic-based studies only focus on a select sample of musculoskeletal issues such as trigger points or levator ani spasm. Furthermore, an antiquated unidimensional perspective on pain pervades many contemporary studies of pelvic pain, thus assigning a diagnosis of musculoskeletal pain only when endometriosis, bladder visceral pain, and irritable bowel syndrome have been ruled out. The current literature probably is inadequate in describing the true epidemiology of musculoskeletal contributions to pelvic pain disorders. Newer diagnostic techniques and more stringent sets of criteria for the

Chronic Pelvic Pain, First Edition. Edited by Paolo Vercellini.
© 2011 Blackwell Publishing Ltd. Published 2011 by Blackwell Publishing Ltd.

diagnosis of CPP and PGP will aid in defining a true scale of incidence.

Anatomy

The musculoskeletal pelvis is a complex anatomic structure with external and internal components. All anatomic structures including the bony pelvis (innominate, sacrum, coccyx), articular structures (sacroiliac joint, pubic symphysis, sacrococcygeal joint), ligamentous structures (long dorsal, sacrotuberous, sacrospinous) and musculature (pelvic floor, piriformis, obturator internus) can be potential pain generators in a patient presenting with CPP. Because of the intimate attachments of the pelvis to both the lumbar spine and hip, it must be examined in light of its connection to other parts of the kinetic chain.

The *kinetic chain* describes the coordinated activation of body segments to perform a function optimally. The pelvis is responsible for both stability and mobility as it absorbs and transmits forces from the spine to the lower extremity. A well-functioning pelvis is the result of form closure where joint surfaces congruently fit together, as well as force closure or the ability of pelvic muscles and ligaments to provide force to withstand the loads of normal daily activities. Motor control, or the timing and sequencing of muscle activation and release, in concert with emotion and awareness are key components in the biomechanically optimal musculoskeletal pelvis.

The pelvic joints

The pelvis is a ring composed of innominate bones that are connected anteriorly by the pubic symphysis and posteriorly to either side of the sacrum by the sacroiliac joints. The female pelvis has more joint space surface area and a higher center of gravity compared to the male pelvis. The sacroiliac joint is a true joint consisting of a synovial component inferiorly. This auricular-shaped joint has the thinner sacral side lined with hyaline cartilage and the thicker ilial side lined with fibrocartilage enveloped by an anterior and posterior capsule that carries proprioceptive and pressure fibers as well as unmyelinated free nerve endings. Primary innervation to this joint is thought to be from S1.

Multiple ligaments stabilize the joint intrinsically (interosseus, anterior sacroiliac ligament, posterior sacroiliac ligament) and extrinsically (sacrotuberous, iliolumbar) to the joint. The anterior and posterior sacroiliac joint ligaments cross from the ilium to the lateral and dorsal sacrum, respectively. The sacrospinous ligament attaches medially from the lateral margins of the sacrum and coccyx to the ischial spine, where it coalesces with the sacrotuberous ligament. Its function is to prevent posterior rotation in a sagittal plane of the ilium with respect to the sacrum. The coccygeus muscle also connects to this ligament.

The pubic symphysis is a nonsynovial amphiarthrodial joint with an intrapubic disc between thin layers of hyaline cartilage. Stability of this joint comes from the surrounding ligaments (inferior, suprapubic, anterior, posterior) and rectus abdominis fascial connections. The innervation of the joint includes branches of the pudendal and genitofemoral nerves. The sacrococcygeal joint is a cartilaginous joint connected by anterior, posterior, and lateral ligaments to the sacrum, with secondary attachments to the pelvis via the sacrospinous ligament; afferents to the sacral plexus and comprising the coccygeal nerve innervating this joint are the target for nerve block treatments for coccydynia (or tailbone pain) Some additional stability to the coccyx comes from an anococcygeal ligament attaching proximally to the external anal sphincter and supporting the lower end of the rectum.

Muscle/fascia

The pelvic floor is composed of layers of muscles connecting the anterior and posterior pelvic ring, and surrounding the urethra, vagina, and anus. The superficial pelvic floor or urogenital diaphragm includes the bulbocavernosus, ischiocavernosus, and transverse perineus muscles. The deep pelvic floor or levator ani includes the puborectalis, pubococcygeus, iliococcygeus, and coccygeus.

The levator ani originates lateral to the pubic symphysis on the posterior surface of the superior ramus and inserts onto the inner surface of the ischium at a condensation of obturator fascia, the arcus tendineus. The muscle fiber orientation of the levator ani is such that the fibers pass inferiorly and posteriorly to the center of the pelvis and attach to the coccyx and anus. The middle fibers insert into the rectum and then blend with the fibers of the sphincter muscles. In women, the anterior muscle fibers insert into the sides of the vagina. The perineal body (the central tendon of the perineum) comprises fibrous tissue and the superficial pelvic floor musculature, lies between the vagina and the anus.

Both fast twitch (30%) and slow twitch (70%) muscle fibers of the pelvic floor facilitate sphincter closure to maintain continence, support the intra-abdominal organs to prevent pelvic organ prolapse, and contract during orgasm to allow for sexual appreciation. Pelvic floor innervation posteriorly is by direct efferents from the S2–4 nerve roots, whereas the anterior pelvis is innervated by the pudendal nerve and its three branches: the dorsal nerve to the clitoris, the perineal branch, and the inferior hemorrhoidal nerve. While these somatic structures may provide primary afferent nociceptive signals to the dorsal horn, afferent stimuli from the pelvic viscera also may modulate information from these structures via viscerosomatic reflexes, as seen with irritable bowel syndrome and painful bladder syndrome.

The "core" is in the middle of the human kinetic chain and serves as a link between the upper and lower extremities. This muscular corset works as a unit to stabilize the body and spine with and without movement. There are both local core (posture, tonic, segmental stabilizers) and global core (dynamic, phasic, torque-producing movers) muscles. No single muscle owns a dominant responsibility for lumbopelvic stability. The pelvic floor is considered a local stabilizer and is often called the "floor of the core." In combination with pelvic floor, the piriformis and obturator internus muscles, which function as movers as well as stabilizers, and the deep transversus abdominis, lumbar multifidi, and diaphragm, all work synergistically to support the dynamic function of the female pelvis.

Pathophysiology

CPP with a musculoskeletal basis is described in the literature as "pelvic girdle pain". PGP is defined as pain between the upper level of the iliac crests and the gluteal folds in the region of the sacroiliac joint in conjunction with or separately from pain in the pubic symphysis and influenced by position and locomotion. The diagnosis can be made once lumbar causes have been ruled out, and by specific clinical tests.

The exact pathophysiology in PGP is not well understood, but likely includes potentiation of algogesic substances released due to neural inflammation or from normal trauma (Table 11.1). The pain generator may be structural, related to bony muscular, tendinous, or ligamentous pathology such tears or edema, or intra-articular in nature (i.e., true sacroiliac joint pain). Connective tissue restrictions may subtly limit the mobility of neural structures and trophic support. Otherwise innocuous mechanical insult or injury to the pelvis in the setting of vulnerable tissue (such as an arthritic spine with posterior pelvic referral) can lead to persistent pain. Hormonal, inflammatory, and central neural sensitivity are all probable factors in the etiology of chronic PGP.

Diagnostics

★ TIPS & TRICKS

Do not discount the patient's history. A woman who has recently had a traumatic injury to the pelvis, even without evidence of ligamentoskeletal injury on imaging, likely has a musculoskeletal etiology to her pain symptoms. All too often, gynecologists blame endometriosis as causing new-onset pain symptoms even when there is another blatantly obvious element to the external history such as a fall.

A simple maneuver for distinguishing between deep visceral/peritoneal pain and abdominal wall pain is to examine the patient while lying down supine, with both areas relaxed, and when doing a "crunch" engaging the rectus abdominis.

Abdominal wall pain usually is still painful during the crunch, while visceral pain will often improve during this voluntary guarding.

Physical examination

External pelvis

A thorough musculoskeletal examination of the lumbar spine and hip along with a good lower

Table 11.1 Differential diagnosis of musculoskeletal causes of pelvic pain

Category	Diagnoses
Muscular/fascia	Pelvic floor myofascial pain, levator ani syndrome, tension myalgia Myofascial pain syndromes of associated extrinsic muscles (iliopsoas, adductor, piriformis) Dyssynergia of the pelvic floor muscles Vaginismus, dyspareunia
Skeletal/joint	Pelvic insufficiency, stress fracture Sacroiliac joint dysfunction Pelvic obliquity or derangement, pelvic asymmetry Pubic symphysitis, osteitis pubis, pubic symphysis separation Coccydynia Lumbar degenerative disc disease, spondylosis or listhesis (with referral to the posterior pelvis (L4–L5–S1) Hip osteoarthritis, hip fracture, acetabular labral tears, chondrosis, developmental hip dysplasia, femoral acetabular impingement, avascular necrosis of the femoral head Bony metastasis
Neurologic	Radiculopathy Plexopathy Peripheral neuropathy—pudendal neuropathy
Viscerosomatic (presumed)	Endometriosis Irritable bowel syndrome Bladder pain syndrome Dysmenorrhea

extremity neurologic examination marks the beginning of an appropriate clinical examination for a patient with PGP. Tests well validated in PGP are described below. Many other tests exist but have not been found to be as sensitive and specific for PGP. This includes examination for pelvic obliquity.

Pelvic joint provocation tests

These tests are designed to provoke a painful response in the pelvic girdle. These can be helpful in identifying PGP structures, as opposed to pelvic visceral structures, as the primary pain generator.

Patrick (Faber) test. With the patient supine, the patient's leg is flexed, abducted, and externally rotated so that the heel rests on the opposite kneecap (Figure 11.1). This test is positive with production of pain in the pelvic joint.

Posterior pelvic pain provocation test (thigh thrust). With the patient supine, the femur is flexed to be perpendicular with the table at 90 degrees, and the knee is flexed to 90 degrees

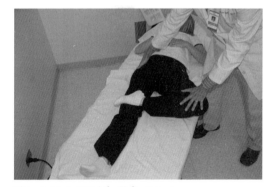

Figure 11.1 Patrick (Faber) test.

(Figure 11.2). A gentle force is applied to the femur in the direction of the examination table. The test is positive when the patient experiences pain in the gluteal region of that leg.

Long dorsal sacroiliac ligament palpation. The subject stands up and the areas above both sacroiliac joints are palpated (Figure 11.3). Specifically, the long dorsal sacroiliac ligament is

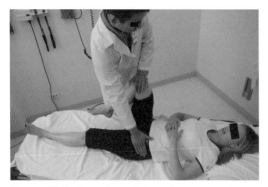

Figure 11.2 Posterior pelvic pain provocation test.

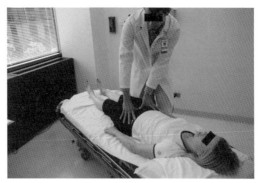

Figure 11.4 Pubic symphysis palpation.

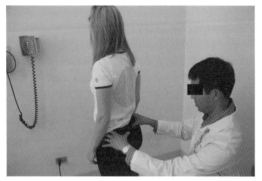

Figure 11.3 Long dorsal sacroiliac ligament palpation.

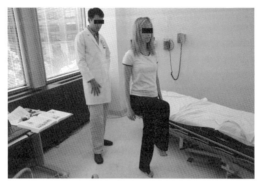

Figure 11.5 Modified Trendelenburg test.

palpated directly caudomedially from the posterior iliac spine to the lateral dorsal border of the sacrum. If palpation causes pain that persists for 5 seconds after removal of the examiner's hand, it is recorded as pain. If the pain disappears within 5 seconds, it is recorded as tenderness. When the identical pain is felt directly in the vicinity but outside the borders of the ligament, the test is deemed negative.

Pubic symphysis palpation. The subject's pubic symphysis joint is palpated while the patient is lying supine to elicit tenderness (Figure 11.4). If palpation causes pain that persists 5 seconds after removal of the examiner's hand, it is recorded as pain. If the pain disappears within 5 seconds, it is recorded as tenderness.

Modified Trendelenburg test. The woman turns her back to the examiner and, standing on one leg, flexes the hip and knee of the other leg to 90 degrees (Figure 11.5). The test is considered positive if pain is experienced in the symphysis.

Functional stability testing
Active straight leg raise test. To globally assess core function with a single test in suspected PGP dysfunction, clinicians perform this test with the patient supine with straight legs extended on the table 20 cm apart. The patient raises each leg one at a time 30 degrees above the table without bending the knee (Figure 11.6). The test is positive when the patient describes a heaviness or difficulty in performing the task. In the second part of the maneuver, posterior compression is applied and the patient is then asked to actively perform a straight leg raise. If there is greater ease in motion, this is considered a positive test.

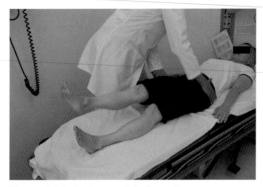

Figure 11.6 Active straight leg raise test.

★ TIPS & TRICKS

In order to get the pelvic floor musculature activated, consider utilizing the natural coactivation pattern of the transversus abdominis. This can be done be asking the patient to draw in her belly button and have her palpate just below her anterior superior iliac spines bilaterally at the same time she is performing a Kegel contraction (voluntary tightening of the pelvic floor); she will feel how abdominal contraction works together with pelvic floor activation. In addition, many patients when asked to perform a pelvic floor contraction actually use a Valsalva maneuver and activate their abdominal musculature instead. Internal palpation of an appropriate Kegel contraction can be highly instructive in order to avoid this.

Internal pelvis (pelvic floor examination)

The pelvic floor examination should be performed both vaginally and rectally. The neurologic component generally includes both sacral sensation testing and the anal wink reflex. The superficial and deep pelvic floor as well as the obturator internus should be assessed for tenderness and trigger points externally and internally, noting side-to-side asymmetry. Voluntary pelvic floor contraction and relaxation, and involuntary contraction (cough, Valsalva maneuver), should be assessed on observation and digital palpation. Manual muscle strength examination using the Modified Oxford scale (0–5, where 0 mean no voluntary strength at all, and 5 means normal strength) for testing of muscle strength and endurance (type 1), as well as "quick flick" or fast-firing testing (type 2), can detect functional weakness. Rectal sphincter, coccyx, and posterior pelvic floor assessment in a side-lying position completes the examination. The pelvic floor findings are often recorded using a pelvic clock, where the 12 o'clock position marks the pubic bone and the 6 o'clock position represents the anus.

★ TIPS AND TRICKS

Finding the obturator muscle and the course of the pudendal nerve transvaginally is easy for gynecologists or other practitioners who routinely conduct pelvic examinations. First find the ischial spine. The thick condensation of connective tissue going all the way distally to the pubic bone at the imaginary sites of 3 o'clock and 9 o'clock of the vaginal introitus from the spines is the arcus tendineus, and this separates the obturator muscle (superior to the arcus) from the levator plate (inferior). The pudendal nerve runs in Alcock's canal inferior to this in a condensation of obturator fascia, and palpation of the nerve's course that elicits pain may suggest involvement of the nerve in pain symptoms.

Imaging and injections

Current evidence supports the physical examination more than diagnostic imaging or nerve blocks in understanding PGP. There is no evidence for the use of radiography, computed tomography, or bone scanning in the diagnosis of PGP. Magnetic resonance imaging is recommended for use in discriminating change in and around the sacroiliac joint. Diagnostic injections (the sacroiliac joint in particular) may have some utility but only account for ruling out articular pathology and not other musculoskeletal causes.

Treatment

Management of musculoskeletal causes of pelvic pain varies with the clinician's diagnostic impression. For conditions such as vaginismus, vulvodynia, and painful bladder syndrome, there is some level III (Agency for Healthcare Research and Quality evidence scoring system) evidence to support the efficacy of physical therapy approaches. One Dutch study incorporated these manual therapies into a multimodal strategy for treating CPP and found that the combined approach was superior to a unidimensional operative laparoscopic strategy in a randomized controlled trial.

The general strategy is to relieve the area of relative ischemia, improve the normal flexion/extension range of the involved muscles and ligaments, and address any imbalances of the unified elements of the kinetic chain encompassing the lumbosacral region, pelvis, hip, and abdomen. If there are areas of neural compression, improvement of connective tissue mobility can also relieve symptoms. Peripherally focused treatments such as selective nerve blocks, trigger point injections, or electrogalvanic stimulation seem most effective in cases where there is isolated muscle spasm or connective tissue restrictions. With generalized or multifocal pain presentations such as painful bladder syndrome, these treatments may best be complemented by systemic therapies such as neuromodulating medications, which are detailed in Chapter 9.

Myofascial release/retraining

A well-trained women's health physical therapist will have experience providing all of the following modalities, although certain therapists emphasize certain aspects more than others. A key skill we believe is mandatory for a successful therapist is comfort with directed internal pelvic floor assessment and manual therapy, and in the United States there are numerous formal training programs that provide this certification. Globally, a physical therapist should address the key elements of the core (rectus abdominis and obliques anteriorly, paraspinals, hip flexors/extensors, levator ani) and determine whether the patient has an imbalance in relative strength. Particularly postpartum, a significant proportion of women with pelvic pain in our practice will present with clear evidence of impaired core strength, which may not be the primary source of their pain but likely makes the pain experience more difficult to manage. Assessment of the ability to perform an abdominal crunch and hold alternating single leg stance are simple approaches for gauging core function.

Physical therapists should be requested to also restore full pelvic joint mobility in these women. With upwards of 80% of women with CPP exhibiting a nonrelaxing pelvic floor, manual therapy to release taut muscle bands throughout the core and adductor muscles is a key aspect of peripherally targeted therapies. This consists primarily of deep tissue massage along the longitudinal plane of the muscle belly, complemented by home exercises designed to open the relevant joint to its full range of motion (such as pigeon prep used in yoga exercise, which helps place the obturator muscles into full extension). Particularly with the pelvic floor, this may run counter to the traditional Kegel exercises historically used to improve stress urinary incontinence, but the goal is to enhance both voluntary contraction and relaxation of the pelvic musculature. Manual therapy is also indicated when patients present with symptoms suggestive of peripheral nerve entrapment including the ilioinguinal nerve anteriorly and the pudendal or sciatic nerves (deep in Alcock's canal) or the nerve to the piriformis (greater sciatic foramen).

✋ CAUTION

Many clinicians will prescribe home therapy with vaginal dilators to help reduce pelvic floor hypertonus. While the use of dilators may seem harmless, the physician should be careful in advising their use in certain women, particularly those with a prior history of radiation to the pelvis, such as for cervical cancer treatment. The authors have witnessed a case of rectovaginal fistula developing within a few weeks of prescribing the use of vaginal dilators for a woman with pain at the vaginal fornix. This complication has not been formally reported and is nevertheless likely a low risk. Similar complications have been described for women undergoing neovaginal expansion in Meyer–Rokitansky–Kuster–Hauser syndrome.

More localized approaches include connective tissue release. Although not well validated, several authors have proposed that fascial restrictions locally in the pelvis can be a source of persistent pain. Some therapists have described "skin-rolling," where the subcutaneous tissue in areas of restrictions is worked repeatedly between the therapist's fingers. This may be worth discussing with the therapist, particularly for incisional pain (episiotomy or abdominal scars), pudendal neuralgia, urethral syndrome, and vulvar pain syndromes.

A subset of women will have overt malalignment issues noted at evaluation. This can be congenital, post-traumatic, or secondary to muscle spasm. For cases refractory to manual release techniques, it may help to use a pelvic lift as with rotated innominate bones, or for a leg length abnormality, a heel lift. Proper muscle retraining can also be helpful.

Energy-based therapy

Application of energy to areas of muscle spasm is used throughout the body by physical therapists to favorably influence cellular, tissue, segmental, and physiologic changes. A thorough discussion is beyond the scope of this chapter, but excellent reviews exist in physical therapy manuals. A transcutaneous electrical nerve stimulator will often be employed in combination with manual therapy using either transvaginal or surface electrodes—the exact selection of the waveform, phase duration (generally 20–200 μs), and pulse rate (2–100 pulses per second) should be determined by the therapist, and each treatment may last up to 45 minutes. Similarly, small studies have described transperineal and transvaginal ultrasound (1–2.5 W/cm²) for both male and female pelvic pain syndromes involving the pelvic floor, with up to three-quarters of patients with uncomplicated pelvic floor pain having good responses.

Medications

Mild cases of pelvic musculoskeletal pain should be treated conservatively, including pelvic rest, moderate use of nonsteroidal anti-inflammatories for 1–2 weeks, and home measures such as warm compresses (where appropriate) or soaking in a warm bath. In patients with persistent abnormal muscle compliance, a wide range of locally acting and systemic medications to reduce muscle spasm or diminish local or central pain sensitivity can be employed. Again, only limited case series exist to estimate their relative efficacy.

Oral muscle relaxants such as cyclobenzaprine (5–10 mg up to three times a day) and benzodiazepines such as clonazepam (0.5–1 mg up to three times daily) have both centrally sedating and direct muscle effects; there is, unfortunately, some risk of dependence. To avoid the central side effects, we have treated some cases of pelvic floor spasm with an off-label vaginal insertion of diazepam (5 mg twice a day) or baclofen (10 mg three times a day) without any significant central side effects. The classic belladonna and opium suppositories (16.2/30 or 16.2/60 mg two or three times a day) used transrectally for ureteral pain also may have some efficacy for persistent pelvic floor pain associated with painful bladder syndrome if inserted transvaginally, while appearing to have less systemic side effects.

With more resistant cases of muscle spasm or focal trigger points, some patients will respond to trigger point injections. We use small volumes (up to 5–7 mL) of buffered 1% xylocaine generally in a weekly or biweekly series of 3–6 injections into both abdominal wall and pelvic floor trigger points. These, in combination with transvaginal pudendal blocks or potentially ambulatory lumbar epidurals, may facilitate the manual work being done by a therapist. Botulinum toxin A (80 U total bilaterally) has been studied in a small randomized controlled trial compared to saline placebo for pelvic floor treatment in CPP but did not show superiority over placebo. As with trigger point injections, certain patients may benefit, and its prolonged effect makes it a promising treatment that requires further investigation.

⚠ CAUTION

If you do not use local anesthetics frequently for nerve blocks or the treatment of trigger points, be mindful that the neurologic and cardiac toxicity of these medications can be serious if not monitored. Dosing for a 70 kg female for 1% xylocaine should generally not exceed 4.5 mg/kg, which is about 30 mL.

Bupivicaine 0.25% strength has also been used and has a longer duration of action (roughly 2–4 hours); no more than about 40 mL of solution of this strength should be used for a similarly sized patient (maximum dose 2 mg/kg).

⚗ SCIENCE REVISITED

Why might botulinum toxin work for myofascial pain? Recall that the mechanism of action of botulinum toxin is at the nerve terminal by blocking the release of acetylcholine. It has been proposed that one likely mechanism is that release of local muscle contraction uncouples the cycle of pain–spasm–pain thought to underlie myofascial trigger points. However, because some patients report relief of pain following injection prior to the muscle relaxant effect, an additional effect may come through the blocked exocytosis of pain neuropeptides such as substance P and calcitonin gene-related peptide. The challenge of using botulinum toxin of course is that efferent neuronal function to these muscles is also likely impacted, and some individuals will run the risk of incontinence until the drug wears off.

As with all chronic pain syndromes, the concomitant use of centrally acting neurologic drugs (antiepileptics, tricyclic antidepressants, or the newer selective serotonin–norepinephrine reuptake inhibitors) may be useful in concert with all the above modalities, and in general we favor multidimensional therapy. This is detailed further in Chapter 14.

★ TIPS & TRICKS

A variety of topical agents are available to facilitate manual therapy, although they do not necessarily have Food and Drug Administration approval for this indication. Consider using topical 20% ketoprofen gel 2–3 times a day, 1 g applied to the areas externally where there is significant musculoskeletal pain. Xylocaine topical patches can be helpful for some women as well.

Home therapy

The antecedents of pelvic musculoskeletal injury should be identified and eliminated if present. Sedentary occupations and lack of regular exercise, coupled with the normal trauma from pregnancy and delivery, are addressable factors. Again, while evidence is lacking, we do encourage our patients to begin programs improving flexibility and endurance, such as yoga or pilates, embrace an improved diet with an anti-inflammatory emphasis, and consider meditation programs such as mindfulness. No doubt there are other equally worthwhile approaches that can bring musculoskeletal balance to the hectic modern lifestyle of many of these patients.

Selected bibliography

Abbott JA, Jarvis SK, Lyons SD, Thomson A, Vancaille TG. Botulinum toxin type a for chronic pain and pelvic floor spasm in women: a randomized controlled trial. Obstet Gynecol 2006;108:915–23.

Akuthota V, Nadler SF. Core strengthening. Arch Phys Med Rehabil 2004;85(3 Suppl. 1): S86–92.

Beales DJ, O'Sullivan PB, Briffa NK. Motor control patterns during an active straight leg raise in chronic pelvic girdle pain subjects. Spine 2009;34:861–70.

Cholewicki J, van Dieen JH, Arsenault AB. Muscle function and dysfunction in the spine. J Electromyogr Kinesiol 2003;13:303–4.

FitzGerald MP, Kotarinos R. Rehabilitation of the short pelvic floor. I. Background and patient evaluation. Int Urogynecol J Pelvic Floor Dysfunct 2003;14:261–8.

Fortin JD, Aprill CN, Ponthieux B, Pier J. Sacroiliac joint: pain referral maps upon applying a new injection/arthrography technique. II. Clinical evaluation. Spine 1994;19:1483–9.

Frahm JD. Physical therapies electrotherapy. In: Carriere B, Feldt CM, eds. Beckenboden, Vol. 1. Stuttgart: Thieme; 2006.

Gamble JG, Simmons SC, Freedman M. The symphysis pubis. Anatomic and pathologic considerations. Clin Orthop Relat Res 1986;(203):261–72.

Mense S. Neurological basis for the use of botulinum toxin in pain therapy. J Neurol 2004;S1:I1–7.

Oyama IA, Rejba A, Lukban JC et al. Modified thiele massage as therapeutic intervention for female patients with interstitial cystitis and high-tone pelvic floor dysfunction. Urology 2004;64:862–5.

Peters AA, van Dorst E, Jellis B, van Zuuren E, Hermans J, Trimbos JB. A randomized clinical trial to compare two different approaches in women with chronic pelvic pain. Obstet Gynecol 1991;77:740–4.

Prather H, Dugan S, Fitzgerald C, Hunt D. Review of anatomy, evaluation, and treatment of musculoskeletal pelvic floor pain in women. PMR 2009;1:346–58.

Travell JG, Simons DG. Myofascial pain and dysfunction: the trigger point manual. Baltimore: Williams & Wilkins; 1992.

Tu FF, As-Sanie S, Steege JF. Musculoskeletal causes of chronic pelvic pain: a systematic review of existing therapies. 2. Obstet Gynecol Surv 2005;60:474–83.

Tu FF, Holt J, Gonzales J, Fitzgerald CM. Physical therapy evaluation of patients with chronic pelvic pain: a controlled study. Am J Obstet Gynecol 2008;198:272 e1–7.

Vleeming A, Albert HB, Ostgaard HC, Sturesson B, Stuge B. European guidelines for the diagnosis and treatment of pelvic girdle pain. Eur Spine J 2008;17:794–819.

Dyspareunia: Causes and Treatments (Including Provoked Vestibulodynia)

Marta Meana[1] and Yitzchak M. Binik[2]

[1]University of Nevada, Las Vegas, Nevada, USA
[2]McGill University, McGill University Health Center, Montreal, Quebec, Canada

Introduction

Recurrent or persistent painful intercourse is a very common presenting (or subsequently discovered) complaint in gynecologic practice. It has been associated with a large number of physical conditions while far more commonly presenting with no evidence of obvious organic pathology. It afflicts women of all ages and engenders significant psychological and relational distress. Much in the same manner as other types of chronic pelvic pain, dyspareunia is thus a complicated disorder to assess and treat, often creating frustration in both healthcare professionals and patients.

general population. On average, intercourse pain accounts for 26% of the sexual difficulties reported by women. Among women with sexual pain, less than 20% reported that the pain had had a recent onset (1 month to less than several months), more than 50% of cases reported an onset that dated from several months to less than 6 months, and close to one third reported that the pain had persisted for 6 months or more. Some studies have found the prevalence to be higher in young women, while others have found it to be higher in older women. Clearly, dyspareunia occurs across the lifespan.

EVIDENCE AT A GLANCE

A recent literature review found the prevalence of dyspareunia to range from a low of 0.4% to a high of 61%. This large range is likely attributable to significant methodologic variations between studies, including study populations, definitions of dyspareunia, and measures used to assess it. A 2006 World Health Organization review of dyspareunia studies reported an incidence of painful intercourse ranging between 8% and 22%. The prevalence of provoked vestibulodynia, the most common type of dyspareunia in premenopausal women, has been estimated at 12% of premenopausal women in the

The International Classification of Diseases 10th revision (ICD-10) distinguishes between organic and nonorganic dyspareunia, while the Diagnostic and Statistical Manual of Mental Disorders 4th revision (DSM-IV) subsumes dyspareunia in the sexual dysfunctions and allows for two types: "due to psychological factors" and "due to combined factors." Both classifications exclude painful intercourse attributable to lack of lubrication or to vaginismus, and the DSM excludes dyspareunia due to a general medical condition.

There are, however, a number of problems with these current formulations that may be interfering with optimal care. First, the distinction between organic and nonorganic is often

Chronic Pelvic Pain, First Edition. Edited by Paolo Vercellini.
© 2011 Blackwell Publishing Ltd. Published 2011 by Blackwell Publishing Ltd.

tenuous, if not impossible. Second, even in cases in which organic pathology appears obvious, the successful treatment of that pathology often fails to result in the eradication of pain during intercourse. Factors responsible for the origination of pain may be different from the ones that are working to perpetuate the pain. Third, lack of lubrication may be a product of the anticipation of pain, not to mention that the assessment of lubrication during sexual activity is at best unreliable. Fourth, the distinction between dyspareunia and vaginismus lacks sufficient empiric validation, with little support for the purported muscle spasm attributed to vaginismus. Finally, the pain of dyspareunia also more often than not occurs in the context of nonsexual vulvar contact (e.g., tampon insertion, gynecologic examinations). It may have only an incidental, albeit distressful, association with sex per se.

EVIDENCE AT A GLANCE

There is currently a debate in the literature about the extent to which dyspareunia is best classified as a sexual dysfunction or as a pain disorder. Its classification as a sexual dysfunction had traditionally led researchers and clinicians in search of psychosexual and relational conflicts that could manifest themselves somatically. This approach had negligible treatment efficacy—as far as anyone could tell from the mostly anecdotal literature. Could it be that, in most cases, the pain associated with dyspareunia is simply the unfortunate and mostly incidental pairing of hyperalgesia in a part of the body that *happens* to get maximally stimulated during sex? Some researchers are proposing that this might be the case most of the time. Although it is important to address the effects of dyspareunia on the couple's sexual life, treatment approaches that consider dyspareunia to be a pain disorder with unfortunate sexual consequences have been more effective than treatment approaches that consider dyspareunia to be a sexual problem that results in pain.

This chapter will thus focus on the assessment and treatment of women who report pain when they attempt to have intercourse (whether or not penetration is possible), without delving into theoretical distinctions and dualisms that can detract from effective patient care. It will also necessarily privilege those cases of dyspareunia in which organic pathology is not obvious, as these are the most common and the most perplexing. The premise here is that the best approach to the treatment of dyspareunia is a multidisciplinary one that assumes a multiplicity of etiologic and/or perpetuating factors. Dyspareunia shares many of these factors with other chronic pain syndromes, while some factors are specific to the sexual context that constitutes the most distressing aspect of this particular pain syndrome.

Causes/correlates of dyspareunia

It is often difficult to ascertain a single causal pathway to dyspareunia. There are, however, a variety of associated physical and psychological factors that may be etiologic or that may work to mediate or maintain the pain, sometimes long after the purportedly offending pathology has been successfully treated. The list of potential physical factors that could conceivably produce dyspareunia is very long, and an investigation of each of these would be beyond the scope of this chapter. The onus will thus be on the most common dyspareunia-associated conditions, which are often divided into those linked to deep dyspareunia and to superficial dyspareunia. Deep dyspareunia refers to pain experienced inside the vaginal canal, at the level of the cervix or in the pelvic/uterine/abdominal region, while superficial dyspareunia refers to pain in the vulvar region and or the vaginal opening (introitus). Psychological and relational problems are also likely to be correlated with either type of pain, especially if its interference with sexual intercourse has been long-standing.

Conditions associated with deep dyspareunia

Deep dyspareunia is usually considered more likely than superficial dyspareunia to be associated with tissue damage or with obvious pathology deep inside the vaginal canal, or of the cervix, bladder, and uterus (although there is actually

Table 12.1 Conditions associated with deep dyspareunia*

Lack of arousal necessary for vaginal lengthening

Chronic cervicitis

Repeated cervical trauma

Pelvic endometriosis

Pelvic adhesions

Uterine fibroids

Pelvic inflammatory disease

Pelvic congestion

Pelvic organ prolapse

Urologic disorders (e.g., interstitial cystitis, painful bladder syndrome)

Bowel disorders (e.g., irritable bowel syndrome, constipation, proctitis)

Postpartum broad ligament laceration

Scar formations associated with surgeries (e.g., total hysterectomy, organ support surgeries)

*Most of these conditions are inconsistently associated with dyspareunia. The majority of women afflicted with these conditions do not report pain specific to sexual intercourse.

little evidence to support this contention). The damage can sometimes be iatrogenic, an unintended result of any number of surgical procedures (Table 12.1).

Although some women report arousal through penile–cervical stimulation, most women experience as painful penile thrusts that make contact with the cervix. This type of contact can occur as a result of inadequate prepenetrative stimulation or size discrepancies, or be a function of certain intercourse positions. The cervix can also become sensitized as a result of chronic cervicitis and repeated diagnostic (e.g., biopsies) and excision procedures (e.g., conization).

In terms of deeper presentations, pelvic endometriosis is one of the most common disorders linked to deep dyspareunia. Many studies, however, fail to show a consistent relationship between pain and the number, size, and location of pelvic adhesions. Pelvic inflammatory disease and pelvic congestion are two additional culprits, although the pain associated with these conditions is unlikely to be experienced exclusively with penetration. Pelvic organ prolapse can also produce deep dyspareunia, but its role is confounded by a number of age-related changes that can contribute to painful intercourse. Deep dyspareunia is sometimes a symptom of a number of bladder and gastrointestinal diseases. Inter-

course pain is reported as one of the most distressing symptoms of interstitial cystitis, despite the fact that the pain of this disorder can be quite generalized. Irritable bowel syndrome can also result in dull, visceral pain during intercourse. It is important to remember that many women with these conditions do not experience pain with intercourse.

Surgery for a number of conditions can leave scar formations that cause discomfort during sex. Some women develop focal pain in the vaginal apex after a total hysterectomy, while some pelvic support surgeries to correct uterine or bladder prolapse can result in painful intercourse.

Conditions associated with superficial dyspareunia

Superficial dyspareunia is the more common type of dyspareunia. Table 12.2 presents conditions considered to be associated with superficial dyspareunia. This list is by no means exhaustive, but the majority of cases presenting in clinical practice are likely to be associated with vulvovaginal atrophy consequent to natural or surgical menopause, and vestibulodynia. Hormonal and vascular changes associated with menopause and aging are thought to result in diminished elasticity of the vaginal canal and a reduced capacity for lubrication. Dyspareunia is

Table 12.2 Conditions associated with superficial dyspareunia

Vestibulodynia (provoked vestibulodynia, general vulvodynia)
Cyclical vulvovaginitis
Vulvovaginal infections (e.g., herpes)
Vulvar dermatoses
Vulvovaginal congenital anomalies (e.g., imperforate hymen)
Obstetric sequelae (e.g., episiotomy scars)
Vulvovaginal atrophy
Neurologic disorders (e.g., pudendal nerve lesions)
Muscular abnormalities (e.g., pelvic floor hyper- or hypotonicity)
Neoplastic vulvar lesions
Urologic disorders
Bowel disorders

menopausal transition. Decreasing sexual function scores correlated with decreasing estradiol but not with androgen levels. In the postmenopausal phase, there was a significant decrease in vaginal lubrication and an increase in dyspareunia. There were also significant declines in sexual interest and frequency of sex.

commonly reported by peri- and postmenopausal women. A significant number of peri- and postmenopausal women, however, experience pain with intercourse that is not caused by estrogen deficiency. It is important to ask postmenopausal women who report painful intercourse whether they experienced the dyspareunia prior to menopause: it is possible that the intercourse pain is a consequence of factors that predated hypoestrogenism.

EVIDENCE AT A GLANCE

A recent review of population-based studies investigating sexual functioning and menopause concluded that that there is an age-related decline in sexual functioning augmented by an incremental decline associated with the menopausal transition. One methodologically sound prospective study that conduced eight annual assessments using a self-report sexual function questionnaire and blood sampling for hormone levels found that sexual dysfunction rose from 42% to 88% from early to late

In premenopausal women, the most common cause of superficial dyspareunia appears to be provoked vestibulodynia (PVD; formerly known as vulvar vestibulitis syndrome). PVD is considered to be a neurosensory disorder characterized by severe pain upon even light touch of the vestibule, tenderness or pressure localized within the vulvar vestibule, and, in some cases, vestibular erythema. It is common for PVD to be misdiagnosed as psychogenic dyspareunia since there is usually no visible tissue damage or evidence of inflammation. For women with PVD, sexual intercourse can be extremely painful, as can other types of vulvar stimulation. Much of the frustration of both doctors and women dealing with dyspareunia emanates from cases of superficial dyspareunia without obvious organic pathology, most of these being cases of PVD.

Psychophysical, sexual, and psychosocial correlates of dyspareunia

The absence of obvious organic pathology often leads healthcare professionals to ascribe dyspareunia to a psychological etiology. This is usually not helpful and is often interpreted by patients as doctors giving up or, worse, as a dismissal of their condition as "all in their head." Considering that the sexual response is inherently both a physiologic and a psychological process, even the absence of observable tissue damage or inferred nerve dysfunction should not lead us to the dualistic assessment of dyspareunia as emanating from a psychological versus a physical etiology. Dyspareunia is not the only pain syndrome for which pathology is often unobservable (e.g., migraine, lower back pain). That, however, does not mean that we should ignore the psychological correlates of dyspareu-

Table 12.3 Psychophysical, sexual, and psychosocial correlates of dyspareunia

Generalized pain sensitivity
Hypervigilance
Pain catastrophization
Somatosensory amplification
Low desire
Low arousal
Decreased orgasmic capacity
Anxiety
Depression
Partner solicitousness
Marital/relationship distress

nia. There is a voluminous literature addressing the psychosocial correlates of chronic pain in general, regardless of its etiology. This literature has also demonstrated how useful it is to target these psychosocial factors in the treatment of chronic pain, again regardless of how the pain originated.

Table 12.3 lists the psychophysical, sexual, and psychosocial correlates of dyspareunia. A number of studies have shown that women with PVD have a hypersensitivity to pain in general, including pain experienced in nongenital sites. They have also been shown to exhibit a hypervigilance for and a catastrophization of pain. Women with PVD and with other types of dyspareunia have also been shown to be somatically preoccupied, with a tendency to attend to and experience anxiety about a variety of somatic experiences. Not surprisingly, women with dyspareunia also report disturbances at all stages of the sexual response cycle, with relatively consistent findings of lower sexual desire, greater arousal difficulties, and less orgasmic capacity than women who do not experience pain with intercourse.

Anxiety and depression are also commonly higher in women with dyspareunia, as is marital or relationship distress. Partner solicitousness, a relational factor associated in the chronic pain literature with higher pain ratings and functional interference has been found in one study to play a role in the experience of persistent painful intercourse. The findings for sexual abuse are mixed, with some studies reporting an association while others find no such link.

Assessment of dyspareunia

History

Despite changing Western social mores about sexuality and media attention to sexual problems, many women continue to find it difficult to report painful intercourse to their healthcare practitioners. It is thus crucial to inquire about dyspareunia as a routine part of a gynecologic visit. A simple question will validate the woman's experience, communicate that this is a problem that the healthcare provider is willing to tackle, and provide hope that some resolution is possible. If the woman confirms that she has persistent pain with intercourse, useful diagnostic follow-up questions include the following:

- *Lifetime onset.* How long have you experienced pain with intercourse? Have you had pain since the first time you had intercourse or did it develop later on?
- *Episode onset.* When does the pain start? Before, during, or after intercourse?
- *Location.* Where exactly does it hurt when you have or attempt to have intercourse? (A diagram or model of the genital/pelvic region is helpful as the pain experienced during intercourse cannot always be reproduced during a pelvic examination.)
- *Intensity.* Describe the pain in terms of intensity (on a 1–10 scale) and quality (descriptors such a "burning," "cutting," or "throbbing" can be useful diagnostic cues).
- *Duration.* How long does the pain last (only during penetration or for some time after)?
- *Conditionality.* Does your experience of pain with intercourse (whether you feel pain and how intense it is) depend on certain conditions (e.g., menstrual cycle, level of arousal, intercourse position, a specific partner, etc.)?
- *Provoked versus unprovoked.* Does the pain that you regularly feel with intercourse ever happen without provocation (e.g., does it happens sometimes when you do not have intercourse or when no other contact is going on that could explain the onset of the pain)?

- *Nonintercourse related pain.* Do you have genital or pelvic pain with other sexual or nonsexual contact (e.g., tampon insertion, pelvic examinations, finger insertion, oral sex, urination)?
- *Lay causal attributions.* Do you have any theory about what could be causing the pain you experience with intercourse?
- *Interference.* How is this intercourse pain interfering with your sex, relationships, and general wellbeing?
- *Previous treatments.* Have you had any treatments for this intercourse pain, what were they, and did they help?

The answers to these questions may be at best diagnostic, in and of themselves, but at the very least they will start to rule out certain possible etiologic factors. For example, research shows that vulvar pain during intercourse that is described as "burning" is highly likely to indicate either PVD or vaginal atrophy. Women's causal attributions for their pain have also been found to be useful indicators of possible etiology and of the woman's psychosocial adjustment.

✋ CAUTION!

Although it is important to communicate to the patient that you are invested in the accurate diagnosis and effective treatment of her intercourse pain, it is important that you do not create false hopes about its resolution. Validating that the pain is real and that you are taking it seriously will be very therapeutic, but be careful not to overreach and create false expectations that will lead to unnecessary disappointment in the patient and frustration in you. The patient should be told that this is a difficult problem to resolve, that you are committed to doing your best to work toward that resolution, but that you cannot promise an eradication of the pain, although it is possible for that to happen. Immediate effects of treatment are rare, and both you and the patient need to prepare for what might be a lengthy process, involving more than one healthcare provider. This stance will go some ways toward discouraging doctor-shopping, which is common in genital pain conditions. In one online study of 428 women with vulvar pain, close to half reported consulting 4–9 physicians, and only 40% trusted their current physician to manage the pain.

Physical examination

Most women with dyspareunia are quite capable of tolerating pelvic examinations, but these can be anxiety-producing and painful for a significant number of patients. It is thus important to proceed giving the woman as much control as possible over the process. One good rule of thumb is to announce what you will be doing next before executing it. Another useful technique is to provide the patient visual access to what is being done (e.g., via a mirror or videocolposcope). Letting the woman know that she can stop the examination at any time is also very important. Some patients may require even more emotional support. In these cases, it can be useful to have an assistant holding the woman's hand or talking her through the examination.

For both diagnostic and rapport-building reasons, the physical examination should be methodically and carefully executed. Visual inspection is important as it can immediately reveal any number of possible culprits, including infection, fissures, inflammation, trauma, and dermatoses. For women reporting vulvar or introital pain with intercourse, sensory mapping of the vulva and vestibule should be performed with a moistened cotton-tipped applicator. It is generally a good idea to start palpation in areas that are not expected to be hyperalgesic, such as the inner thigh or mons pubis. This eases the patient into the procedure and distinguishes between painful and nonpainful stimulation. Women with PVD will generally report exquisite pain very specifically located in the vestibule. Women with conditions affecting the general anogenital region (e.g., infection, dermatoses, neuropathic processes) will report pain in a more diffuse region, including the labia majora and perineum.

★ TIPS & TRICKS

A systematic routine should be adopted for the cotton-swab palpation part of the physical examination. Start by applying pressure in areas that are not expected to be painful—the medial thigh, the buttocks, and the mons pubis. Then proceed to the labia majora, clitoral prepuce, perineum, and intralabial sulci. Next, gently palate the labia minora, lateral to Hart's line, which borders on the vulvar vestibule. Finally, gently palpate the vestibule at seven sites: at 11 and 1 o'clock, at 3 and 9 o'clock, at 4 and 8 o'clock, and at 6 o'clock.

The next step in the examination should involve a vaginal evaluation with index finger insertion just past the introitus. Care needs to be taken to insert the finger through the hymenal ring with as little vestibular contact as possible. The index finger is then used to palpate the lateral, anterior, and posterior walls of the vagina, the urethra, and pelvic floor muscles. The patient should be asked to contract and relax the muscles. A narrow and generously lubricated speculum can then be inserted, again with minimal vestibular contact, to assess the vaginal mucosa, the presence of fissures or other abnormalities, vaginal atrophy, and vaginal depth. Gentle palpation of the cervix and cervical fornices with the cotton swab is also indicated as it can reveal cervical allodynia, endometriosis, and pelvic inflammatory disease. After this comprehensive single-digit examination, the abdominal hand can then be added to the procedure to further assess the condition of the pelvic viscera.

★ TIPS & TRICKS

Add the abdominal hand to palpate only after you have completed a comprehensive single-digit transvaginal palpation of the adnexal areas on each side. If you add the abdominal hand too early in the process, you may confound nociceptive signals from the myofascial structures of the abdominal wall with signals that may be emanating from the uterus and adnexa.

Throughout these manipulations, the patient should be asked if the pain or discomfort experienced resembles the pain she feels during sexual intercourse. Cultures, vulvovaginal biopsies, and serum testing for hormonal abnormalities can be performed as indicated by the findings from the physical examination and patient history.

✋ CAUTION!

Even if you do not find any pathology during the physical examination or in any of the other diagnostic tests, never intimate to the patient that you think the dyspareunia is psychogenic in origin. First of all, you are not in a position to make that dualistic determination but, most importantly, women with dyspareunia are often told that the pain is "in their heads." This is universally experienced as invalidating, blaming, and an indication that the physician has given up trying to help them. Pain is pain, and it is your job to try to alleviate it. Also resist the temptation to make superficial suggestions such as "you need to relax" or "have a glass of wine" before sex. You can be assured that women with chronic pain during sex have already tried the obvious, to no avail. Dyspareunia is a complex condition that is unlikely to be impacted by simple directives.

Treatment of dyspareunia

Because dyspareunia is a heterogeneous disorder that can have a variety of causes, treatment will vary, to some extent, as a function of the physical pathology suspected to be playing a role in the generation of pain. However, research is increasingly indicating that dyspareunia is multidetermined, with only rare cases in which physical pathology and psychosocial factors can be reliably disentangled. It is thus likely that almost all types of long-standing dyspareunia will share some features that need addressing in treatment. These may include pelvic floor dysfunction developed as a function of reactions to intense, recurrent pain in the genital region, generalized sexual dysfunction, cognitive sets that exacerbate pain, behavioral avoidance, emotional distress, and relationship discord. Furthermore and as mentioned above, the most common cases of dyspareunia presenting in gynecologic practice will have no obvious pathology. The sensory dysfunction associated with PVD will usually have no consistent manifestation, other than the hyperalgesia of the vestibule.

For these reasons, the recommended treatment for dyspareunia is multidisciplinary, combining the expertise of gynecologists, physical therapists, and mental health professionals specialized in sex therapy and pain management. Furthermore, it is recommended that this multidisciplinary effort be a concurrent one rather than a sequential one. The point is not to refer patients out to other professionals but to work in tandem with these other professionals in a team effort to simultaneously target all factors reasonably associated with the experience of pain with intercourse.

★ TIPS & TRICKS

Become acquainted with pelvic floor physical therapists and sex therapists in the community. You will often need to refer to these professionals, or you will receive referrals from them. Pelvic floor physical therapists can be accessed using online national databases, and sex therapists can be accessed through the membership directories of sex therapy professional associations. Ideally, you will not just refer patients to these individuals but be in regular communication with them in order to provide coordinated care.

Targeting obvious pathology

It is beyond the scope of this chapter to review treatments for all the physical problems possibly associated with dyspareunia. Each of the potential physical etiologies has its own indicated treatment. Estrogen therapy is often indicated for vaginal atrophy (depending on the specific woman's risk factors), and there are also nonhormonal alternatives that have a direct impact on vaginal dryness; antimicrobial and antifungal treatments are appropriate for the treatment of infections and cyclical vulvovaginitis; a variety of topical corticosteroids (and doses), as well as antihistamines, are indicated for dermatoses, again depending on type; pharmacologic or surgical treatment are employed in the case of endometriosis; and surgery is a likely option for fibroids, adhesions, or prolapsed pelvic organs.

Although the aforementioned pathologies have been associated with dyspareunia, women with these conditions who do not concurrently experience pain with intercourse are more numerous than women who have intercourse pain. Dyspareunia is not an inevitable result of most of these problems. Gynecologists have long been treating these conditions without the frustration associated with the treatment of painful intercourse. That is because eradication of physical pathology, when possible, will often fail to result in the resolution of intercourse pain. If the intercourse pain has been experienced for a considerable period of time, it is likely that the patient has become classically conditioned to pair pain with sex, and this conditioning is not amenable to medical or surgical interventions. That is why dyspareunia stands out as a particularly thorny problem that often escapes the straightforward treatment of physical pathology. Although addressing the physical problems that might be playing a role in the experience of pain is necessary, it is often insufficient. Coordinated treatment will require the incorporation of other treatment approaches such as physical therapy, sex therapy, and pain management.

Targeting provoked vestibulodynia

Although the cause of PVD remains largely unknown, most researchers agree that neuropathic pain is the common end result. Although there are treatment algorithms that recommend a standard strategy with all women who have PVD, these are based on expert opinion. There have been very few randomized trials of treatment for any kind of vulvodynia. Some vulvar specialists recommend a customized approach to PVD, depending on the prominence of pelvic floor dysfunction, hormonal changes, acquired neuronal proliferation, or congenital neuronal hyperplasia.

When pelvic floor hypertonicity is present, as assessed through palpation during the physical examination, pelvic floor physical therapy is an essential treatment component. Physical therapists who specialize in the treatment of pelvic floor dysfunction use a variety of manual therapy techniques, electromyography biofeedback, vaginal dilators, vibrators, and electrical stimulation to retrain muscular control, with excellent results in women with dyspareunia. Muscle relaxants can also be added to treatment, although there are concerns over dependence, especially given the distress many of these women experience. Some studies have reported success with intralevator injections of botulinum toxin type A, while others have found no effect.

If hormonal factors are suspected, as assessed by low levels of serum estradiol and testosterone, some suggest that women should stop taking hormonal contraceptives and that a compound of estradiol and testosterone be applied to the vestibule daily. If laboratory findings indicate acquired or congenital neuronal proliferation, as assessed by the density of C afferent nociceptors in a vestibular biopsy, suggested treatments boasting some (although inconsistent) empiric support include oral tricyclic antidepressants (starting at 25 mg and increasing to 100 mg), capsaicin cream (0.25%), topical lidocaine (5% prior to intercourse), xylocaine, ketoconazole (2%), interferon injections, and steroid injections. There is, however, no pharmacologic intervention that has been empirically shown to consistently outperform placebo.

The one treatment for PVD that has received the strongest and most consistent empirical support is surgery—more specifically, vestibulectomy with vaginal advancement.

⚛ SCIENCE REVISITED

In a vestibulectomy, the epithelium of the posterior vestibule is excised, the excision usually bordering on the junction with the external skin, usually up to the 3 o'clock and 9 o'clock positions (although some prefer to excise higher, at 1 o'clock and 11 o'clock), and into the cephalad margin of the posterior hymen. The epithelium of the lower vagina is then detached only as far as necessary to cover the excised part of the vestibule without tension. Two-week dissolvable sutures are commonly used, and postoperative care ranges from topical estrogen to lidocaine to physical therapy 1 month to 6 weeks after surgery. Research has shown that surgical outcomes are enhanced by postoperative cognitive behavioral therapy.

Not surprisingly, the invasiveness of this treatment option generally makes it a last resort option, after more conservative approaches have failed. It is important to note, however, that it boasts a higher success rate than all other approaches. Complications from this surgery are infrequent and minor, although it can cause iatrogenic harm in a minority of cases. Considering the superior efficacy of vestibulectomy compared to other treatments for PVD, as well as the understandable impatience of many women to finally hit on a successful treatment, one can only guess that the reticence to opt for the surgical route is related to an equally understandable risk aversion in physicians.

EVIDENCE AT A GLANCE

Results at a 6-month follow-up in a randomized study comparing group cognitive-behavioral therapy (CBT; weekly 2-hour sessions for 8 weeks), biofeedback, and vestibulectomy for the treatment of provoked vestibulodynia demonstrated that women in the vestibulectomy treatment arm had experienced the greatest pain reduction (as assessed clinically). Sixty-eight percent of women who had had a vestibulectomy reported significant pain reduction, compared to 39% of the women in the CBT condition and 35% of those in the biofeedback condition. It is important to note, however, that 9%

of the women who had a vestibulectomy reported higher pain intensity post treatment. There were also significantly more women randomized to the vestibulectomy condition who refused to undergo the procedure compared to the other two treatment conditions. This tells us that despite the higher rate of pain reduction with vestibulectomy, the procedure may have lower palatability and higher risk than other less invasive treatments. In a 2.5-year follow-up, vestibulectomy participants still had the lowest clinically assessed pain levels of the three treatment conditions, but the incidence of self-reported pain during intercourse was no lower than for the CBT condition.

Targeting common factors in many types of dyspareunia

As already mentioned, it is likely that a woman who has been experiencing painful intercourse for a significant period of time, regardless of its etiology, has also developed certain cognitive sets and behaviors that at best interfere with the improvement or resolution of her pain problem, and at worst exacerbate it. In addition, she is likely to be experiencing difficulty at the desire, arousal, and orgasm stages of the sexual response, which also adds to the pain difficulty. Last, but not least, mood disturbances characterized by anxiety and depression are not unusual given how profoundly dyspareunia can affect the woman's sense of wellbeing, as well as her current relationship or relationship prospects. If these psychosocial processes have been at play for a significant period of time, they will have to be addressed in treatment, in addition to and concurrently with the treatment of any physical problem.

Rarely in a position to address these problems in any depth, gynecologists need to add mental health professionals who specialize in sex therapy and pain management to their multidisciplinary treatment team. Dyspareunia assessment and treatment do not involve an either/or, physical/psychological dualistic determination. With very few well-justified exceptions, the assumption should be that women with dyspareunia are likely to need the concurrent services of a gynecologist, a physical therapist, and a sex therapist/psychologist with an expertise in sexual function and pain management. In certain cases, dermatologists can also be very helpful.

Cognitive-behavioral therapy (CBT), in conjunction with physical therapy, has been shown to be helpful in the treatment of dyspareunia. CBT first aims to educate women and their partners about dyspareunia as a pain syndrome impacted by cognitive, emotional, behavioral, and relationship factors, regardless of physical pathology. It then proceeds to re-educate patients to think differently about intercourse pain (decatastrophize), regulate emotions associated with the pain and its interference (reduce anxiety), reinstate desire and arousal through a modified sexual repertoire that is not exclusively focused on penetration, and modify intimacy avoidant behaviors.

Treatment techniques include pain diaries, relaxation techniques, systematic desensitization using vaginal dilatation, cognitive restructuring exercises, distraction techniques using sexual imagery, the rehearsal of coping self-statements, and communication skills training focused on the expression of emotional needs and sexual preferences. The ultimate aim of all of these techniques is to encourage changes in the patient's cognitive set, emotional regulation, behavioral repertoire, and relational dynamic so as to decrease the fear of pain and penetration, which usually decreases the intensity of pain experienced. Physical therapy augments the effort by also using systematic desensitization through its pelvic floor manipulations and exercises. Both can also be useful in helping the patient to adhere to treatment regimens prescribed by their gynecologists.

The referral of a patient to CBT should not be a last resort when all other medical or surgical treatments have been exhausted. CBT is most helpful when it is concurrent with these other treatments as it can increase their effectiveness, in addition to contributing its own unique benefits. In studies pitting CBT against biofeedback, corticosteroid cream, and vestibulectomy for women with PVD, CBT performed as well as or better in reducing pain with intercourse. Importantly, CBT targets areas related to sexual functioning and relational adjustment that can have a significant impact on the experience of pain and on general quality of life.

Sometimes patients with dyspareunia will be referred to gynecologists by sex therapists. In these cases, the gynecologist will not be in a position of having to promote CBT to the patient but rather to possibly communicate (given a release of information) with the therapist. Details regarding diagnostic findings or medical/surgical treatment outcomes can be helpful to the CBT process. In either case, it is important that the gynecologist consider CBT part of an overall multidisciplinary treatment effort rather than a referral out for a psychogenic problem. CBT functions as a pain management program that seeks primarily to address pain and the factors, psychological, relational and otherwise, that mediate its intensity. The patient needs to know that pain management is an integral component of the treatment of any variety of pain syndromes that do not have the psychogenic stigma traditionally associated with dyspareunia.

☆ TIPS & TRICKS

Cognitive-behavioral therapy (CBT) for dyspareunia is ideally delivered to the couple rather than just to the woman herself. When recommending CBT, encourage the patient to include her partner in the therapy as much as possible as participation of the partner in treatment accomplishes a number of important goals. First, it communicates that dyspareunia is not just the woman's problem but the couple's problem, solutions to which require a team effort. Second, partners sometimes have their own sexual dysfunction that can interfere with treatment, and this dysfunction can be addressed in therapy. Third, partners can also learn to modify attitudes and behaviors that can be counterproductive and work against treatment strategies. Finally, involving the partner in therapy is likely to engender closeness and increase partner patience with the often lengthy process. Not all patients, however, will have willing or regular partners, and thus this recommendation cannot be communicated as a necessary requirement of CBT for dyspareunia.

Alternative treatments

There are now a handful of studies with small samples indicating that both acupuncture and hypnotherapy may be useful in the treatment of vulvar pain. Hypnotherapy has shown significant pain reduction in two studies of women with PVD. The data available on acupuncture indicate that pain relief may be short term, but more research is necessary to determine the effectiveness of either of these two interventions. Referral to these alternative treatments would have to be made with the assurance that their practitioners were familiar with dyspareunia.

Conclusions

Dyspareunia is a multidetermined pain disorder that optimally requires a concurrent multidisciplinary treatment approach, a large dose of sensitivity to patient distress, meticulous assessment of the pain and associated pathology, and the patience to consider as many treatments as are empirically supported and/or theoretically reasonable. In addition, the treatment of dyspareunia is likely to be greatly enhanced (if not sometimes determined) by the involvement of a pelvic floor physical therapist and a psychologist or other mental health professional specializing in sex therapy and pain management. The coordination of the treatment team can be complicated by the availability of professionals, challenges in interdisciplinary communication, and the financial burden on the client. Flexibility in the face of constraints is necessary, and hopeful endurance through the typically long treatment process is important.

Selected bibliography

Bergeron S, Binik YM, Khalifé S et al. A randomized comparison of group cognitive-behavioral therapy, surface electromyographic biofeedback, and vestibulectomy in the treatment of dyspareunia resulting from vulvar vestibulitis. Pain 2001;91:297–306.

Binik YM. The diagnostic criteria for dyspareunia. Arch Sex Behav 2010;39:292–303.

Dennerstein L, Alexander J, Kotz K. The menopause and sexual functioning: a review of the population-based studies. Annu Rev Sex Res 2003;14:64–82.

Desrochers G, Bergeron S, Landry T, Jodoin M. Do psychosexual factors play a role in the etiology of provoked vestibulodynia? J Sex Marital Ther 2008;34:198–226.

Ferraro S, Ragni N, Remorgida V. Deep dyspareunia: causes, treatments, and results. Curr Opin Obstet Gynecol 2008;20:394–9.

Goldstein AT, Klingman D, Christopher K, Johnson C, Marinoff SC. Surgical treatment of vulvar vestibulitis syndrome: Outcome assessment derived from a postoperative questionnaire. J Sex Med 2006;3:923–31.

Goldstein AT, Pukall CF, Goldstein I, eds. Female sexual pain disorders. Oxford: Wiley-Blackwell; 2009.

Gordon AS, Panahian-Jand M, McComb F, Melegari C, Sharp S. Characteristics of women with vulvar pain disorders: Responses to a web-based survey. J Sex Marital Ther 2003;29(s): 45–58.

Haefner HK, Collins ME, Davis GD et al. The vulvodynia guideline. J Low Genit Tract Dis 2005;9:40–51.

Harlow BL, Wise LA, Stewart EG. Prevalence and predictors of chronic lower genital tract discomfort. Am J Obstet Gynecol 2001;185: 545–50.

Hayes RD, Bennett CM, Fairley CK, Dennerstein L. What can prevalence studies tell us about female sexual difficulty and dysfunction. J Sex Med 2006;3:589–95.

Hayes RD, Dennerstein L, Bennett C, Fairly CK. What is the true prevalence of female sexual dysfunction and does the way we assess these conditions have an impact? J Sex Med 2008;5: 777–87.

Kao A, Binik YM, Kapuscinski A, Khalife S. Dyspareunia in postmenopausal women: a critical review. Pain Res Manag 2008;13:243–54.

Landry T, Bergeron S, Dupuis M-J, Desrochers G. The treatment of provoked vestibulodynia: a critical review. Clin J Pain 2008;24:155–71.

Latthe P, Latthe M, Say L, Gulmezoglu M, Khan KS. WHO systematic review of prevalence of chronic pelvic pain: a neglected reproductive health morbidity. BMC Public Health 2006;6: 177–83.

Meana M, Binik YM, Khalife S, Cohen D. Dyspareunia: sexual dysfunction or pain syndrome? J Nerv Mental Dis 1997;185:561–9.

Pukall CF, Binik YM, Khalifé S, Amsel R, Abbott FV. Vestibular tactile and pain thresholds in women with vulvar vestibulitis syndrome. Pain 2002;96:163–75.

Steege JF, Zolnoun DA. Evaluation and treatment of dyspareunia. Obstet Gynecol 2009;113: 1124–36.

Sutton KS, Pukall CF, Chamberlain S. Pain ratings, sensory thresholds, and psychosocial functioning in women with provoked vestibulodynia. J Sex Med 2009;35:262–81.

Management of Chronic Pelvic Pain in the Adolescent Woman

Luigi Fedele, Giada Frontino, and Stefano Bianchi

University of Milan, Milan, Italy

Introduction

In adolescent girls, dysmenorrhea is one of the most common pain-related complaints, with a prevalence of 40–90%. Not infrequently, pelvic pain is one of the first symptoms of the beginning of a woman's fertile age. The first menstrual cycles are not usually particularly painful as they mostly represent anovulatory cycles. While adult patients are commonly evaluated for pelvic pain, an adolescent poses a more complex diagnostic approach due to the absence of a relevant past pain history and the more difficult interaction with the patient, which can be worsened by distressed parents.

Evaluation

When an adolescent patient presents with pelvic pain, several issues will need to be evaluated, other than the symptoms, that are related to the medical and psychosocial history. It will be necessary to evaluate the family history of endometriosis and the past surgical history, as well as excluding renal tract or other congenital anomalies. Establishing good communication with the young patient will increase the likelihood of being able to explore relevant issues and identify risk factors such as depression, sexual activity, and drug or alcohol intake. A student who is being bullied may be avoiding school and may thus be simulating menstrual pain for this reason.

> ☆ **TIPS & TRICKS**
>
> Adolescents may have concerns regarding confidentiality that limit their reliability for revealing risky sexual behaviors, making it difficult for the clinician to assess the patient's risk for having pelvic inflammatory disease. Furthermore, many adolescent girls are new to pelvic examinations and may be unwilling or unable to cooperate with a good clinical examination. It is particularly prudent that clinicians provide the most comfortable and safe environment possible when evaluating an adolescent for pelvic inflammatory disease.

> ☆ **TIPS & TRICKS**
>
> An adolescent patient will possibly be embarrassed to spontaneously disclose details regarding her menstrual cycle, such as intermenstrual spotting, so it is essential that the clinician suggest specific points to be discussed.

Nongynecologic causes of chronic or recurrent pelvic pain

Pelvic pain presenting in a woman of any age requires ruling out nongynecologic causes.

Chronic Pelvic Pain, First Edition. Edited by Paolo Vercellini.
© 2011 Blackwell Publishing Ltd. Published 2011 by Blackwell Publishing Ltd.

Nongynecologic causes of chronic pelvic pain include cystitis, irritable bowel syndrome, Crohn's disease, ulcerative colitis, infectious enterocolitis, diverticulitis, intestinal obstructions, bowel cancer, hernias, recurrent appendiceal colic, and intestinal endometriosis.

Irritable bowel syndrome is probably the most common cause of abdominal pain. Such pain can be intermittent and cramp-like or even constant, lasting from a few minutes to weeks. Usually, such pain worsens after meals and is not associated with weight loss. Diagnosis is suggested by the intermittency of pain, the patient's good general conditions, and the relation between the symptoms and the environmental conditions and stress.

Crohn's disease is characterized by a triad of symptoms that includes diarrhea, pain in the right iliac fossa and rarely fever. The pain is unrelenting or has the typical characteristics of a colic and is cramping in nature. The disease is chronic and is characterized by the periodic exacerbation and remission of symptoms. In ulcerative rectocolitis, pain is almost always associated with bloody diarrhea, and in severe cases with fever and weight loss. The clinical picture can be variable in relation to the extension and course of the disease.

Gynecologic causes of chronic pelvic pain in adolescents

Gynecologic causes of chronic pelvic pain specific to adolescents that should be taken into consideration include ovarian cysts, pelvic inflammatory disease, primary dysmenorrhea, endometriosis, and congenital müllerian anomalies.

The majority of cases of dysmenorrhea in adolescents and young adults are primary (or functional), are associated with a normal ovulatory cycle and with no pelvic pathology, and have a clear physiologic etiology based on prostaglandins and leukotrienes mediating the inflammatory cascade following progesterone withdrawal before menstruation. In primary dysmenorrhea, the pain is usually cramp-like, is referred to the lower abdominal quadrants, and often radiates to the thighs and lumbosacral region. The pain generally starts a few hours before the menstrual flow, being severe during the first day and lasting from a few hours to 1 day, but not normally for more than 2 days. When dysmenorrhea is severe, requiring pain medication, nonsteroidal anti-inflammatory drugs (NSAIDs) such as naproxen can be used on a short-term basis during the menstrual cycle. An oral contraceptive is considered as a valid option in sexually active patients or especially when gastritis may complicate the chronic use of NSAIDs.

Pelvic endometriosis should be considered also in adolescents, and an ultrasound is mandatory, especially in those young patients with persistence of symptoms not responding to treatment with an oral contraceptive. This should also rule out adnexal masses such as ovarian cysts and hemorrhagic cysts or corpora lutea. Nonendometriotic ovarian cysts are seldom a cause of chronic intermenstrual pelvic pain and, regardless of size, the symptoms are of pressure and heaviness in the hypogastric or iliac fossa region.

While the scientific literature has not shown that the early diagnosis and treatment of pelvic endometriosis limits disease progression, most studies confirm that it is reasonable to start with a first-line treatment of a low-dose oral contraceptive pill, in either a cyclic or a continuous regimen, and NSAIDs. Other medical treatments commonly used for symptoms of pelvic endometriosis are progestins, such as norethisterone acetate and medroxyprogesterone acetate, and gonadotropin-releasing hormone agonists. Both have shown important side effects due to the prolonged hypoestrogenemia, such as a progressive decrease in the bone mineral density.

Laparoscopy can be necessary when a pelvic mass is suspected and when symptoms are not controlled by the medical therapy. In a recent review, almost 50% of adolescents with endometriosis confirmed by biopsy at laparoscopy showed a severe stage of the disease. Each case should be assessed carefully, and surgery should be indicated in specific conditions, when all options have been undertaken and discussed. Surgery offered as a first-line diagnostic tool and treatment has not been proven to limit disease progression or the impact on reproductive prognosis and will possibly predispose to repeat surgeries in the future.

When assessing a sexually active adolescent patient, a vaginal swab is essential to exclude ascending vaginal infections. Subacute and chronic pelvic inflammatory disease is considered to be a frequent cause of pelvic pain. The subacute variant is due to an incomplete recovery from a first episode or a reinfection. The pain may be severe and is usually associated with nausea, vomiting, abdominal bloating, fever, and leukocytosis. There is diffuse pelvic tenderness, which is worsened by mobilization of the cervix. Adnexal masses can be palpated, and the uterus is usually fixed and immobile. The pain reported by the patient is due to the tubo-ovarian and Douglas pouch abscesses that are found in this variant.

Patients with chronic pelvic inflammatory disease do not present with the typical pelvic inflammatory signs but still have pelvic pain that worsens in the premenstrual and menstrual phases, as well as dyspareunia. Menstrual cycles are also often irregular. The pelvic examination can reveal adnexal masses, a fixed uterine retroversion, and tenderness in the posterior parametrium. Such findings can be explained by the presence of tubo-ovarian fibrotic thickenings of variable degree and their adhesion to the posterior uterine wall, the broad ligament, and the lateral pelvic wall.

⚘ SCIENCE REVISITED

Pelvic inflammatory disease is a highly preventable cause of significant reproductive morbidity in young women and adolescents. Sexually active adolescents are at increased risk for developing pelvic inflammatory disease compared to older women because of both anatomic and behavioral factors. The immature cervix has a wider surface area of columnar epithelium on the ectocervix for microorganisms to infect, and the cervical mucus may be altered due to the persistent hyperestrogenic state in anovulatory cycles, therefore decreasing the local defense mechanisms against the upper tract ascension of microorganisms. Higher exposure rates in adolescents are also due to unprotected sex in relationships of short duration and high frequency.

Obstructive müllerian anomalies, which typically cause dysmenorrhea due to retention of menstrual blood, can usually be diagnosed within a year from menarche, thereby limiting the risk of developing pelvic endometriosis. Congenital imperforate hymen is probably the most common obstructive anomaly of the female reproductive tract. Many young women with imperforate hymen may reach menarche before the diagnosis is made. In these cases, the patient is premenarchal despite pubertal development, and presents with intermittent lower abdominal pain and a hymenal bulge. Patients may seldom present with a suprapubic mass that can, in severe cases, lead to acute urinary retention with secondary hydronephrosis and constipation. A gentle pressure on the suprapubic mass while inspecting the perineum will reveal that the hymenal membrane will bulge. Treatment requires surgical stellate incision of the hymen.

Differential diagnosis should include a transverse vaginal septum and vaginal and/or cervical atresia, which are not characterized by a hymenal bulge. Both a transverse vaginal septum and cervical agenesis or vaginal atresia can be variably associated with other congenital anomalies, including those of the urinary tract, lumbar spine, and heart. Ultrasound and a magnetic resonance imaging (MRI) scan are mandatory in order to assess the pelvic anatomy and to exclude the presence of renal anomalies such as a pelvic kidney.

Vaginal atresia requires surgical excision and anastomosis of the margins of the vaginal mucosa in order to avoid stenosis. Cervical dysgenesis with a normal uterine corpus can result from complete agenesis or partial atresia; it can be solitary or associated with absence of variable portions of the vagina. Transabdominal and transrectal ultrasound as well as MRI aid in appropriate study and surgical planning, although the preoperative diagnosis of cervical dysgenesis is usually difficult. Although in the past many authors have recommended hysterectomy as the only treatment that eliminates the cause of pelvic pain, hematometra, endometriosis, and sepsis, scientific literature has shown that in these young patients a recanalization with an anastomosis between the distal supracervical uterine portion and the vaginal mucosa can be attempted, with a relatively good possibility of restoring menstrual function and reproductive potential.

Another obstructive müllerian anomaly is represented by a double uterus with an obstructed hemivagina. In this condition, menstrual blood cyclically partially accumulates inside the hemivaginal pouch while partially draining from the contralateral canalized hemivagina. A certain anatomic variability within this anomaly not infrequently causes difficulties in promptly recognizing the presence of an obstructed hemivagina. One of the variables that should necessarily be assessed is whether the double uterus is characterized by a midline septum or a bicornuate morphology, since both can be associated with an obstructed hemivagina.

Ultrasound and MRI scanning will be important in the diagnostic work-up of these cases, despite the fact that the hematocolpos will occasionally not be recognized but may actually be mistaken for an adnexal mass when the blood-filled hemivagina reaches a considerable diameter. Additional assessment of the upper urinary tract should be performed since associated renal and ureteral anomalies are a relatively frequent finding in patients with a double uterus and obstructed hemivagina. Yet another variable that can affect the timing of the diagnosis is the possible presence of fistulae in the vaginal septum, which may limit the distension and pain but can be suspected when postmenstrual spotting is reported by the patient.

A laparoscopic exploration of the pelvis will establish the diagnosis and confirm the uterine morphology, and the vaginal septum can be excised using a vaginal approach. Hysteroscopic metroplasty of the uterine septum should not be performed at a perimenarchal age but will, after adequate counseling, be postponed to an age when the woman seeks to have children.

A rudimentary horn with a functional cavity but absence of communication with the vagina will cause cyclic pain due to the presence of cryptometra and/or hematosalpinx. Although in the majority of cases the rudimentary horn is non-cavitated, this can be confirmed with an ultrasound performed in the premenstrual phase, which will determine the presence of not only a rudimentary bulb, but also a cavity within it. Again, urinary tract anomalies need to be excluded due to a strong association with a uni-

cornuate uterus. Hysteroscopic recognition of a single tubal ostium will confirm the noncommunicating nature of the rudimentary horn, which can be subsequently removed via laparoscopy.

> **⚠ CAUTION**
>
> Hysteroscopic metroplasty of a uterine septum should not be performed at a perimenarchal age but instead, after satisfactory counseling, postponed to an age at which the woman wishes to have children.

> **SCIENCE REVISITED**
>
> **Differential diagnosis of causes of chronic pelvic pain in adolescents**
> Endometriosis—endosalpingosis
> Adenomyosis
> Constipation
> Depression
> Diarrhea
> Pelvic inflammatory disease
> Cystitis
> Hernia
> Irritable bowel syndrome
> Müllerian anomalies

Selected bibliography

Emans J, Laufer MR, Goldstein DP. Pediatric and adolescent gynecology, 5th ed. Philadelphia: Lippincott Williams & Wilkins, 2005.

Fedele L, Bianchi S, Frontino G et al. Laparoscopically assisted uterovestibular anastomosis in patients with uterine cervix atresia and vaginal aplasia. Fertil Steril 2008;89:212–6.

Harel Z. Dysmenorrhea in adolescents and young adults: from pathophysiology to pharmacological treatments and management strategies. Expert Opin Pharmacother 2008;9:2661–72.

Miller RJ, Breech LL. Surgical correction of vaginal anomalies. Clin Obstet Gynecol 2008;51: 223–36.

Reese KA, Reddy S, Rock JA. Endometriosis in an adolescent population: the Emory experience. J Pediatr Adolesc Gynecol 1996;9:125–8.

Multidisciplinary Management of Chronic Pelvic Pain Without Obvious Pathology

Liza Marie Colimon, David Ashley Hill, and Georgine Lamvu

Florida Hospital, Orlando, Florida, USA

Introduction

Chronic pelvic pain (CPP) is a common but complex symptom that can result from multiple urologic, gastroenterologic, musculoskeletal, or gynecologic etiologies. For some patients, the pain has no clear identifiable cause or persists in spite of treatment for a known (one or multiple) underlying disorder. Persistent pain in this setting can cause significant long-term distress and disability. Generally, for this group of patients, traditional clinical investigations are negative, focused unidimensional treatments are not helpful, and eventually frustration and mistrust ensue, leading to a complete breakdown of the patient–provider relationship. It is in this environment that CPP usually becomes identified as the primary disease rather than an acute symptom that can be easily cured. When a provider is faced with this type of challenging patient, the treatment paradigm must change to incorporate the following concepts:

- Management of CPP can focus on treating the pain itself or the underlying cause, but preferably both.
- Treatment of CPP should focus more on therapies that help manage the pain rather than on curing the pain; thus, the focus becomes improving quality of life and finding ways of coping with the pain.
- Managing CPP involves addressing multiple biologic, psychological, and environmental factors that may affect pain levels; thus,

therapy for CPP often involves a multidisciplinary approach.

Modern definitions of pain describe it as a symptom with two essential components: first, the physical sensation arising from pathology or disturbed physiology (the sensory experience), and second, the patient's beliefs about that symptom and associated behavior (the emotional experience). Focusing only on the sensory aspect of pain neglects the needs of patients with chronic pain of unknown etiology. For patients with intractable pain and without obvious pathology, we suggest that managing the emotional aspects of pain perception and behavior is as important as controlling the sensory aspects of the pain experience. This chapter will focus on the important aspects of multidisciplinary treatment for the different facets of CPP. The goal of the information provided here is to allow healthcare providers to develop a patient-centered agenda that focuses on long-term pain management *and* on improving measures of quality of life.

The initial encounter: special considerations when evaluating women with CPP without an identifiable cause

Research shows that most women with CPP have negative perceptions of their interactions with healthcare providers, especially gynecologists. Women receiving gynecologic care often feel like they do not receive personal care, that they are

Chronic Pelvic Pain, First Edition. Edited by Paolo Vercellini.
© 2011 Blackwell Publishing Ltd. Published 2011 by Blackwell Publishing Ltd.

not understood or taken seriously, and that they are frequently dismissed without reassurance or an explanation for their pain. Chronic pain patients also have difficulty understanding and accepting normal test results and often express disappointment with the overall quality of the consultation. These findings are unfortunate, given that the a better quality of the initial gynecologic consultation (as perceived by the patient) has been shown to be associated with better recovery and treatment outcomes.

Most pelvic pain experts emphasize the importance of the initial gynecologic consultation. This initial encounter should involve a comprehensive review of the history and physical examination. The physician should begin the interview with open-ended questions that allow the patient to express her main concern. Questions should focus on how the pain impacts her daily function, quality of life, and social relationships, and define which emotional states are a consequence of her chronic pain (e.g., depression, anxiety). Identifying what the patient perceives is most distressing about her pain enables the provider to achieve three main goals:

1. to tailor interventions that target specific components *identified by the patient* as being important pain generators or potentiators;
2. to identify patient expectations for treatment outcome that may be unrealistic (i.e., a cure or complete elimination of the pain) and would contribute to noncompliance or viewing of the treatment as unsuccessful;
3. to generate a clinical environment that focuses on building a relationship of trust through patient-centered and personalized care.

To establish a relationship of trust during the initial interview, providers must convey interest, listen with attention, validate the patient's experience, and explain to their patients that they will do their best to help. Within this framework, the provider should obtain a detailed chronologic pain history, and determine the presence of any aggravating or alleviating factors, as well as the results of previous attempts at treatment. The clinician must also assess for symptoms that indicate possible involvement of the gastrointestinal,

urinary, musculoskeletal, and reproductive systems. Next, the clinician needs to determine the current pain regimen that the patient is using, its effectiveness, and the impact of the residual pain on the patient's quality of life. Although we encourage the use of open-ended questions when initiating the interview, eventually the clinician must carefully guide the patient through specific questions assessing the above organ systems.

> **⚠ CAUTION**
>
> To establish trust during the initial patient interview, providers must convey interest, listen with attention, validate the patient's experience and explain to the patient that they will do their best to help. Occasionally, the physical examination may have to be delayed until the second visit.

Admittedly, the initial interview can become quite lengthy and sometimes cannot be performed in a single office visit, especially when a through physical examination also needs to be completed. When office visits are limited by time, it has been our experience that patients do not object to being scheduled for additional visits, especially if the provider explains that the problem is complex and requires a more thorough and lengthy work-up. Patients may respond less well if they feel they are being rushed through the evaluation; cramming everything into the first visit for the sake of completing it on time is therefore not recommended.

A brief psychosocial assessment will provide clues to the patient's function in her social and home environment, her daily activity levels, her sexual function, and her interactions with her partner. All these factors will enable the provider to gain insight into the patient's emotional state and ability to cope with her pain. Sometimes a more in-depth psychosocial assessment is necessary, but we caution against conducting this type of questioning on the first visit. Asking about psychiatric dysfunction during the first encounter many times makes patients feel like the provider thinks that they are "crazy" or that the provider does not believe their pain. If this is the case, a breakdown of the patient–provider relationship may occur. To avoid this scenario, we recommend that a brief screen for abuse and safety be conducted at the first visit, while the more in-depth psychosocial assessment be completed at subsequent visits (or by a health psychologist), after a sense of trust and open communication has already been established with the patient.

The physical examination in patients with CPP is markedly different from the routine gynecologic evaluation. Sometimes, patients are so distressed by their pain or by retelling their history that the examination needs to be deferred to the second visit. This can be done safely in patients with chronic pain, especially if they have had multiple previous evaluations and diagnostic tests. If the patient appears too distressed, it is always best to reassure the patient, describe the steps of the physical examination, and give her the option of rescheduling her visit for a full examination. If the patient chooses to continue with the examination, it is important to give her a sense of control by explaining that she may stop the examination any time.

The physical examination should be methodical and directed at identifying the specific location of the pain as well as replicating the patient's pain. Chronic pain patients can sometimes have multiple sources of pain, so it is important to educate the patient about describing the pain in terms of intensity (many providers use a numeric scale) and determining whether the pain she feels is the same as the chronic pain she usually has when she is not being examined. As the examination is being conducted, the provider should give feedback about the steps of the evaluation as they are being performed.

Because the speculum and bimanual examination are the most uncomfortable and often the most anxiety-provoking aspects of the physical assessment, it is recommended that they be performed last. Instead, the examination should begin with an evaluation of the general appearance, mood, affect, mobility, and posture, followed by a supine and standing musculoskeletal evaluation of the lower back and abdomen. These tend not usually to be performed in the realm of routine gynecologic practice, but for women with CPP are an essential part of the evaluation (see Chapter 11). During the abdominal examination, a superficial inspection of scars and skin will identify areas of allodynia or hypersensitivity, while deep palpation will identify musculoskeletal trigger points, organomegaly, and other abdominal and pelvic masses.

Mood, affect, posture, musculoskeletal condition, and levels of activity are important factors to follow as patients with CPP of unknown etiology progress through treatment. Numerical pain scales that describe sensory levels of pain are often utilized, but they may be difficult to interpret: they may vary from visit to visit, and they lack measure for the affective component of the pain, which assesses how much the pain actually bothers the patient. In these cases, an additional evaluation of the patient's physical ability, activity levels, and demeanor may be more helpful when monitoring progress.

> ### ⚛ SCIENCE REVISITED
>
> Numerical pain scales describing sensory levels of pain are often used but may be difficult to interpret as the responses may differ between visits and they also lack any measure for the affective component of pain, which assesses how much the patient's pain actually bothers her. In such cases, it may be more helpful to undertake an additional evaluation of the patient's physical ability, activity level, quality of life, and general demeanor when monitoring her progress.

The pelvic examination should start with a gentle evaluation of the external genitalia. Beginning with a sensory examination, particular attention should be paid to identifying vulvovaginal disorders that are associated with CPP, such as vulvodynia, localized vestibulodynia (or vestibulitis), and vaginismus. If possible, a single-digit examination should be performed next to assess the pelvic floor musculature, bladder, urethra, vaginal walls, and cervix. For women with CPP of unknown origin, this is an important part of the internal evaluation. Many patients have painful spasms of the pelvic floor musculature, including the levator ani, obturator, pubococcygeus, and deep transverse perineal muscles, that go unrecognized for years. Musculoskeletal dysfunction can be the primary cause of pain or an effect of pathology elsewhere, so it is important that it is evaluated during both the external and internal examination of the patient.

Last, a bimanual and speculum examination can be performed, but only if the patient tolerates the initial portions of the vaginal examination. The bimanual examination can help identify cervical tenderness, uterosacral nodularities, and uterine tenderness. A rectovaginal examination is especially helpful in patients with suspected pudendal neuropathy as this allows the examiner to evaluate perineal hypoesthesia, paresthesias, and rectal tone. The speculum examination should be avoided in patients with vaginismus. However, in patients who can tolerate it, the speculum allows visualization of mucosal or cervical lesions, infections, and rarely endometrial implants. In patients with a previous hysterectomy, the vaginal cuff should be carefully probed for painful areas that may represent trigger points, neuromas, or painful granulation tissue. The speculum examination must be modified to allow visualization of all vaginal walls, especially in women who have previous vaginal scars (e.g., surgical scars, episiotomy) or pelvic organ prolapse.

> ### ✋ CAUTION
>
> The speculum examination should be avoided in patients with vaginismus. Musculoskeletal dysfunction can be the primary cause of pain and must be evaluated during both the external and internal examination. A bimanual and speculum examination may be performed only if the patient can tolerate the initial portions of the vaginal examination.

In general, women with CPP move from provider to provider and undergo a variety of gynecologic examinations and diagnostic tests that are often negative. In spite of this, it is essential to avoid omitting portions of the history and examination, even if this takes several visits. Often, a previously unrecognized or a new source of pain is identified only when a thorough examination has been completed. More importantly, a thorough review of the history and physical examination allows the provider to determine which

physical and psychosocial components are primary determinants of the patient's pain. This information can then be incorporated into a multidisciplinary treatment regimen that is specific to each patient.

Multidisciplinary pain management

Multidisciplinary pain treatment integrates therapies that target both the biologic and psychosocial aspects of pain (Figure 14.1). For patients with CPP, the multidisciplinary treatment approach can involve combinations of any of the following:

1. specific therapies that target the viscera with identifiable pathology (e.g., surgical excision of endometriosis);
2. physical therapy and rehabilitation that target somatic structures when musculoskeletal and/or neuropathic dysfunction is present;
3. psychosocial interventions directed at alleviating stress and moderating the pain experience through improved coping and social functioning;
4. treatment of concurrent psychiatric disorders (e.g., anxiety, depression);
5. pharmacologic and adjuvant therapies to manage pain.

Some research is available on the effectiveness of the multidisciplinary care model for treating women with CPP. The available data are reassuring that this treatment approach is more effective than the traditional treatment provided by a single provider, at least in women with a history of previous negative evaluations by a gynecologist. As a result, therapy incorporating multiple treatment options or referral to a multidisciplinary treatment center is recommended for women with CPP of unknown origin.

Pharmacologic management of pain

When CPP becomes the disease process, optimization of oral analgesic and pharmacologic therapy is an essential part of the patient's treatment and rehabilitation process. Pain perception involves an intricate relationship between neurotransmitters and chemical pathways in the peripheral and central nervous systems. Analge-

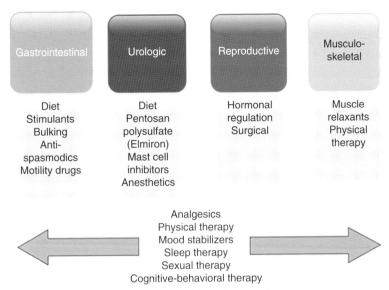

Figure 14.1 Multimodal therapies for chronic pelvic pain disorders.

sics of different properties may interrupt this pathway to decrease transmission of pain and lessen perceived pain.

Different pharmacologic treatment options will be discussed in this section. However, regardless of the preferred treatment modality, the patient's response will be optimized by adhering to a scheduled regimen, avoiding short-acting preparations, scheduling regular follow-up intervals, and establishing expectations early in the treatment process. As a healthcare provider, it is essential to be familiar with all pharmacologic therapies being prescribed and their side effect profiles, dosing, and half-life. Patient education regarding potential adverse side effects is fundamental to reduce anxiety, encourage compliance, and establish trust. The patient's pain symptoms and effectiveness of analgesia, medication requirements, adverse side effects, and activity level must be documented at every visit.

★ **TIPS & TRICKS**

Pharmacologic therapy for chronic pelvic pain includes the following:
• Schedule regular follow-up visits.
• Avoid "as required" (prn) dosing.
• Make long-term treatment goals (over 3–6 months).

• Follow and record the patient's progress.
• Use sequential pain scales and examinations.
• Start pharmacologic therapy at the lowest dose.
• Do not stop medications abruptly.
• Avoid managing pain exacerbations over the phone without physical evaluation.

Nonsteroidal anti-inflammatory drugs
Peripherally acting analgesics such as aspirin, acetaminophen, and nonsteroidal anti-inflammatory drugs (NSAIDs) are considered to be first-line therapy and have been shown to be effective in treating chronic pain and dysmenorrhea. Like nonselective inhibitors of cyclo-oxygenase (COX-1 and COX-2), they inhibit prostaglandin and thromboxane synthesis. These are key mediators in the inflammatory pathway that can result in pain. Given the large variability in patient response to the different NSAIDs available, even when they are structurally and chemically similar, it is recommended to try several regimens prior to abandoning therapy. It is also important to optimize dosing and frequency intervals because most patients use NSAIDs incorrectly.

⚛ SCIENCE REVISITED

Aspirin, acetaminophen, and nonsteroidal anti-inflammatory agents are considered to be first-line therapy and are effective in treating chronic pain and dysmenorrhea. They inhibit the synthesis of prostaglandin and thromboxane, which are key mediators in the inflammatory pathway and can result in pain; the NSAIDs therefore act in the same way as nonselective inhibitors of cyclooxygenase (COX-1 and COX-2). It is important to try several regimens prior to abandoning therapy as there a wide range of variability in patient response to these agents.

Patients should be educated about the risk of dyspepsia, a common side effect often requiring the use of H_2 receptor antagonist therapy with prolonged use of NSAIDs. A potential more serious side effect can be gastric or intestinal ulceration resulting in an acute or chronic gastrointestinal bleed. Although less common, patients may also experience salt and fluid retention causing edema, hypertension, and renal failure. Peripheral neuropathy has also been reported and may have an insidious onset. Prolonged use at high doses may also result in pathologic bleeding due to platelet inhibition. NSAID therapy should be avoided in patients using diuretics or angiotensin-converting enzyme inhibitors. NSAIDs should also be avoided in the first and third trimester of pregnancy.

To minimize side effects, therapy may be initiated with scheduled ibuprofen. However, for long-term therapy, sustained release or long-acting NSAIDs such as diclofenac and naproxen are preferred. Due to the increased potential for side effects, therapy with profens and COX-2 inhibitors should not be combined. Several classes of commonly prescribed NSAIDS are outlined in Table 14.1.

Opioid analgesics

Opioid analgesics act centrally, primarily on the μ receptors, to inhibit nociceptive pain. Although opioids can be beneficial and powerful pain control substances, use of opioids for the management of CPP remains controversial given the lack of randomized control trials to support their efficacy in long-term pain control. Besides having analgesic and sedative properties, opioids can also cause euphoria, drowsiness, dizziness, nausea, vomiting, pruritus, urinary retention, respiratory depression, lethargy, and decreased gastrointestinal motility. However, the main concerns with opioid therapy are the risks for tolerance, dependence, and addiction; therefore, opioid therapy should be considered only in select patients after other therapies to control pain have failed.

Opioid use is contraindicated in patients with a current or prior history of drug abuse or addiction. It is important to prescribe opioids on a scheduled basis and avoid a pain-mandated pharmacologic approach, which is encouraged by "prn" ("as required") dosing. Patients initiating opioid therapy should be extensively educated about the risks of opioid therapy and be asked to agree to an opioid contract. This contract can be a formal written agreement or just a discussion documented in the patient's record. To ensure compliance and monitor the potential for substance abuse, we also ask patients in our clinical practice to participate in random urine drug testing during the course of their treatment.

★ TIPS & TRICKS

Written contracts for opioid management should cover the following:
• Establish yourself as the sole provider of opioids.
• Refill opioids at subsequent office visits (and avoid over-the-phone refills).
• Patient must agree to comply with the specified dosing regimen.
• Patient must agree to participate in alternative therapies.
• Document the risks for dependence and side effects that have discussed.
• Use random drug screens to confirm proper use.

Close patient follow up at regularly scheduled visits is key to successful management in CPP patients on opioid therapy. Each visit should address the extent of pain relief, presence of side effects, degree of restoration of an acceptable

Table 14.1 Commonly prescribed pharmacologic therapy for chronic pelvic pain

Class	Drug	Half-life (hours)	Common side effects
Nonsteroidal anti-inflammatory drugs	Diclofenac	1.9	Dyspepsia, nausea, abdominal pain, constipation, headache, dizziness, rash, elevation in liver transaminases
	Ibuprofen	1.8–2.0	Dyspepsia, gastritis
	Indomethacin	4.5	Dyspepsia, nausea, somnolence
	Ketorolac	2.1	Headache, nausea dyspepsia, somnolence, gastrointestinal bleed, gastrointestinal ulcers
	Meloxicam	15–20	Dyspepsia, abdominal pain, nausea
	Naproxen	12–17	Dyspepsia, nausea, constipation, abdominal pain
	Piroxicam	50	Dyspepsia, nausea, constipation, abdominal pain
Opioids	Morphine	3.8	Nausea, vomiting, constipation, decrease oxygen saturation, pruritis, hypotension, urinary retention
	Codeine	2.5–4.0	Nausea, vomiting, sweating, dry mouth, constipation, sedation, dizziness
	Methadone	8–59	Nausea, vomiting, sweating, light-headedness, constipation, sedation
	Fentanyl	3.7	Somnolence, asthenia, confusion, nausea, vomiting, constipation
	Oxycodone	3.2–4.5	Constipation, nausea, vomiting, headache, pruritis, insomnia
	Tramadol	6.5	Constipation, dizziness, somnolence, pruritis, headache, seizure, serotonin syndrome
Tricyclic antidepressants	Amitriptyline	10–26	Drowsiness, dry mouth, constipation, blurred vision, palpitations, tachycardia
	Nortriptyline	18–44	Drowsiness, dry mouth, dizziness, constipation, blurred vision, palpitations
	Imipramine	11–25	Drowsiness, dry mouth, dizziness, constipation, blurred vision, palpitations
	Doxepin	6–8	Drowsiness, dry mouth, dizziness, constipation, blurred vision, palpitations, tachycardia
Muscle relaxants	Robaxin (methocarbamol)	1–2	Somnolence, light-headedness, pruritis, uticaria

(Continued)

Table 14.1 (*Continued*)

Class	Drug	Half-life (hours)	Common side effects
	Carisoprodol	10	Drowsiness, dizziness, headache
	Cyclobenzaprine	18	Drowsiness, dry mouth, fatigue, headache, abdominal pain
Neuroleptics	Neurontin (gabapentin)	5.7	Dizziness, somnolence, ataxia, fatigue, peripheral edema, nystagmus
Anxiolytics	Clonazepam Diazepam Lorazepam Alprazolam	11–60	Drowsiness, fatigue, muscle weakness, ataxia, venous thrombosis, phlebitis (intravenous, intramuscular), depression, impaired coordination, ataxia, nervousness, confusion, dependency, abuse, withdrawal

level of functioning, improvement of quality of life measures, and emotional stability. Providers should look for signs of tolerance and withdrawal such as hyperalgesia in spite of increasing doses, irritability, restlessness, insomnia, abdominal cramping, generalized muscle or joint pain, tachycardia, and hypertension. These symptoms may develop as early as after 10 days of use. Addiction or abuse may be suspected in patients who exhibit loss of control over drug use, use the drugs in spite of evident harm (side effects), or develop a preoccupation with use for nonpain-relief purposes. In these cases, patients should be weaned off opioids and alternative therapies initiated.

Using an NSAID in conjunction with an opioid may increase the analgesic effect as they act in synergy. Tramadol is an alternative to traditional opioids because of its mild opioid as well as nonopioid properties. It binds to mu receptors and also inhibits serotonin and norepinephrine (noradrenaline) reuptake. Multiple sustained-release preparations are available facilitating a longer dosing interval and it is also produced in combination with acetaminophen. Tramadol is better tolerated as patients experience less nausea, vomiting, and constipation, and a decreased risk of dependence. Table 14.1 summarizes the commonly prescribed opioids that may be used for short- or long-term pain therapy.

Antidepressants

Tricyclic antidepressants (TCAs) can be efficacious in reducing depressive symptoms, improving sleep patterns, and increasing pain tolerance. TCAs such as imipramine, desipramine, doxepin, and amitriptyline have been shown to be superior to placebo in improving pain tolerance and pain levels in various chronic pain syndromes. In general, when TCAs are used, pain relief effect is noted at lower doses than give rise to the antidepressant effect. Consequently, in the treatment of chronic pain, TCAs can be prescribed at lower doses, avoiding typical side effects such as sedation, dry mouth, and constipation.

⚙ SCIENCE REVISITED

Tricyclic antidepressants have been shown to help reduce symptoms of depression, improve sleep patterns, and increase tolerance to pain. Tricyclic agents such as imipramine, desipramine, doxepin and amitriptyline are better than placebo at improving pain tolerance and pain levels in various chronic pain syndromes. They can also be prescribed at lower doses, thus decreasing the risk for typical side effects such as sedation, dry mouth, and constipation.

In our practice, TCA therapy is usually initiated at low doses nightly and titrated weekly until pain relief is achieved or side effects are noted. Patients should be educated regarding possible side effects including, but not limited to, lethargy, dizziness, loss of libido, and anticholinergic effects. Secondary amines such as nortriptyline and desipramine tend to have fewer side effects when compared to tertiary amines such as amitriptyline and imipramine.

Like any other pharmacologic therapy, patients are carefully selected for TCA therapy. We prefer to use TCAs in patients with neuropathic-type pain or in patients who have pain with some symptoms of depression. For patients who show no symptom improvement within 6–8 weeks of therapy, the initial TCA may be replaced with another; up to 50% of patients may respond to a different TCA when a prior one has failed to alleviate their symptoms. When therapy needs to be discontinued, we recommend a titrated dose decrease instead of abruptly stopping the medication as patients can experience withdrawal symptoms from TCA therapy.

Selective serotonin and norepinephrine reuptake inhibitors (SSNRIs) such as venlafaxine and duloxetin are alternative antidepressants that show promise in adjunctive treatment for chronic pain.

Anticonvulsants

Anticonvulsants inhibit excessive secondary neuron stimulation in the spinal cord, leading to inhibition of pain transmission. Anticonvulsants such as gabapentin, carbamazepine, phenytoin, clonazepam, lamotrigine (Lamictal), levetiracetam (Keppra), and topiramate (Topamax) are typically used to treat seizure disorders and neuropathic pain arising from postherpetic or pudendal neuralgia. More recently, this class of drug has been thought to be particularly useful in patients with CPP (especially those with vulvodynia or interstitial cystitis). Side effects of anticonvulsant therapy may include sedation, lethargy, memory loss, cognitive impairment, nightmares, weight gain, menstrual cycle abnormalities, and skin rashes. Therefore, slow dose titration is recommended until pain relief has been achieved or side effects are noted.

> ### ⚠ CAUTION
>
> The side effects of anticonvulsant therapy may include sedation, lethargy, cognitive impairment, memory loss, nightmares, weight gain, menstrual cycle abnormalities and rash. It is therefore recommended that the dose be slowly titrated until pain relief is achieved with minimal side effects.

Muscle relaxants

Muscle relaxants are a heterogeneous group of compounds used to treat spasticity from upper motor neuron syndromes and muscular pain or spasms from peripheral musculoskeletal disorders. In CPP, muscle relaxants are particularly useful when the pain is associated with pelvic floor muscle dysfunction, myalgias, or dyspareunia. Cyclobenzaprine, tizanidine, carisoprodol, methocarbamol, and baclofen are examples of muscle relaxants commonly used in practice. In general, muscle relaxants may cause dry mouth, constipation, sedation, weakness, and rarely hepatotoxicity.

Fair evidence is available demonstrating the efficacy of muscle relaxants over placebo in the treatment of spastic disorders of the neck or lower back. However, there is insufficient evidence to determine the relative efficacy or safety of one muscle relaxant over another. Therefore, careful patient selection and a slow increase in dosing is crucial when initiating muscle relaxant therapy.

Hormonal manipulation

Thresholds for pain perception vary across the menstrual cycle; decreased pain thresholds and increased pain sensitivity have been demonstrated in the time period just before and during menses. Traditionally, cyclic pelvic pain has been associated with reproductive sources of pain such as endometriosis and adenomyosis. However, the finding that pain perception and sensitivity may vary across the menstrual cycle in normal female physiology suggests that reproductive-aged women who are menstruating and have chronic pain may experience exacerbation in their pain even if the origin of their pain is not gynecologic. Indeed, the impact of the menstrual cycle on other clinical pain syndromes such as fibromyalgia, irritable bowel syndrome, and interstitial cystitis has already been documented.

Patients with CPP who report cyclic exacerbation of their pain during the menstrual cycle should be offered menstrual suppression. This can be achieved with oral combination contraceptives, continuous progestins, or intermittent gonadotropin-releasing hormone agonist therapy. Long-term suppressive therapy can be beneficial in some patients: oral combination contraceptives, oral progestins, and even the levonorgestrel intrauterine device are routinely used in our practice.

Adjuvant therapies

> ### ⭑ TIPS & TRICKS
>
> Adjuvant treatments to consider for chronic pelvic pain include:
> - physical therapy;
> - trigger point injections;
> - anesthetic nerve blocks;
> - denervation procedures;
> - acupuncture;
> - cognitive-behavioral therapy;
> - surgery.

Trigger point injections

Myofascial trigger points are taught bands of muscle that are associated with chronic abdominal or pelvic pain. Although the exact pathway by which they cause pain is not well understood, trigger point injections have emerged as an alternative therapy for managing myofascial pain. A thorough physical examination is key to identify focal taught bands of muscle, often found on the abdominal wall or in the pelvic floor musculature. The tender areas are first identified by palpation (abdominal, intravaginal) and then with the needle before injection; eliciting a twitch response ensures proper placement of the injection.

Various techniques and anesthetic combinations are described. Generally, small amounts of anesthetic (1–2 mL) are injected into the muscle using a small syringe and a 21–25-gauge needle. Although saline injections have been shown to have some efficacy, a long-acting local anesthetic such as bupivacaine is preferred. Botulinum toxin A has also been used for abdominal wall trigger point injections because local temporary muscle paralysis is believed to reduce neurogenic inflammation and has been shown to produce significant reductions in pain scores.

Nerve blocks

Nerve blocks using a variety of long-acting anesthetic combinations may be effective in a select group of patients with CPP whose pain follows a more distinct nerve distribution pattern. For example, patients who have a suspected pudendal nerve injury may benefit from a pudendal nerve block. Likewise, a genitofemoral or ilioinguinal nerve block may be beneficial in patients who have groin pain after undergoing a hysterectomy or trauma. A superior hypogastric plexus block may be more appropriate for patients with central pelvic pain.

Physical therapy

Pelvic physical therapy can be highly beneficial in patients with CPP both for general rehabilitation and an overall improvement in daily function, and also for pain control. Pelvic floor myalgia and muscle spasms resulting in CPP, dyspareunia, or bladder or bowel dysfunction can be treated by an experienced physical therapist. Therapy is individualized to each patient based on the location and severity of dysfunction.

Electrotherapy, biofeedback, manual therapy of myofascial trigger points, pelvic floor exercises, and vaginal dilators can all be employed to improve the vaginal and pelvic floor muscle tone, decrease patient anxiety and stress with vaginal penetration, and provide patients with home exercises that help with pain relief and minimize pain exacerbations. Other techniques employed by a specialized physical therapist include mobilization of nerves or muscles believed to be under tension, connective tissue manipulation, and myofascial release of both external and internal muscle groups. When selecting a physical therapist, it is important to identify a specialist who is comfortable performing both internal and external myofascial manipulation.

Before initiating physical therapy, the provider should explain to the patient that therapy may involve internal manipulation through the vagina or rectum. Patients should be assessed regarding their willingness to participate in both the physical therapy sessions and the maintenance home exercises. For CPP, physical therapy involves several treatment sessions spaced out over a long period of time. Initiation of therapy may cause a temporary increase in pain that requires additional analgesics, but patients should be reassured that pain relief is usually achieved after several sessions of treatment. During therapy, patients may be also asked to abstain from certain activities that worsen pain and cause significant anxiety, such as lifting heavy objects, prolonged activity, or vaginal intercourse.

Acupuncture and neurostimulation

Acupuncture has been found to be superior to placebo for treatment for primary dysmenorrhea but not as beneficial for nonmenstrual CPP. The mechanisms through which acupuncture affects the pain pathways is not clear, but it may provide pain relief in patients with low back pain and pelvic pain in pregnancy. In our experience, individual results vary, and the decision to initiate acupuncture therapy is usually based on patient choice.

Sacral nerve electrical stimulation via implantable devices is emerging as a potential therapy for CPP, especially in patients with concurrent bladder symptoms such as urgency, frequency, or retention. This therapy is available to a highly select group of patients with intractable pain who have failed multiple other therapies and who are willing to undergo a surgical procedure to have an electrical stimulation device implanted. Long-term efficacy for pain relief is reported at less than 50%, and complications include lead migration and infection at the surgical site.

Combination therapy

For many patients with CPP, combination therapy that uses multiple therapies with different mechanisms of action may improve their chances of obtaining pain relief. For example, centrally acting and peripherally acting pharmacotherapy may be combined—such as NSAIDs and opioids.

Antidepressants may be combined with opioids or NSAIDs, especially if pain is present with depressive symptoms. Muscle relaxants can be added to NSAIDs or opioids if muscle tension is present. Finally, additional therapy such as trigger point injections or neural blocks can be, and often is, combined with analgesic therapy and physical therapy. Regardless of the combination, oral pharmacotherapy should be combined with caution. Medication regimens must be administered on a scheduled basis before severe pain ensues. Most therapies are not effective once pain levels are too high, so patients should be encouraged to use oral therapies for pain prevention. This discourages "prn" use and reduces the chances of developing maladaptive pain behaviors.

Addressing psychopathology and improving quality of life

Psychological, behavioral, and social factors are known to modulate pain levels in women with CPP. Initial studies conducted among patients with chronic low back pain show that up to 59% of these patients have a concurrent psychiatric diagnosis, the most common diagnoses being depression, substance abuse, and anxiety disorders. This was noted to be much higher than baseline lifetime rates of similar mental disorders in the general population, which were reported at 5–17%.

However, the causal relationship between the development of pain and psychopathology is not well understood. Proponents of a causal link between pain and mental disorders are supported by studies showing that nociceptive and affective neural pathways share anatomic space and neurotransmitters, namely norepinephrine and serotonin. That there is a causal link between pain and psychopathology is further strengthened by data showing that antidepressants can be effective in the treatment of some patients with chronic pain. However, others argue that there is no causal link between chronic pain and psychopathology, citing that in many instances each condition can exist without the other. Furthermore, if depression is considered as an example, depression may coevolve with CPP but is rarely the primary cause of pain. Finally, depression may be important in baseline levels of pain, but is not always associated with a poor response to treatment for pain.

Regardless of whether psychopathology causes pain or vice versa, it is clear that it is important to identify and treat psychopathology in patients with chronic pain for several reasons. Psychopathology can alter pain intensity, perception, and coping, and can also exacerbate disability. Besides interfering with successful rehabilitation, psychologic and behavioral factors can also lead to other physical symptoms such as autonomic arousal, vigilance, or somatic amplification. Additional emotional states that modulate pain perception include anger, frustration, and mismatch between provider and patient expectations. Although not characterized as mental disorders, these states must also be identified, validated, and addressed during the patient encounter.

Psychological assessment can be conducted by a health psychologist, psychiatrist, or any other provider involved in the care of the patient, such as a gynecologist or family physician. The main purpose of this assessment is to determine the level of disability associated with pain, emotional distress, and impairment of quality of life. Although extensive standardized pain and psychological tests can be administered, providers can identify women who will likely benefit from extensive psychosocial assessment and treatment by asking the following brief screening questions:

1. How has your pain affected your ability to function and your daily activities, such as work, relationships, sleep, or sexual function?
2. How has your pain affected your mood? Are you feeling irritable or depressed? Are you feeling anxious or tense?
3. How much stress do you have in your life— very little, a moderate amount, or a high level? If the level is high, how do you feel that you are coping with the pain and the stress?
4. Have you ever been a victim of physical, emotional, or sexual abuse? If you have, please explain. Are you currently being abused, or are you concerned about your safety or the safety of your children?
5. Who is there to support you as you cope you your pain (or stress or abuse)?
6. Are you interested in counseling for pain-coping skills, depression, or stress management, couples/marital counseling, sexual therapy, or counseling for unresolved abuse?

It has been our experience that patients are more responsive to this line of questioning after comfort and trust has been established with the provider. Although these questions can be administered at the initial interview, responses may vary as the patient may not reveal much information if she is not comfortable with the provider. Thus, we recommend that these questions be introduced to the patient at several visits if needed, but especially after the patient has been educated that cognitive-behavioral therapies: (1) are usually a successful adjunct rather than a replacement for medical therapy; and, (2) improve overall quality of life and decrease suffering and disability.

Screening will sometimes reveal various forms of psychopathology such as depression, anxiety, personality disorders, and substance use/abuse disorders, all conditions that are overrepresented in patients with severe long-standing CPP. Treatment of mild to moderate symptoms of depression or anxiety can be initiated by any provider, but patients with severe symptoms and those with personality or abuse disorders should be referred to or evaluated in collaboration with a mental health specialist.

Various pharmacologic agents are available for the treatment of depression, including heterocyclic antidepressants, selective serotonin reuptake inhibitors (SSRIs), and the newer SSNRIs. All agents are available in variable doses, and we recommend starting at the lowest dose and increasing slowly until the desired effect is achieved. If no therapeutic effect is attained within 6–8 weeks, a change in agents is recommended. However, it is important to note that 30–50% of patients who do not respond to one drug may respond to another drug of the same class. Patients may develop tolerance and withdrawal to antidepressants as they can to analgesics. Potential side effects include drowsiness, dizziness, dry mouth, and constipation with heterocyclic agents; nausea, diarrhea, headaches, and loss of libido with SSRIs (loss of libido may be avoided with bupropion, a selective norepinephrine and dopamine reuptake inhibitor); and anxiety or mania with bupropion or venlafaxine.

Anxiolytic therapy is helpful when pain flare-ups are made worse by anxiety with an excessive focus on pain. Although relaxation exercises and stress management may be helpful in reducing tension and anxiety, oral antianxiety agents should be considered when nonpharmacologic therapy is not enough. Anxiolytic therapy may help potentiate analgesic effects when combined with opioids, but great care must be taken to avoid sedation, drowsiness, apathy, and respiratory depression. Long-term use and withdrawal from anxiolytic therapy may also be associated with worsening anxiety, disorientation, memory impairment, sleeplessness, abdominal pain, headaches, slurred speech, easy crying, and changes in blood pressure and pulse. Rebound symptoms can be easily confused with pain flare-ups, and there is significant potential for dependence and addiction. To avoid these complications, we recommend starting therapy at the lowest dose, avoiding "prn" dosing, and using anxiolytics with a medium to long half-life while avoiding those with short half-life properties. As with opioids, anxiolytic therapy should be avoided in patients with a history of (or potential for) substance abuse; immediate referral to a mental health specialist is recommended.

Patients exhibiting emotional states such as anger, frustration, and other maladaptive personality reactions may have difficulty complying with recommended therapy. In addition, these patients may be labeled as "difficult" patients or mistakenly diagnosed with a personality disorder. In general, these patients evoke strong negative reactions from healthcare professionals. It is important to recognize that these emotional states can be a reflection of several factors, such as years of chronic pain and untreated maladaptive behaviors, a potential more acute pain flare, or more serious psychiatric dysfunction. Regardless of the cause, it is important when negative emotional states are encountered that providers monitor their emotional reactions to patients. In other words, providers must avoid potentiating patient anger, frustration, or anxiety with negative emotions of their own. Instead, the focus should be on listening to the patient, validating her concerns, and providing reassurance. When serious psychiatric dysfunction is suspected, it is important to explain to the patient why she may benefit from psychological support.

Cognitive-behavioral therapy

The goal of cognitive-behavioral therapy in pain management is to teach self-management techniques, improve coping abilities and sense of control, reduce disability, and promote behavior against relinquishing to pain. The overall goal is to lessen the impact of chronic pain on quality of life. Relaxation techniques, attention diversion, distraction techniques, and external focus on other activities may heighten a patient's sense of control and coping abilities and decrease her primary focus on pain symptoms. Promoting wellness to improve overall lifestyle is an important aspect of cognitive-behavioral therapy. Although there are few studies from which to make evidence-based recommendations about dietary modifications that may improve pelvic pain, encouraging and facilitating nutritious eating habits may be beneficial. Other lifestyle modifications such as adequate sleep and physical exercise may also improve one's ability to cope with pain.

Among patients presenting with symptoms of pain, underlying social factors often determine the extent of suffering and degree of disability. Therefore, it is important to obtain information regarding the patient's relationship with her spouse or significant other. If there is a history of physical, emotional, or sexual abuse, the patient should be strongly encouraged to seek counseling. If the patient is in an unsafe, abusive environment, her willingness to continue with the relationship should be assessed, and a plan should be implemented to ensure her safety. If the patient is in a supportive relationship, involving her partner in the treatment plan may also be helpful.

CPP can have significant negative effects on sexual function. Fear of worsening pain experienced during intercourse can be the source of stress, anxiety, and marital or relationship discord, all of which will decrease the patient's ability to cope with pain. In such cases, a marital or sexual therapist is an integral part of the patient's therapy.

Conclusions

For patients with CPP of unknown origin, the focus of therapy begins with an extensive pain history, physical examination, and review of psychosocial factors that may influence pain. Instead of therapy directed at a single cause, pain management requires a combination of therapies including medical, physical, interventional, and cognitive-behavioral. Healthcare providers who treat women with CPP need to have a significant amount of knowledge about available therapies and potential side effects. Extensive patient education and follow-up must be undertaken to ensure compliance with therapy and to avoid misuse of medications. Moreover, patient education should emphasize the need for long-term care that focuses on pain management (and not cure), enhanced coping, improved function, and better quality of life.

Selected bibliography

ACOG Practice Bulletin No. 51. Chronic pelvic pain. Obstet Gynecol 2004;103:589–605.

Boardman LA, Cooper AS, Blais LR, Raker CA. Topical gabapentin in the treatment of localized and generalized vulvodynia. Obstet Gynecol 2008;112:579–85.

Borg-Stein J, Stein J. Trigger points and tender points: one and the same? Does injection treatment help? Rheum Dis Clin North Am 1996;22:305–22.

Chou R, Clark E, Helfand M. Comparative efficacy and safety of long-acting oral opioids for chronic non-cancer pain: a systematic review. J Pain Symptom Manage 2003;26:1026–48.

Chou R, Peterson K, Helfand M. Comparative efficacy and safety of skeletal muscle relaxants for spasticity and musculoskeletal conditions: a systematic review. J Pain Symptom Manage 2004;28:140–75.

Dersh J, Polatin PB, Gatchel RJ. Chronic pain and psychopathology: research findings and theoretical considerations. Psychosom Med 2002;64:773–86.

Eriksen J, Sjogren P, Bruera E, Ekholm O, Rasmussen NK. Critical issues on opioids in chronic non-cancer pain: an epidemiological study. Pain 2006;125:172–9.

Grace VM. Problems women patients experience in the medical encounter for chronic pelvic pain: a New Zealand study. Health Care Women Int 1995;16:509–19.

Gunter J. Chronic pelvic pain: an integrated approach to diagnosis and treatment. Obstet Gynecol Surv 2003;58:615–23.

Howard FM. Chronic pelvic pain. Obstet Gynecol 2003;101:594–611.

Howard FM, Perry CP, Carter JE, El-Minawi A. Pelvic pain: diagnosis and management. Philadelphia: Lippincott Williams & Wilkins; 2000.

Jamison RN, Raymond SA, Slawsby EA, Nedeljkovic SS, Katz NP. Opioid therapy for chronic noncancer back pain. A randomized prospective study. Spine (Phila Pa 1976) 1998;23:2591–600.

Jarrell JF, Vilos GA, Allaire C et al. Consensus guidelines for the management of chronic pelvic pain. J Obstet Gynaecol Can 2005;27:781–826.

Lamvu G, Robinson B, Zolnoun D, Steege JF. Vaginal apex resection: a treatment option for vaginal apex pain. Obstet Gynecol 2004;104:1340–6.

Lamvu G, Williams R, Zolnoun D et al. Long-term outcomes after surgical and nonsurgical management of chronic pelvic pain: one year after evaluation in a pelvic pain specialty clinic. Am J Obstet Gynecol 2006;195:591–8; discussion 598–600.

The Role of Definitive Surgery in the Management of Chronic Pelvic Pain and Posthysterectomy Pain

Brett A.H. Schultz[1] and Tommaso Falcone[2]

[1]St. Elizabeth Medical Center, New York , USA
[2]Cleveland Clinic, Cleveland, Ohio, USA

Introduction

Chronic pelvic pain (CPP) is defined as nonmenstrual pelvic pain, of at least 6 months' duration, that is severe enough either to cause functional disability or to require treatment. The etiology of CPP may be gynecologic, nongynecologic (gastrointestinal, genitourinary, musculoskeletal, neurologic, psychiatric), or a combination of the two. Women with pain related to more than one organ system display pain at a greater intensity than women with pain related to only one organ system. CPP is a common condition, with a prevalence of approximately 15–20% in women aged 18–50 years. It is estimated that 10% of all outpatient gynecologic office visits are for CPP complaints.

Many CPP patients have been seen by multiple physicians and have undergone surgeries for the treatment of their pain. To be successful in treating women with CPP, the physician must first earn the patient's trust. A systematic and comprehensive history and physical examination must be performed, which may be aided by an intake questionnaire such as the one provided on the International Pelvic Pain Society website at www.pelvicpain.org. Adequate time should be allotted in order to perform these tasks and to allow for a discussion of assessment and treatment options. One study has demonstrated that this is best accomplished by providing personalized care by actively listening to the patient's complaints, showing understanding and taking her pain complaints seriously, providing an explanation for the pain, and providing reassurance and a commitment to attempt to alleviate her pain.

The management of CPP is based on the underlying diagnosis. To arrive at the best treatment plan for an individual patient, the physician and patient need to have a comprehensive discussion regarding her goals, preferences, desires regarding medical versus surgical treatments, and plans for future fertility. CPP often presents a diagnostic dilemma and is frequently difficult to cure or treat, often leading to surgical intervention.

Most patients with CPP of gynecologic origin will be best served initially with a trial of medical therapy, followed by conservative surgical treatment. Diagnostic laparoscopy is the most common surgical means for evaluating CPP and is able to offer patients a means for treatment in a substantial proportion of cases. Women with CPP of gynecologic origin who do not benefit from conservative therapy may benefit from hysterectomy with or without oophorectomy as means of definitive treatment. Of the 590,000 hysterectomies performed annually in the United States, 10% list CPP as the indication. Sometimes there is not a clear etiology for the

Chronic Pelvic Pain, First Edition. Edited by Paolo Vercellini.
© 2011 Blackwell Publishing Ltd. Published 2011 by Blackwell Publishing Ltd.

pain, and treatment must be directed at alleviating symptoms.

Large prospective cohort studies, the Maine Women's Health Study and the Maryland Women's Health Study, showed significantly improved pain outcomes 1 year after hysterectomy. The Maine and Maryland Women's Health Studies are the largest prospective studies of outcomes of hysterectomies performed for benign conditions on women from the United States. These two studies provide strong evidence that in women with significant symptoms related to gynecologic disorders (i.e. leiomyomas, CPP, endometriosis, dysfunctional uterine bleeding, etc.), hysterectomy substantially improves symptoms. However, both studies had patients whose symptoms did not improve, whose symptoms got worse, who developed new symptoms, or who had additional problems after surgery. A further study looked at the Maryland data to identify factors associated with the lack of symptom relief. Factors significantly associated with poor outcomes after hysterectomy were an annual household income of US$35,000 or less, depression, and being in therapy for a psychiatric indication at the time of hysterectomy. In addition, it is important to realize that hysterectomy in young women (less than 30 years old) is associated with a higher incidence of regret, sense of loss, and persistent symptoms compared to older women (over 40 years old).

General principles of hysterectomy

Most hysterectomies for CPP can be performed by laparoscopy. A laparoscopic approach can exclude or treat pelvic pathology such as endometriosis or lyse adhesions before proceeding to remove the uterus and possibly the adnexa. If the route of hysterectomy to be attempted is laparoscopic, it should be discussed with the patient prior to surgery that conversion to laparotomy is not necessarily a complication but a decision made in best judgment to carry out the intended surgery in the safest manner possible. Generally, we do not advocate leaving the cervix, nor does the evidence support any proposed benefit from supracervical hysterectomy. In patients with CPP, leaving the cervix may increase the incidence of persistent or residual pain, especially in patients with endometriosis. Consideration should be

given to keeping the ovaries of young women who undergo hysterectomy for CPP. General principles that are important to follow in patients undergoing hysterectomy are listed in the "Tips & tricks" box.

☆ TIPS & TRICKS

Before proceeding to a hysterectomy, the following should be discussed with the patient and documented in her medical record:
- informed consent;
- a review of her health history;
- an assessment of the need for medical preoperative consultation, laboratory evaluation, and/or imaging;
- that the patient has completed childbearing;
- that an adequate trial of medical or nonsurgical treatment for CPP has been attempted, offered, or refused;
- the route of hysterectomy agreed upon by the patient and physician;
- the likelihood of pain relief after surgery;
- the risks and benefits of oophorectomy;
- an assessment of the potential need for blood products;
- a review of the cervical cytology.
Perioperative recommendations are as follows:
- use prophylactic antibiotics;
- use first- or second-generation cephalosporins;
- initiate antibiotics within 1 hour before the incision to prevent infection of the surgical site;
- redose the antibiotics in procedures lasting two times the half-life of the antibiotic (i.e., more than 3 hours for cefazolin) or with an estimated blood loss greater than 1,500 cm³;
- discontinue prophylactic antibiotics within 24 hours after surgery;
- administer prophylaxis for venous thromboembolic events;
- perform a pregnancy test in reproductive-aged women.

The role of definitive surgery in specific gynecologic conditions

Endometriosis

Endometriosis is a complex disease that typically manifests itself as a chronic pain disorder. It is characterized by the presence of endometrial glands and stroma outside the uterine cavity. A definitive diagnosis is made from surgical biopsy with histologic confirmation. Endometriosis is most commonly found in the pelvis (the left hemipelvis being more frequently affected than right) and adnexa. The most frequent locations for endometriotic implants are on the ovaries, the anterior and posterior cul-de-sac, the broad ligament, and the uterosacral ligaments.

In the general female reproductive-aged population, the prevalence of endometriosis is estimated to be approximately 10%. In women who undergo a diagnostic laparoscopy for evaluation of CPP, the prevalence of endometriosis is about 33%. Among adolescents with severe pelvic pain or dysmenorrhea, up to 70% have endometriosis. In addition, approximately 70–75% of women with endometriosis have pelvic pain. The association between endometriosis and CPP is supported by studies showing an improvement in pain scores after treatment of endometriosis. On the other hand, it has been observed that the severity of pain related to endometriosis does not correlate with the severity of disease.

Treatment of endometriosis is either medical or surgical and is based on the woman's age, her desire for future fertility, previous treatments, the degree to which symptoms affect her quality of life, and the location and severity of disease. The medical and conservative management of endometriosis are discussed in Chapter 4. When medical and/or conservative management has failed, hysterectomy with or without bilateral salpingo-oophorectomy may be the next option for treatment as long as the patient has completed childbearing.

☆ TIPS & TRICKS

The gynecologist performing surgery for endometriosis should be knowledgeable in pelvic anatomy, especially retroperitoneal dissection, as most hysterectomies in women with advanced endometriosis require this approach. Preoperative evaluation prior to hysterectomy mandates a thorough examination to assess for deeply infiltrating endometriosis (DIE). Ultrasonography can also help to detect DIE. In addition to the hysterectomy, all disease needs to be excised at the time of surgery to obtain an optimal outcome. A laparoscopic approach should be used if the surgeon is skilled. Surgeons uncomfortable with repairing the bowel, bladder, or ureter should obtain the assistance of a consulting service when necessary.

Endometriosis is the second leading cause of hysterectomy in the United States, accounting for 18% of the procedures. At the time of hysterectomy, it is important to focus on complete excision or destruction of all visible disease, including peritoneal lesions, endometriomas, and endometriosis of the bowel or bladder. For this reason, it is the author's preference to attempt total laparoscopic hysterectomy with or without bilateral salpingo-oophorectomy and laparoscopic resection of endometriotic implants. Laparoscopy can provide better visualization of endometriotic implants via its magnification properties. Excision or destruction of implants can be performed via electrical, mechanical, thermal, or laser energy. No studies have shown one method of removal or destruction to be superior to another. Therefore, surgeons should choose the energy source with which they are most knowledgeable and competent. As long as full exposure is obtained, full-depth resection or destruction of endometriotic implants should be attempted. Excised lesions should be sent to pathology for histologic confirmation of the diagnosis.

Supracervical hysterectomy, both laparoscopic and open, has been increasing in popularity over the past few decades and has been the subject of much debate. We do not recommended performing a supracervical hysterectomy in women with CPP related to endometriosis because endometriosis can harbor itself within the cervix, requiring reoperation to excise the cervical stump (trachelectomy). In a retrospective study of 70 patients who underwent supracervical hysterectomy, 17 women (24.3%) required trachelectomy due to symptoms related to their cervical stump. Of the 17 women requiring trachelectomy, 14 (82.3%) had a history of prior treatment for endometriosis.

There is no consensus on the advisability of removal of both ovaries if one or both are not directly involved by endometriosis. A retrospective study has evaluated patients undergoing conservative versus definitive surgery for endometriosis-associated pain and their requirement for further surgery after a 7-year period. The study populations included 120 women with laparoscopic excision of endometriotic lesions only and 120 women undergoing hysterectomy with or without oophorectomy. The findings for surgery-free percentages at 2, 5, and 7 years were as follows: in women with laparoscopic excision of endometriotic lesions only 79.4%, 53.3%, and 44.6%; in women with hysterectomy with ovarian preservation (at least one ovary preserved), 95.7%, 86.6%, and 77.0%; and in women with hysterectomy without ovarian preservation (both ovaries removed), 96.0%, 91.7%, and 91.7%, respectively. The most important variables in determining outcome were found to be surgical procedure and age.

The authors speculate that the reason hysterectomy is associated with a lower reoperation rate is because most patients with endometriosis have pain during their menses. Once the uterus has been removed, there is no further menstrual bleeding, leading to a decrease or absence of pain. Regardless of surgery type, women with only one ovary had a lower risk of reoperation than those with both ovaries. Hysterectomy with bilateral salpingo-oophorectomy reduced the risk of reoperation by 2.44 times. The benefit of bilateral salpingo-oophorectomy is seen primarily in women 40 and older, whereas there is no substantial reduction in reoperation rates in women aged 30–39. Therefore, definitive treatment with hysterectomy is associated with a low reoperation rate, and ovarian preservation remains a viable option, especially in women less than 40 years old.

Preoperative suppressive medical therapy utilizing gonadotropin-releasing hormone (GnRH) agonists is not recommended because they have not been shown to make surgery less difficult or to improve surgical outcome. After conservative surgery, most studies have shown significant pain relief from definitive surgery; however, it is important for the surgeon to remember that the diagnosis of endometriosis in women with CPP does not guarantee that treatment will result in pain relief. Although uncommon, endometriosis has been reported to recur in 5–10% of patients after hysterectomy and bilateral salpingo-oophorectomy. There is controversy regarding the role of hormone replacement therapy after bilateral salpingo-oophorectomy, as the possibility of symptom or disease recurrence exists and there have been no high-quality studies to evaluate the risks and benefits.

Leiomyomas

Uterine leiomyomas, also known as fibroids, fibromas, or myomas, are benign tumors of smooth muscle cell origin. They are the most common tumors of the female pelvis. Although over 50% of leiomyomas are asymptomatic, they may also cause symptoms that affect quality of life and require treatment. The major clinical symptoms of uterine leiomyomas are pelvic pain or pressure (bulk symptoms), abnormal uterine bleeding, anemia, and reproductive dysfunction. The patient's complaints are often related to the size and location of the fibroid(s)—submucosal, intramural, subserosal, pedunculated, or combined locations.

The treatment of leiomyomas depends on their location and can be medical or surgical. Medical treatment for leiomyomas is discussed further in Chapter 8. Surgical/radiologic treatment of leiomyomas includes myomectomy (hysteroscopic, abdominal, vaginal, laparoscopic), endometrial ablation, uterine artery embolization (UAE), high-intensity magnetic resonance imaging (MRI)-guided focused ultrasound therapy (HIFU), cryomyolysis, laparoscopic uterine artery ligation, or hysterectomy. Although UAE is an acceptable method of treating women with symptomatic fibroids, there is a high recurrence rate of symptoms, and approximately 25% of patients will require further intervention. Surgery is the mainstay of therapy, and hysterectomy is the definitive treatment for symptomatic uterine leiomyomas. Please refer to Chapter 8 for a further discussion of the treatment options for leiomyomas.

Hysterectomy is recommended for treatment of symptomatic fibroids in:

- patients with acute blood loss not responding to other treatments;
- women who have completed childbearing and desire definitive treatment of their leiomyomas due to either significant symptoms, a uterus greater than 12–14 weeks' size, or multiple leiomyomas;
- women who have failed other treatments for leiomyomas;
- patients with a suspicion for uterine malignancy;
- women who have completed childbearing and have another disorder or increased future risk for a disorder that would be decreased or eradicated by hysterectomy (i.e., abnormal cervical cytology, symptomatic pelvic organ prolapse, endometriosis, adenomyosis, endometrial hyperplasia, ureteral compression causing moderate or severe hydronephrosis, carrier of a *BRCA1* or *BRAC2* mutation, a strong family history of gynecologic carcinoma, a history of breast cancer on tamoxifen therapy, or a carrier of hereditary nonpolyposis colorectal cancer syndrome (Lynch syndrome type II);
- postmenopausal women with a new or rapidly enlarging pelvic mass, bleeding, or pelvic pain.

The advantages of hysterectomy over other forms of treatment are that it eliminates symptoms and the possibility of recurrence.

Symptomatic uterine fibroids are the leading cause of hysterectomy in the United States, accounting for 30% of such procedures. The preoperative work-up is dependent on symptomatology and may include laboratory studies (complete blood count, type, and screen, iron studies), endometrial biopsy, tumor markers, or imaging modality (pelvic ultrasound, computed tomography [CT], MRI). Discussion with the patient should be performed prior to surgery regarding her desires if the need arises for a blood transfusion, including allogeneic blood transfu-

sion, autologous blood donation, and use of a cell saver. The route of hysterectomy (abdominal, vaginal, laparoscopic) should be based on surgeon familiarity/comfort level, the size of the uterus, the degree of prolapse, the presence of associated pathology, and patient preference.

☆ TIPS & TRICKS

The surgeon may consider giving gonadotropin releasing-hormone (GnRH) agonists prior to hysterectomy if the patient has significant anemia that has not responded to iron therapy or it is believed that a reduction in the uterine volume could change the surgical approach or ease of the procedure. Prior to major surgery, a 2–3-month preoperative course of GnRH agonists has been shown to improve preoperative blood counts, decrease hospital stay, decrease intraoperative blood loss, decrease operative time, and decrease postoperative pain. However, no studies have demonstrated a decrease in blood transfusion risk or an improvement in quality of life. Therefore, the risks and benefits of GnRH agonist use must be weighed given their substantial cost and side effect profile.

Adenomyosis

Adenomyosis is defined as endometrial glands and stroma present deep within the myometrium. The ectopic endometrial tissue is presumed to cause smooth muscle cell hyperplasia and hypertrophy, leading to a uniformly enlarged uterus. Clinical symptoms of adenomyosis are dysmenorrhea, abnormal uterine bleeding, CPP, dyspareunia, and an enlarged, tender uterus on bimanual examination. The etiology, pathogenesis, and incidence of adenomyosis are unknown. Many cases of adenomyosis are associated with leiomyomas, which may make it difficult to distinguish which disorder is causing the patient's symptoms. A diagnosis may be presumed in a patient with clinical symptoms, physical examination findings, endometrial biopsy, imaging modalities (ultrasound, MRI), or hysteroscopic findings suspicious for adenomyosis. However, a definitive diagnosis of adenomyosis can only be made by histologic evaluation of the uterus at time of hysterectomy.

Conservative treatments of adenomyosis are discussed in Chapter 8 and may consist of medical therapy (oral contraceptive pills, progestin therapy, GnRH agonists, aromatase inhibitors, danazol) or surgery (endomyometrial ablation or resection, laparoscopic myometrial electrocoagulation, excision of adenomyosis, UAE, HIFU). There are no sufficient studies evaluating the efficacy of medical or conservative surgical therapy for adenomyosis. The only guaranteed treatment for alleviating the symptoms of adenomyosis is hysterectomy. Hysterectomy is the recommended treatment for women with significant symptoms related to adenomyosis who have completed childbearing. The route of hysterectomy (abdominal, vaginal, laparoscopic) should be based on surgeon familiarity/comfort level, the size of the uterus, the degree of prolapse, the presence of associated pathology, and patient preference. Because adenomyosis is a disorder of the uterus, ovarian conservation is a viable option unless there are contraindications or patient preference indicating otherwise.

Adhesions

Adhesions are fibrous tissue band connections, often the result of previous surgery, infection, or endometriosis, by which anatomic structures pathologically adhere to one another. Adhesion formation is usually an unavoidable outcome of surgery, especially in abdominal and pelvic surgery. Laparoscopy has been associated with a markedly reduced rate of adhesion formation. At the time of surgery, the surgeon should take steps to help minimize the chance of forming new adhesions by observing the rules of microsurgery. The tenets of microsurgery include: minimal, atraumatic tissue handling with use of magnification, utilization of microinstruments, maintaining hemostasis, using fine nonreactive sutures, precise approximation of tissues with no tension, limiting thermal injury, continuous irrigation to avoid desiccation, and avoiding foreign body contamination from laparotomy sponges, glove powder, etc. Refer to Chapter 7 for a further discussion regarding adhesions and CPP.

EVIDENCE AT A GLANCE

The role of adhesions in causing chronic pelvic pain (CPP) is controversial. Observational studies have shown a substantial improvement in CPP scores after adhesiolysis, signifying that adhesions may play a role in CPP. However, the best evidence available suggests that adhesiolysis is not useful for relieving chronic pain in most women with chronic pelvic or abdominal pain.

This conclusion is based on two randomized controlled trials. Peters et al. performed a randomized controlled study in which 48 women with a prior diagnosis of CPP and adhesive disease diagnosed by laparoscopy were randomly assigned laparotomy with adhesiolysis or expectant management. Follow-up between 9 and 12 months demonstrated no difference pain score improvement between women who underwent surgery versus expectant management (odds ratio 1.54, 95% confidence interval 0.81–2.93, $n = 148$) except in a small subset of patients with severe adhesions. This small subset had severe adhesions, noted to be dense vascular adhesions involving the bowel and peritoneum, which did demonstrate significant benefit from surgery (odds ratio 16.59, 95% confidence interval 2.16–127.2, $n = 15$).

The other study is a randomized double-blinded controlled study performed by Swank et al. in which 121 participants (88% female, 12% male) with a history of chronic abdominal pain and adhesive disease diagnosed by laparoscopy were randomized to laparoscopic adhesiolysis versus diagnostic laparoscopy only. At 12 months, no difference existed in quality of life or visual analog scores.

The two randomized control trials of patients with chronic pelvic or abdominal pain and adhesive disease suggest no improvement in pain scores in patients undergoing surgical adhesiolysis, except for those with dense vascular adhesions. There are a few explanations for why patients may not receive improvement after surgical adhesiolysis: (1) the adhesions are not the cause of the CPP; (2) the adhesions reform after the surgery; and/or (3) new adhesions are formed as a result of the surgery. The most recent Cochrane Review concluded that "there is still uncertainty about the place of adhesiolysis among patients presenting to gynecologists and the conclusion of this review is that there is no evidence of benefit, rather than evidence of no benefit." The authors of the Cochrane Review conclude that there is a need for either further large trials of adhesiolysis in gynecologic patients with CPP, or careful observational studies that include a psychological and sociocultural investigation, laboratory evaluation of adhesions, and physiologic analysis of intraperitoneal inflammatory and nociceptive processes of adhesive disease.

Symptomatic extensive pelvic adhesive disease involving the uterus may be definitively treated with hysterectomy. The route of hysterectomy may be selected based on the patient's anatomy and the surgeon's skill level. The surgeon may elect to use an adhesive barrier to attempt to decrease the reformation or new formation of adhesions.

EVIDENCE AT A GLANCE

A 2008 Cochrane Review evaluated the effect of adhesive barriers used during gynecologic surgery on pelvic pain, postoperative adhesion reformation, and pregnancy rates. Sixteen randomized control trials—10 trials with laparotomy and 6 trials with laparoscopy—of adhesion barriers versus no treatment were included. Following laparotomy, Interceed (Ethicon, Blue Ash, OH, United States) and Gore-Tex (W.L. Gore & Associates, Inc., Neward, DE, United States) were effective in preventing new adhesion formation and reformation. Gore-Tex was found to be superior to Interceed in preventing adhesion formation, but its use is limited because it requires suturing and is permanent, with the recommendation of reoperation for later removal. Only limited evidence supported the effectiveness of Seprafilm (Genzyme, Cambridge, MA, United States), and no evidence supported the use of fibrin sheet. Following laparoscopy, Interceed has been found to be effective in preventing new adhesion formation and reformation. Adept (icodextrin 4% solution; Baxter, Deerfield, IL, United States) is currently the only Food and Drug Administration-approved adhesion barrier for use during laparoscopy in the United States. A multicenter, prospective, double-blind randomized control study of 402 patients comparing Adept with lactated Ringer's solution demonstrated a higher clinical success rate (a reduction in 30% of adhesions at time of second-look laparoscopy) with Adept solution. In addition, safety was comparable in both groups.

Chronic pelvic pain without pathology at the time of surgery

Obtaining an accurate diagnosis of the etiology for CPP is a complex and challenging task. It is common for a gynecologist to take a patient to surgery for a diagnostic laparoscopy for presumed CPP of gynecologic origin but, at the time of surgery, for no pathology to be observed. In women with CPP without a gynecologic pathologic diagnosis, hysterectomy is not recommended as first-line treatment. Hillis et al. performed a prospective, multicenter cohort study of 308 women who had a hysterectomy performed as treatment for CPP. In patients without pathology found at the time of hysterectomy, they found a recurrence rate of CPP up to 40%. This finding is of particular relevance because a large collaborative review series found that, in hysterectomies performed for CPP, over 60% of the uteri and adnexa were histologically normal. Other factors that increase the probability of persistent pain after hysterectomy are age under 30 years, being uninsured or covered under Medicaid, a history of pelvic inflammatory disease (PID), and having had two or more pregnancies.

It is the authors' preference to take several pictures at time of laparoscopy to document the patient's disease or lack of disease. We have found this to be helpful in the patient's understanding of the etiology of her pain, what has been done surgically, and further treatment(s) necessary. A randomized control trial evaluated the effects of photographic reinforcement of laparoscopic findings and its effect on pain scores at 3- and 6-month follow-up. Photographic reinforcement after surgery did not show a clear benefit in pain scores, nor did it lead to perceived benefit on the part of the patient or physician. Unfortunately, the intervention group had a trend toward greater pain intensity preoperatively compared to the controls, which may have confounded the results of this trial. In addition, the enrollment target was for 450 patients and only 233 patients were enrolled; thus, the final comparisons were different from those originally intended.

The finding that women without pelvic pathology at the time of hysterectomy are more likely to have persistent CPP emphasizes the need for a careful evaluation of gynecologic as well as non-gynecologic (urologic, gastrointestinal, musculoskeletal, psychological) causes of CPP. It is important to keep in mind that the etiology of CPP may be multifactorial. In patients in whom no diagnosis can be made, a multidisciplinary approach to treatment is recommended. In the reports of a large pain specialty center, approximately 90% of patients had a prior unsuccessful gynecologic surgery prior to being evaluated in their facility. The reports also found that non-gynecologic disorders were more frequently the cause of CPP (37% irritable bowel syndrome, over 23% musculoskeletal). The authors of this study report that their ability to diagnose interstitial cystitis was limited, and that recent studies show up to 24–80% of patients with CPP may have interstitial cystitis. Therefore, it is imperative to evaluate nongynecologic sources of pain prior to performing gynecologic surgery for CPP. See the section entitled "Hysterectomy performed for the wrong indication" for a further discussion of CPP without pathology.

Pelvic inflammatory disease

PID is a serious infection of the pelvic that which may cause devastating sequelae including CPP, infertility, ectopic pregnancy, and death. Acute PID is most often attributed to an ascending gynecologic infection with gonorrhea, *Chlamydia*, or polymicrobes and is treated with antibiotic therapy. Chronic PID is usually due to aerobic and anaerobic bacteria or a prior chlamydial infection. If ongoing or subclinical infection is suspected, antibiotic therapy is necessary. Refer to Chapter 5 for a further discussion of PID.

Studies have established an increased prevalence of developing CPP after an acute episode of PID. About 20% of patients with a history of an acute pelvic infection develop CPP versus 5% of controls without a history of pelvic infection. The CPP may be related to a hydrosalpinx or pelvic adhesive disease. All women with CPP thought to be due to a history of PID should undergo laparoscopy to rule out other pathology. Signs and symptoms of chronic PID that may require surgical intervention include persistent and severe CPP, repeat exacerbations of PID requiring medical treatment and hospitalization, progressive enlargement of a tubo-ovarian mass, and severe dyspareunia.

The surgical management for chronic PID is usually determined at the time of surgery based on the surgical findings as well as the patient's history, age, risk factors, surgical preference, and childbearing status. Conservative management for patients wishing to maintain their childbearing status usually consists of salpingectomy if hydrosalpinx is present. Patients with chronic PID often have problems with infertility and require the help of assisted reproductive technology such as in-vitro fertilization.

In most cases, definitive management of chronic PID causing CPP is with hysterectomy and bilateral salpingo-oophorectomy, but published data documenting this treatment for CPP are lacking. The route of hysterectomy (usually abdominal or laparoscopic) should be based on surgeon familiarity/comfort level, the extent of the adhesions, the size of the uterus, the presence of associated pathology, and patient preference. In one study, 40 women with chronic PID who underwent oophorectomy had pathology showing that approximately 50% of the ovaries were free of inflammatory processes and had normal follicular activity. The authors concluded that, in patients without a history of abnormal uterine bleeding, ovarian histology is usually normal. Therefore, it is recommended to conserve normal ovarian tissue unless the patient has a history of dysfunctional uterine bleeding or there is a contraindication to ovarian preservation. When both adnexa are to be removed, it is advisable to also perform hysterectomy at the same time. In addition, adhesions should be lysed, any abscesses found drained, and diseased tissue removed.

It is important for the surgeon to keep in mind that women with a history of PID have a higher likelihood than women without a history of pelvic infection to have persistent CPP after hysterectomy. In the Hillis et al. study referenced above, 31.6% versus 23.2% of woman had continued but decreased pain, and 8.9% versus 1.4% had unchanged or increased pain in women with a history of PID versus no history of pelvic infection, respectively.

Pelvic congestion syndrome

Pelvic congestion syndrome (PCS), also known as ovarian vein incompetence, is a condition characterized by vascular pelvic engorgement or pelvic varicosities and CPP. The diagnosis remains controversial, but evidence exists that some women with pelvic varicosities and venous stasis diagnosed via pelvic venography have CPP that cannot be related to other pathology. PCS is more common in multiparous, reproductive-aged women. The etiology and pathophysiology of the disorder are unknown. Venographic studies propose that the main mechanism for dilatation of the pelvic veins and congestion of the surrounding tissues is related to retrograde flow in incompetent ovarian veins (ovarian varicocele), which in turn leads to pelvic pain. Other mechanisms that may lead to this disorder are pregnancy, absence of ovarian venous valves, ovarian valvular incompetence, retroaortic left renal vein, compression of the left renal vein by the superior mesenteric artery, right common iliac vein compression, portal hypertension, and acquired inferior vena cava syndrome.

The PCS pelvic pain is usually a dull, achy pain in the pelvis that is often premenstrual, unilateral, and exacerbated by prolonged standing. Other symptoms may include dysmenorrhea, dyspareunia, postcoital ache, low back pain, sacrodynia, dysuria, vulvar pain, rectal pain, headache, fatigue, and psychiatric disturbances. On physical examination, the examiner may find the following:

- the external genitalia: vulvar varices that may extend to the thigh and buttock;
- on abdominal examination: tenderness at the ovarian point (on a line drawn from the anterior superior iliac spine to the pubic symphysis, the point that lies at the intersection of the upper and middle thirds);
- on speculum examination: excessive clear mucoid cervical discharge and a cervix that is bluish in color;
- on bimanual examination: cervical motion tenderness, uterosacral ligament tenderness, parametrial tenderness, ovarian and adnexal tenderness, and increased uterine volume.

Diagnostic laparoscopy is frequently performed on these patients due to their history of CPP. At time of laparoscopy, the high intra-abdominal pressure and Trendelenburg position may lead to venous drainage, thus diminishing evidence of venous congestion. If there is no pathology found at the time of laparoscopy to explain the patient's pain and PCS is suspected, attempt to visualize pelvic varicosities by decreasing the intra-abdominal pressure and reversing the Trendelenburg position. In addition, a uterus affected by PCS may appear mottled and/or dusky blue in color.

Pelvic venography (selective retrograde ovarian venography, transuterine venography) is the "gold standard" in the diagnosis of PCS as it displays a visualization of retrograde blood flow into the dilated, tortuous pelvic veins, and ovarian venous congestion as evidenced by reduced venous clearance of contrast medium. However, venography is rarely used due to its invasive nature and exposure to ionizing radiation. Less invasive modalities such as ultrasound, CT, and MRI are often used in place of venography to assist in the diagnosis of PCS. Transvaginal color Doppler ultrasound may be useful in helping to make the diagnosis of PCS by displaying the following criteria: (1) tortuous pelvic veins with a diameter greater than 4 mm, (2) slow blood flow (approximately 3 cm per second), and (3) a dilated arcuate vein in the myometrium that communicates between bilateral pelvic varicose veins. Women with PCS may have ovaries containing cystic components, resembling a polycystic ovarian syndrome-type picture. CT and

MRI will display dilated, tortuous pelvic veins that may extend into the broad ligament, pelvic sidewall, and/or paravaginal venous plexus.

The physician treating PCS should be open to multiple approaches, including medical therapy, psychotherapy, and surgery. Medical therapy and psychotherapy have been discussed in Chapter 6. To date, there have been no randomized controlled clinical trials of surgical treatment for PCS. Possible surgical or interventional treatments for PCS include ovarian vein ligation, embolization of the ovarian and/or internal iliac veins, sclerotherapy, and hysterectomy with or without bilateral salpingo-oophorectomy. Randomized controlled trials are desperately needed to compare medical, interventional, and surgical treatments for CPP associated with PCS.

Ovarian vein ligation is one of the original treatments for PCS, dating back to the early 1900s. It has been performed via laparotomy as well as laparoscopically, and small studies have shown a significant improvement in pain. Ovarian vein occlusion has been performed with the use of stainless steel coils or glue (Enbucrilate; B. Braun, Melsungen, Germany), with an average success rate from all documented trials after embolotherapy with coils of 89% (range 74–100%) and after embolotherapy with glue of 68%. Likewise, in a small prospective pilot study, ovarian vein sclerotherapy was found to be safe and effective in providing symptomatic treatment in most patients with PCS. Please refer to Chapter 6 for a further discussion of these treatment modalities.

Treatment of PCS with hysterectomy is controversial. A retrospective study evaluated the outcome after hysterectomy in 99 patients who by history and examination had symptoms suggestive of PCS. After a period of 22 months, the authors found that 22% of the patients had persistent pelvic pain. On the other hand, a prospective nonrandomized trial of hysterectomy with bilateral salpingo-oophorectomy was performed on 36 women with demonstrated PCS, 33 of whom had failed medical treatment. After a 12-month follow-up period, a significant improvement in pain scores and quality of life, and an increased frequency of sexual activity, was reported. It is possible that failure to remove the ovaries may have contributed to the continued pain in patients in the former study. The data on hysterectomy for PCS remain mixed, and further trials are necessary to evaluate the usefulness of hysterectomy with or without bilateral salpingo-oophorectomy.

Pain that remains after hysterectomy

Hysterectomy performed for the wrong indication

CPP is often a multifactorial disease and commonly has more than one underlying problem. The treatment of CPP in patients with multiple problems is challenging, and the goals of treatment need to be realistic. Patients may give a history of a diagnosis of endometriosis or surgery for the treatment of endometriosis by another physician, complain of "pain in my uterus or ovaries," or frankly demand a hysterectomy to "fix my pain." It is important to perform a thorough history and physical examination and to request all records from a patient's prior work-up or surgical evaluation for CPP. The use of an intake questionnaire such as the one provided on the International Pelvic Pain Society website may be helpful and save time during the office evaluation. Adequate time should be allotted in order to perform these tasks and to have a discussion with the patient of assessment and treatment options. Patients with CPP can consume a large amount of time and energy in terms of their work-up and evaluation, and education for their illness.

Although up to 95% of patients who undergo hysterectomy for CPP have an improvement or resolution of their pain, approximately 25% of patients report persistent pain within 1 year after surgery. The finding that women without pelvic pathology at the time of hysterectomy are more likely to have persistent CPP emphasizes the need for careful evaluation of gynecologic as well as nongynecologic (urologic, gastrointestinal, musculoskeletal, psychological) causes of CPP. The high incidence of patients whose pelvic pain was reduced but not resolved by hysterectomy may also indicate the multifactorial interplay between the physiologic and psychological facets of CPP.

In patients with CPP, the pain itself may become the disease. Studies have shown that the longer a woman has experienced pain, the less likely it is that treatment of the underlying condition(s) will provide long-term resolution of the pain. In addition, multiple studies have confirmed that patients with CPP who receive a multidisciplinary approach to treatment (medical, surgical, psychological, pain therapy), are more likely to experience an improvement in their pain than are patients who receive only medical or surgical therapy.

Residual or recurrent pain after hysterectomy and bilateral salpingo-oophorectomy in endometriosis patients

Women with recurrent symptoms after hysterectomy and bilateral salpingo-oophorectomy for endometriosis often have residual endometriosis in the cul-de-sac and perirectal areas. The disease was most likely present at the time of surgery but not removed because of the location. Endometriosis expresses its own aromatase activity, resulting in an estrogenic microenvironment from the conversion of androgens to estrogens. In these patients, GnRH agonists have no role since they are already hypogonadal. However, the use of an aromatase inhibitor such as letrozole has resulted in decreased pain. Patients that fail medical management will require surgical excision of any residual disease.

Ovarian remnant syndrome

Ovarian remnant syndrome is the presence of pelvic pain, pelvic mass, or dyspareunia caused by a residual amount of ovarian tissue left behind after intended oophorectomy. In most cases, this happens when dissection has been difficult due to extensive pelvic adhesive disease, endometriosis, PID, or neoplasm. The ovarian remnant is usually plastered to the pelvic side wall and is in close proximity to the external iliac vessels, ureter, bladder, infundibulopelvic ligament, both small and large bowel, and/or omentum. The residual ovarian tissue is encased in adhesions and has a variable blood supply, which may be the cause of the pelvic pain.

The diagnosis of ovarian remnant syndrome can be challenging. Follicle-stimulating hormone level can be checked and, if in the premenopausal range, may facilitate the diagnosis. The GnRH agonist stimulation test can be performed to identify the presence of functioning ovarian tissue—as treatment with a GnRH agonist is continued, the patient may experience pain relief. In addition, imaging modalities such as pelvic ultrasound with use of color Doppler imaging, CT scan, or MRI may assist in the diagnosis and help define the surrounding structures in preparation for surgical intervention.

Medical management with analgesics and/or hormonal suppression utilizing oral contraceptive pills, progestins, or GnRH agonists may be attempted, but data on their effectiveness are limited. Definitive treatment of ovarian remnant syndrome is excision of the residual ovarian tissue via laparoscopy or laparotomy. Surgical intervention will likely also include extensive adhesiolysis and ureterolysis, and may include excision or destruction of endometriosis. The surgeon should be well versed in pelvic anatomy, especially retroperitoneal dissection. Special care should be taken during the dissection since there will likely be adhesive disease and the ovarian tissue may be intimately involved with vital organs or vessels. Complications can and do occur and must be recognized and repaired at the time of the surgery. Some surgeons prefer to consult a urologist to place a ureteral stent on the affected side prior to the start of the surgery.

In the excision of an ovarian remnant, retroperitoneal entry along the affected pelvic side wall is performed. The ovarian remnant is dissected from the pelvic side wall and any other structures it may be involved with (e.g., external iliac vessels, ureter, infundibulopelvic ligament bowel), taking special care not to damage those structures. The ovarian remnant is removed, and the peritoneal defect is repaired.

Conclusions

Hysterectomy has been shown to significantly improve pain outcomes in patients with CPP. This is especially true in patients with endometriosis. However, some patients do get worse, and there is a high incidence of regret in women less than 30 years of age. We recommend removing the cervix in patients with chronic pain because of the higher incidence of recurrence of symptoms. The value of removing the normal ovaries at the time of hysterectomy for endometriosis-associated pain is not clear if all the endometriosis implants are removed, so consideration should be given to keeping normal ovaries. Hysterectomy for leiomyoma, adenomyosis, and chronic PID associated with pain is quite effective.

In patients with no identifiable pathology, it is important to exclude non-gynecologic causes before considering definitive surgery. Hysterectomy for PCS is more controversial as the diagnosis is more subjective. Nonresolution or recurrence of chronic pain after hysterectomy mandates a reassessment of the cause. These patients require a multidisciplinary team to execute an appropriate treatment regimen. Persistent or recurrent symptoms after hysterectomy for endometriosis may be due to residual disease that was not removed at the time of definitive surgery. Residual ovarian tissue can also cause pain in some women. Surgery for this condition is complex.

Selected bibliography

Ahmad G, Duffy JMN, Farquhar C et al. Barrier agents for adhesion prevention after gynaecological surgery. Cochrane Database Syst Rev 2008, Issue 2. Art. No.: CD000475.

Beard RW, Kennedy RG, Gangar KF et al. Bilateral oophorectomy and hysterectomy in the treatment of intractable pelvic pain associated with pelvic congestion. Br J Obstet Gynaecol 1991;98:988–92.

Brown CB, Luciano AA, Martin D et al. Adept (icodextrin 4% solution) reduces adhesions after laparoscopic surgery for adhesiolysis: a double-blind, randomized, controlled study. Fertil Steril 2007;88:1413–26.

Carlson KJ, Miller BA, Fowler FJ, Jr. The Maine Women's Health Study. I. Outcomes of Hysterectomy. Obstet Gynecol 1994;83:556–65.

Clayton RD, Hawe JA, Lovee JC et al. Recurrent pain after hysterectomy and bilateral salpingo-oophorectomy for endometriosis: evaluation of laparoscopic excision of residual endometriosis. Br J Obstet Gynaecol 1999;106:740–4.

Falcone T, Walters MD. Hysterectomy for benign disease. Clinical Expert Series. Obstet Gynecol 2008;111:753–67.

Hillis SD, Marchbanks PA, Peterson HB. The effectiveness of hysterectomy for chronic pelvic pain. Obstet Gynecol 1995;86:941–5.

Howard FM. The role of laparoscopy in chronic pelvic pain: promise and pitfalls. Obstet Gynecol Surv 1993;48:357–87.

Kjerulff KH, Langenberg PW, Rhodes JC et al. Effectiveness of hysterectomy. Obstet Gynecol 2000;95:319–26.

Kjerulff KH, Rhodes JC, Langenberg PW, Harvey LA. Patient satisfaction with results of hysterectomy. Am J Obstet Gynecol 2000;183:1440–7.

Lamvu G, Williams R, Zolnoun D et al. Long-term outcomes after surgical and nonsurgical management of chronic pelvic pain: one year after evaluation in a pelvic pain specialty clinic. Am J Obstet Gynecol 2006;195:591–600.

MacDonald SR, Klock SC, Milad MP. Long-term outcome of nonconservative surgery (hysterectomy) for endometriosis-associated pain in women <30 years old. Am J Obstet Gynecol 1999;180:1360–3.

Okaro EO, Jones KD, Sutton C. Long term outcome following laparoscopic supracervical hysterectomy. Br J Obstet Gynaecol 2001;108:1017–20.

Price J, Farmer G, Harris J et al. Attitudes of women with chronic pelvic pain to the gynaecological consultation: a qualitative study. Br J Obstet Gynaecol 2006;113:446–52.

Shakiba K, Bena JF, McGill KM et al. Surgical treatment of endometriosis: a 7-year follow-up on the requirement for further surgery. Obstet Gynecol 2008;111:1285–92.

Stones W, Cheong YC, Howard FM. Interventions for treating chronic pelvic pain in women. Cochrane Database Syst Rev 2005, Issue 2. Art. No.: CD000387.

Stovall TG, Ling FW, Crawford DA. Hysterectomy for chronic pelvic pain of presumed uterine etiology. Obstet Gynecol 1990;75:676–9.

Alternative Treatments for Chronic Pelvic Pain

Cindy Farquhar

University of Auckland, Auckland, New Zealand

Introduction

The management of women with chronic pelvic pain (CPP) is often challenging for both patients and their doctors. There are several reasons for this. One is that the underlying causes of CPP are poorly understood and thought to be multifactorial. Another is that there are few well-designed randomized controlled trials (RCTs) of women with CPP. For example, a Cochrane Review identified only 19 RCTs of a variety of pharmaceutical, psychological, and surgical interventions, which is relatively few for such a disabling condition. Furthermore, many of the recommended treatments involve surgery or medications, which have a potential for harm in a proportion of women. Faced with such a lack of evidence for effectiveness, many of the conventional treatments are empirical and pragmatic, depending upon experience or observation alone.

With such a poor evidence base, many women with CPP seek alternatives to conventional medicine as such alternative approaches are considered more attractive. Around 30–50% of adults in Western countries have been found to use some form of complementary medicine to prevent or treat health-related problems. Complementary therapies are more commonly used by women of reproductive age, with almost half (49%) reporting their use. However, in order to recommend any treatment, including complementary and alternative treatments, evidence from well-designed studies is required.

Complementary medicine has been defined as "practices and ideas that are outside the domain of conventional medicine in several countries," which are defined by its users as "preventing or treating illness, or promoting health and wellbeing." Complementary medicine is used together with conventional medicine. An example of a *complementary* therapy is using a natural remedy such as arnica to help lessen a patient's discomfort following surgery. An *alternative* medicine, however, is used in place of conventional medicine. An example of an alternative therapy is using a treatment instead of undergoing a therapy that has been recommended by a conventional doctor.

Many different therapies are considered as complementary therapies; these include treatments people can administer themselves (e.g., botanicals, nutritional supplements, health food, meditation, magnetic therapy), treatments that providers administer (e.g., acupuncture, massage, reflexology, chiropractic and osteopathic manipulations), and treatments people can administer under the periodic supervision of a provider (e.g., yoga, biofeedback, Tai Chi, homoeopathy, Alexander therapy, ayurvedic medicine).

Sources for this chapter have included the Cochrane Library (2009, Issue 3), the Allied and Complementary Medicine Database (August 2009), Embase (July 2009), and Medline (July 2009). The following terms were used: chronic pelvic pain, complementary and alternative, acupuncture, spinal manipulation, herbal, dietary, traditional Chinese medicine (TCM), vitamins, and magnesium. A summary of the treatments is provided in Table 16.1.

Chronic Pelvic Pain, First Edition. Edited by Paolo Vercellini.
© 2011 Blackwell Publishing Ltd. Published 2011 by Blackwell Publishing Ltd.

Table 16.1 A summary of the alternative therapies for women with chronic pelvic pain (CPP)

Alternative therapy	Description	Mechanism of action	Effectiveness	Adverse effects	Conclusions and recommendation for use
Acupuncture	Fine needles are inserted into specific points on the skin according to meridian points as defined by traditional Chinese medicine	Modulation of endogenous opioids such as beta-endorphins, serotonin, and dopamine. Anti-inflammatory actions via the prostaglandins is also likely	No studies in women with CPP. In women with dysmenorrhea, three months of weekly acupuncture for 3 out 4 weeks was found to be more effective for the outcome of pain relief	Nil	Acupuncture is considered to be safe and can be used, although it does required repeated treatments and the effects are unlikely to be long-lasting
Acupuncture with stimulation either by moxa or pressure	Burning of moxa (the plant *Artemisia vulgaris* or mugwort) close to the skin to induce a warming sensation. Acupressure is the application of pressure to certain points	Unknown	Unknown	Skin warming and, rarely, burns	Not recommended as no studies
Spinal manipulation	Involves mobilization and manipulation, which are techniques applied to a joint or articulation to normalize function	Vertebral mechanical dysfunction affecting blood supply to the pelvic viscera. Manipulation may improve spinal mobility and pelvic blood flow. It may also work through neural networks or by decreasing prostaglandin F2 alpha levels	No studies in women with CPP. In women with dysmenorrhea, there are four RCTs but only one small study suggested benefit. One larger study with sham acupuncture as a control group concluded there was no evidence for the use of spinal manipulation for women with dysmenorrhea	Severe adverse reactions, including fractures and cauda equina syndrome (nerve compression), have been reported infrequently with manipulation of the lower spine	Spinal manipulation is not recommended as there are safety concerns and there is no evidence of effectiveness in the studies comparing it with sham acupuncture

Chinese herbal medicine	A range of herbs are used according to the principles of CHM and tailored to the patient's needs.	Most CHM preparations contain more than one active compound. One study has reported that there are improvements in haemocytologic parameters	No studies in women with CPP: In women with dysmenorrhea, no benefit was found when compared to placebo. However, Chinese herbal medicine was found to have better pain relief than acupuncture and heat compression	No safety issues have been identified	There are no safety concerns with CHM, but effectiveness is yet to be established_
Vitamin B$_1$	Tablets and systemic use. The usual adult dose to treat deficiency is 5–30 mg daily either as a single dose or in divided doses	Vitamin B$_1$ deficiency is characterized by fatigue, muscle cramps, various pains and a reduced tolerance to pain	No studies in women with CPP: In women with dysmenorrhea, some benefit was suggested in small RCTs	Generally considered safe	Vitamin B$_1$ can be used although evidence of benefit is limited. There are no safety concerns
Vitamin B$_6$	Tablets with dosages from 25 to 100 mg daily	Vitamin B$_6$ is involved in the production of prostaglandin E2 (which contributes to myometrial relaxation) and in the utilization of magnesium	No studies in women with CPP: In women with dysmenorrhea, some benefit was suggested in small RCTs	Well-known sensorineural adverse effects in dosages greater than 100 mg per day	Vitamin B$_6$ can be used although there is only limited evidence of effectiveness, and there are safety concerns at higher doses
Vitamin E	Tablets of 150–400 IU per day	Vitamin E has analgesic and anti-inflammatory properties, which result in prostaglandin formation by inhibiting arachidonic acid release	No studies in women with CPP: Reduction in pain reported in three RCTs in women with dysmenorrhea	Doses greater than 400 IU per day are associated with a slight increase in mortality and heart failure	Vitamin E can be used although there is only limited evidence of effectiveness, and there are safety concerns at higher doses
Magnesium	Magnesium is available in oral, transdermal, and systemic preparations. It is unclear what dose or regimen of treatment should be used for magnesium therapy	Magnesium may have a role in pain reduction by inhibiting calcium entry into the cell, which may be important in the mechanisms of antinociception	No studies in women with CPP: In women with dysmenorrhea, magnesium was reported to reduce pain in three RCTs of women with dysmenorrhea	Generally considered safe	Magnesium can be used although only limited evidence of effectiveness. No safety concerns

CHM, Chinese herbal medicine; RCT; randomized controlled trial.

Acupuncture

Description

Acupuncture is a form of therapy that sits within the complex framework known as traditional Chinese medicine and has been practiced for thousands of years. In recent years, there has been increasing interest in acupuncture in Western countries. In China, acupuncture is an accepted treatment for endometriosis. Acupuncture involves inserting fine needles into specific points on the skin in order to stimulate corresponding meridian points, as defined by TCM theory. Other methods of stimulation of these points are also traditionally used, such as the burning of moxa (the plant *Artemisia vulgaris* or mugwort) close to the skin to induce a warming sensation and applying pressure (acupressure). Other methods developed more recently include electronic stimulation and laser acupuncture.

Mechanism of action

There are several possible explanations for the effects of acupuncture. However, emerging literature demonstrates acupuncture-mediated analgesia and an alteration of specific hormone levels. Acupuncture appears to influence the experience of pain by modulating the endogenous opioids such as beta-endorphins. Increases of endogenous opioids and the neurotransmitters serotonin and dopamine have been shown to cause analgesia, sedation, and recovery of motor function. An anti-inflammatory signal via both humoral and neural mechanisms has also been reported, and in women with dysmenorrhea the levels of prostaglandin F2 alpha in menstrual levels are improved. Recent data suggest that acupuncture has regionally specific, quantifiable effects on relevant brain structures. Acupuncture may also stimulate the gene expression of neuropeptides.

Benefits in chronic pelvic pain

Although the mechanism of action of acupuncture remains unclear, there may be potential benefits for women with CPP. However, there are problems with the evaluation of acupuncture, and ideally a sham procedure should be used on a control group. No studies in women with CPP were found, although there was a report of two cases suggesting benefit. As there were no studies in women with CPP, it was necessary to consider effectiveness in women with dysmenorrhea, but only one RCT on this has been found. This small RCT of 43 women reported that acupuncture once a week for 3 weeks a month, for 3 months, was more effective than placebo acupuncture and effect in two control groups (a standard waiting list control group and a control group with extra visits to medical investigators) for the outcome of pain relief. There was no difference between the two control groups, the placebo acupuncture group, and the acupuncture group in the use of additional medication.

Adverse events

There do not appear to be safety concerns for acupuncture.

Spinal manipulation

Description

Spinal manipulation therapy involves mobilization and manipulation, which are techniques applied to a joint or articulation to normalize function. Mobilization uses passive movement applied in a rhythms or oscillatory manner, whereas manipulation uses long or short lever thrust movements to impart a bigger impulse of force of short duration and low amplitude. In theory, the thrust should move the joint just beyond its normal range. Both mobilization and manipulation are used by chiropractors to treat conditions of the spine.

Mechanism of action

There is controversy over the use of spinal manipulation use to treat visceral conditions such as endometriosis and CPP. There are several ways that spinal manipulation could theoretically assist in the management of CPP. It is possible that mechanical dysfunction in the lumbar vertebrae results in decreased spinal mobility. This could in turn affect the sympathetic nerve supply to the blood vessels supplying the pelvic viscera, leading to dysmenorrhea as a result of vasoconstriction. Manipulation of these vertebrae may improve spinal mobility, leading to improved pelvic blood flow.

Another possible explanation is that dysmenorrhea is the result of referred pain arising from musculoskeletal structures that share the same pelvic nerve pathways. There is some evidence for musculoskeletal causation from a controlled study of 19 women with CPP and 20 healthy control subjects, in which there was a higher frequency of positive musculoskeletal findings in the CPP group. A decrease in the circulating plasma levels of prostaglandin F2 alpha is a further explanation. This decrease has been reported in conjunction with a decrease in menstrual pain but occurs at the same rate in both the treatment and sham manipulation treatment groups, with no difference in prostaglandin levels between the two groups. These physiologic measures add to our overall knowledge about the effects of spinal manipulation but are not necessarily related to the pain levels experienced by patients and are considered surrogate end points.

Benefits in chronic pelvic pain

There are few well-designed studies of spinal manipulation for gynecologic conditions. Issues exist in studying the effectiveness of spinal manipulation as it is difficult to find a satisfactory placebo intervention and it is difficult to maintain blinding unless the patients are naive to the treatment. Sham manipulation has been developed in which a nontherapeutic level of torque is used in the sham treatment arm. Such peak forces are in the sham procedure are substantially less than the peak forces delivered during true spinal manipulation therapy.

No RCTs were found involving women with CPP. In the Cochrane Review of spinal manipulation for women with primary and secondary dysmenorrhea, only four RCTs were identified for women and only had two had data that could be considered to be useful for clinical decision-making. Meta-analysis combining results from all the trials was not feasible due to differences in the treatments, measurement, timing, and reporting of pain outcomes. One small study of only 10 patients suggested a benefit. In the one trial to use a sham manipulation as a control group, manipulation was shown to be no more effective than the sham procedure, although the level of pain was reduced in both treatment arms. The one trial with an adequate sample size ($n = 137$) and the best methodologic rating also found no difference between manipulation and sham treatment.

Adverse effects

Although withdrawals from treatment were uncommon, the reporting of adverse events was not considered by most studies. Severe adverse reactions, including death and paralysis, have been reported with spinal manipulation. However, these extreme effects are usually related to cervical spinal manipulation and occur at the rate of 1 in 1 million manipulations. Manipulation of the lower spine, the area that would commonly be targeted in CPP, is associated with much lower risks, with fractures and cauda equina syndrome (nerve compression) being the most serious reactions.

Chinese herbal medicine

Description

TCM embraces Chinese herbal medicine (CHM) and acupuncture. CHM is a system of medicine that has been described for more than 2,000 years. In recent years, there has been increasing integration of CHM into Western medicine in China, and this interest has spread into many Western countries.

Although CPP was not described in CHM, a range of pelvic symptoms were described that included dysmenorrhea, dysuria, dyschezia, and menorrhagia. CHM describes stagnation of the blood and *Qi* (vital energy), which may cause localized obstructions and lead to pain. This is remarkably similar to the understanding of the central role that pelvic congestion may play in the causal mechanisms of CPP.

CHM is not all that dissimilar to Western medicine in many aspects. For example, a key primary requirement of traditional treatment with CHM is that the treatment needs not only to be tailored at the outset to the individual, but should also be modified at different stages of the patient's recovery or illness. This is familiar in Western medicine, where the choice of drug, length of treatment, and dosage are all generally tailored according to the patient's symptoms and disease. However, CHM is broader in its approach, taking interest in other associated complaints such as the feeling of coldness, whether pain is relieved by warmth, psychological status, and so on, all of which impact on the final CHM diagnosis. These associated symptoms form a syndrome with a distinct label, such as "retention of Cold" or "stagnation of *Qi* and Blood." Treatment generally differs according to the identified and diagnosed syndrome.

Although CHM is currently used in public hospitals in China for the treatment of primary dysmenorrhea and there are case studies suggesting benefit in primary dysmenorrhea, there are no studies that focus specifically on CPP.

The range of herbs used in CHM and gynecologic conditions is considerable. *Danggui* (Radix Angelicae Sinensis, Chinese angelica root), *Chuanxiong* (Rhizoma Chuanxiong, Szechuan lovage root), *Chishao* (Radix Paeoniae Rubra, red peony root), *Baishao* (Radix Paeoniae Alba, white peony root), *Yimucao* (Herba Leonuri, Chinese motherwort), *Puhuang* (Typhae Pollen, cat-tail pollen), *Wulingzhi* (Trogopterori Faeces, flying squirrel feces), *Niuxi* (Radix Achyranthis Bidentatae, achyranthes root), *Danshen* (Radix Salviae Miltiorrhizae, salvia root), *Chaihu* (Radix Bupleuri, Chinese thorowax root), *Xiangfu* (Rhizoma Cyperi Rotundi; nutgrass rhizome), *Yanhusuo* (Rhizoma Corydalis Yanhusuo, corydalis rhizome), *Aiye* (Folium Artemisiae Argyi, mugwort leaf), *Wuzhuyu* (Fructus Evodiae, evodia fruit), *Huixiang* (Fructus Foeniculi, fennel fruit), *Rougui* (Cortex Cinnamomi, cinnamon bark), *Dihuang* (Radix Rehmanniae, rehmannia root), *Gouqizi* (Fructus Lycii, lycium fruit), *Dangshen* (Radix Codonopsis, codonopsis root), *Baizhu* (Rhizoma Atractylodis Macrocephalae, atractylodes rhizome), and *Gancao* (Radix Glycyrrhizae, liquorice root). Such a wide range of herbal preparations makes assessment of the beneficial role challenging.

Mechanism of action

Most CHM preparations contain more than one active compound, and it is therefore difficult to establish what the pharmacotherapeutic action might be. Most the preparations have not been fully investigated. In TCM, "stagnation of the blood" is considered to be central to the mechanisms of dysmenorrhea, and high levels of blood viscosity have been found at both high and low shear rates. One study reported improvements in haemocytologic parameters as well as in period pain.

Benefits in chronic pelvic pain

No studies specifically addressed the role of CHM in women with CPP. A Cochrane Review of CHM in women with primary dysmenorrhea has been published. Thirty-nine RCTs involving a total of 3,475 women with primary dysmenorrhea were included in the review. A number of the trials were of small sample size and considered to have methodologic problems. Not surprisingly, few conclusions were reached. When CHM was compared to placebo, there was no evidence of benefit. When CHM was compared to pharmaceutical drugs, there was some evidence of improvements in pain relief for women with primary dysmenorrhea. Other approaches included self-designed Chinese herbal formulae, which were more effective in improving pain outcomes than the more commonly used Chinese herbal health products. CHM also resulted in better pain relief than acupuncture and heat compression. Overall, the review concluded that the use of CHM for primary dysmenorrhea was useful but that interpretation of the results was limited by the poor methodologic quality of the included trials.

Adverse effects

In the Cochrane Review, the measurement and report of adverse effects from the included trials was considered to be poor as only eight out of the 39 included trials mentioned adverse effects in their reports. Only seven trials detailed the number of incidents, and there was no evidence of harm in the CHM groups. Generally, CHM is considered safe when compared to conventional medicines. However, the data are limited, and more trials that monitor possible adverse effects are needed.

Herbal and dietary therapies

Description

Perhaps the most popular complementary medicines are herbal and dietary therapies. For example, 30% of all drugs sold in German pharmacies are herbal medicines. In the United States, over US$3 billion are spent on herbs and natural products every year, and in Australia over AUD $600 million are spent on alternative medicines a year, which is 70% more than the patient contribution towards pharmaceuticals. A telephone survey of Americans found that herbs and other natural products (not including vitamins and minerals) were used by almost 20% of Americans in 2002.

There are a number of reasons for the appeal of these products. Many consumers believe that, because of their "natural" status and their ease of access, they have fewer side effects than prescription drugs. For the more common recurring disorders such as dysmenorrhea, the easy accessibility of herbal and dietary therapies is considered a bonus as they can be self-administered and are usually available from health shops, pharmacies, and supermarkets.

Although there is a widespread perception that herbal therapies are safe, unfortunately this is not universally true, and there are many reports of allergic reactions, toxicity, and drug interactions. There is also the likelihood that adverse events are not properly being reported because these substances are classified as food or dietary products and therefore are not adequately assessed. By classifying them as such, no therapeutic claims can be made, but this also means that these products can be promoted without safety data.

A complete description of herbal and dietary therapies is beyond the scope of this chapter as it is complex and varies from country to country. It is worth noting that, in the United States, phytomedicines (medicines made from plants) have been legally classified as dietary supplements since 1994, while in Europe phytomedicines are regarded as drugs and as such a large number of herbal remedies are integrated into conventional medicine and pharmacy in Europe.

Mechanism of action

There is some evidence that nutritional intake and metabolism may play an important role in the cause and treatment of menstrual disorders. For example, an epidemiologic study of diet and menstrual pain has demonstrated that levels of polyunsaturated fatty acids (PUFAs) are correlated with menstrual pain, with higher levels of n-3 PUFAs being associated with milder menstrual symptoms. The n-6 PUFAs are metabolized into the specific prostaglandins associated with dysmenorrhea, and it appears that the ratio of n-3 to n-6 PUFAs is associated with menstrual symptoms. One small trial showed fish oil (n-3, or more popularly omega-3, fatty acids) to be more effective than placebo for pain relief in women with dysmenorrhea.

Another small RCT investigating the effects of different dietary levels of calcium and manganese showed that increasing calcium intake reduced mood and pain symptoms associated with menstruation. Another finding was that low dietary manganese increased mood and pain symptoms during the premenstrual phase. Magnesium is thought to have a role in pain reduction by inhibiting calcium entry into the cell, which may be important in the mechanisms of antinociception.

The role of vitamins and the experience of painful symptoms arising from a wide range of conditions has been the focus of research for some time. It has been suggested that vitamin E has analgesic and anti-inflammatory properties. A randomized trial of vitamin E for rheumatoid arthritis has shown a significant reduction in pain, which lends further support to this theory. Vitamin B_6 is involved in the production of prostaglandin E2 (which contributes to myometrial relaxation) and in the utilization of magnesium; therefore, higher levels of vitamin B_6 could also influence dysmenorrheal cramps. Vitamin B_1 plays an important role in metabolism, vitamin B_1 deficiency being characterized by fatigue, muscle cramps, various pains and a reduced tolerance to pain, all factors that could be associated with dysmenorrhea. The mechanism of vitamin E is unclear but may involve a reduction in prostaglandin formation by inhibiting arachidonic acid release.

Benefits in chronic pelvic pain

No studies were found that specifically included women with CPP, and a new search did not identify any further studies. With this limitation in mind, the evidence for dysmenorrhea was considered in order to gain some insight into the role of magnesium. A Cochrane Review has summarized the evidence on magnesium from RCTs of women with dysmenorrhea. Overall, magnesium was found to be more effective than placebo for pain relief in three RCTs. A search for more recent studies did not identify any new RCTs for women with either CPP or dysmenorrhea.

Magnesium is available in oral, transdermal, and systemic preparations. It is unclear what dose or regime of treatment should be used for magnesium therapy. There was also evidence from a small number of RCTs suggesting some benefit with vitamin B_1 and B_6 compared to placebo. There is some evidence of effectiveness with vitamin E in women with dysmenorrhea from three RCTs using between 50 and 150 IU per day.

Adverse events

Adverse events are generally inadequately reported in herbal and dietary treatments. Vitamin B_1 adverse events are rare. Vitamin B_6 has well known sensorineural adverse effects in dosages greater than 100 mg per day. Vitamin E has antiplatelet properties and should be used cautiously in women on anticoagulation, and doses greater than 400 IU per day are associated with a slight increase in mortality and heart failure. Magnesium does not appear to have any adverse effects and is generally considered safe.

★ TIPS & TRICKS

- Be open to the idea that your patient with chronic pelvic pain (CPP) may prefer alternative therapies to conventional interventions, especially when conventional medicine may have little to offer, and that evidence for benefit is lacking for both medical interventions and alternative therapies in women with CPP.
- Do not discourage women with CPP from seeking alternative therapies as self-management is important for such patients, and finding their own solutions may prove more useful than medical care, which for women with CPP is largely empiric and has the potential for harm.
- Caution women with CPP about the lack of evidence for any of the alternative therapies in women with CPP.
- Caution women with CPP about the potential for harm with alternative therapies such as spinal manipulation and vitamins B_6 and E in higher doses.
- Discuss the cost of the alternative therapies as in some cases women may

not be in a position to afford alternative treatments and they may find suitable funded pharmaceutical products equally as useful.

Conclusions

There are no well-designed studies of alternative therapies in women with CPP, so making recommendations is challenging with such a paucity of information. This chapter has drawn on the studies of alternative therapies in women with dysmenorrhea, and the results of the studies may not generally apply to women with CPP, which is usually a more severe and persistent condition.

To summarize, acupuncture is considered to be safe, although it does required repeated treatments and the effects are unlikely to be long-lasting. Spinal manipulation is not recommended as there are safety concerns, and there is no evidence of effectiveness in the one large study comparing it with sham acupuncture. There are no safety concerns with CHM but its effectiveness is yet to be established. Vitamin B_1 can be used although there is only limited information, and there are no safety concerns. Vitamin B_6 can be used although there is only limited evidence of effectiveness, and there are safety concerns at higher doses. Magnesium can be used although there is only limited evidence of effectiveness, and there are no safety concerns.

Overall, this chapter has found a paucity of studies for treatment of women with CPP, but it has reported on several alternative therapies that are promising. Where there is no evidence of effectiveness of a treatment in women with dysmenorrhea, it seems unlikely that that treatment has any potential as a treatment for women with CPP. Future research should focus on establishing the effectiveness of acupuncture, vitamins B_1, B_6 and E, and magnesium, using well-designed studies.

Selected bibliography

Assendelft WJ. Bouter LM. Knipschild PG. Complications of spinal manipulation: a comprehensive review of the literature. J Fam Pract 1996;42:475–80.

Astin JA, Marie A, Palletier KR, Hansen E, Haskell WL. A review of the incorporation of complementary and alternative medicine by mainstream physicians. Arch Intern Med 1998;158: 2303–10.

Deng HX, Zhu NS, Wang CW, Qing HX, Xu YZ. Clinical observation on the use of Jia Wei Muo Jie Pian in the treatment of primary dysmenorrhoea. Zhong Guo Zhong Yi Ji Chu Yi Xue Za Zhi [Chinese Journal of Basic Medicine in Traditional Chinese Medicine] 2003;9:57–8.

Dennehy CE. The use of herbs and dietary supplements in gynecology: an evidence-based review. J Midwif Womens Health 2006;51: 402–9.

Eisenberg DA, Davis RB, Ettner SL, Appel S, Wilky S, Van Rompay M. Trends in alternative medicine use in the United States, 1990–1997: results of a follow up national survey. JAMA 1998;280: 1569–75.

Ernst E. Harmless herbs? A review of the recent literature. Am J Med 1998;104:170–8.

Flower A, Liu JP, Chen S, Lewith G, Little P. Chinese herbal medicine for endometriosis. Cochrane Database Syst Rev 2009, Issue 3. Art. No.: CD006568.

Fugh-Berman A. Kronenberg F. Complementary and alternative medicine (CAM) in reproductive-age women: a review of randomized controlled trials. Reprod Toxicol 2003;17:137–52.

Gay RE, Bronfort G, Evans RL. Distraction manipulation of the lumbar spine: a review of the literature. J Manipulative Physiol Ther 2005;28: 266–73.

Hurwitz EL, Aker PD, Adams AH, Meeker WC, Shekelle PG. Manipulation and mobilisation of the cervical spine. A systematic review of the literature. Spine (Phila Pa 1976) 1996;21: 1746–59.

Lin J, Chen W. Acupuncture analgesia: a review of its mechanisms of actions. Am J Chin Med 2008;36:635–45.

Lysakowski C, Dumont L, Czarnetzki C, Tramèr MR. Magnesium as an adjuvant to postoperative analgesia: a systematic review of randomized trials. Anaesthes Analges 2007;104: 1532–9.

Proctor M, Murphy PA. Herbal and dietary therapies for primary and secondary dysmenorrhoea. Cochrane Database Syst Rev 2001, Issue 2. Art. No.: CD002124.

Proctor M, Hing W, Johnson TC, Murphy PA. Spinal manipulation for primary and secondary dysmenorrhoea. Cochrane Database Syst Rev 2006, Issue 3. Art. No.: CD002119.

Stones W, Cheong YC, Howard FM. Interventions for treating chronic pelvic pain in women. Cochrane Database Syst Rev 2005, Issue 2. Art. No.: CD000387.

Zhu X, Proctor M, Bensoussan A, Wu E, Smith CA. Chinese herbal medicine for primary dysmenorrhoea. Cochrane Database Syst Rev 2008, Issue 2. Art. No.: CD005288.

Index

Chronic Pelvic Pain, First Edition. Edited by Paolo Vercellini.
© 2011 Blackwell Publishing Ltd. Published 2011 by Blackwell Publishing Ltd.